D0208369

Pediatric Occupational Therapy and Early Intervention

Jane Case-Smith, EdD, OTR

Assistant Professor
Division of Occupational Therapy
School of Allied Medical Professions
The Ohio State University
Columbus, Ohio

With 9 Contributing Authors

Andover Medical Publishers
Boston London Oxford Singapore Sydney Toronto Wellington

To my husband, Greg, and sons, David and Stephen—
their love, support, and patience made this book possible.

Andover Medical Publishers is an imprint of Butterworth–Heinemann.

Copyright © 1993 by Butterworth–Heinemann, a division of Reed Publishing (USA) Inc.
All rights reserved.

Recognizing the importance of preserving what has been written, it is the policy of
Butterworth–Heinemann to have the books it publishes printed on acid-free paper, and
we exert our best efforts to that end.

Library of Congress Cataloging-in-Publication Data

Pediatric occupational therapy and early intervention / [edited by]
    Jane Case-Smith, with 9 contributing authors.
        p.   cm.
    Includes bibliographical references and index.
    ISBN 1-56372-026-4 (alk. paper)
    1. Occupational therapy for children.   2. Developmentally disabled
children—Rehabilitation.   I. Case-Smith, Jane, 1953–
    [DNLM: 1. Child Development Disorders—therapy.   2. Occupational Therapy—in
infancy & childhood.   WS 350.6 P3708 1993]
    RJ53.025P43   1993
    618.92'85889'06515—dc20
    DNLM/DLC
    for Library of Congress   92-48408
                                                                        CIP

British Library Cataloguing-in-Publication Data

A catalogue record for this book is available from the British Library.

Butterworth–Heinemann
313 Washington Street
Newton, MA 02158

10 9 8 7 6 5 4 3

Printed in the United States of America

□ □ □
□ □ □
□ □ □

Contents

10 Sensory Integration: Assessment and Intervention with Infants   309

Susan Stallings-Sahler, MS, OTR

11 Assistive Technology in Early Intervention: Theory and Practice   342

Yvonne Swinth, MS, OTR
Jane Case-Smith, EdD, OTR

Appendixes

Index   381

Contributing Authors

Janice Posatery Burke, MA, OTR, FAOTA, is an Assistant Professor in the Department of Occupational Therapy at Thomas Jefferson University in Philadelphia. She has served as the Project Director for a federally funded training grant designed to provide early intervention training to master's level occupational therapists and as a consultant and participant in Family Centered Care Workshops.

Jane Case-Smith, EdD, OTR, is an Assistant Professor in the Division of Occupational Therapy, School of Allied Medical Professions, The Ohio State University. She has worked with children as a therapist for 12 years and has been involved in training therapists to work with children during these years. She has been a faculty member for 8 years, first at the Virginia Commonwealth University and, most recently, at The Ohio State University. Her research has focused on the development of an instrument to measure the quality of movement in young infants and on the examination of in-hand manipulation in preschoolers. She is chairperson of the Developmental Disabilities Special Interest Section of the American Occupational Therapy Association (AOTA) and of the Special Interest Section Steering Committee. She currently serves on the editorial boards of *Physical and Occupational Therapy, Occupational Therapy in Pediatrics,* and the *American Journal of Occupational Therapy.*

Debra Galvin Cook, MS, OTR, is an Assistant Professor in the Department of Occupational Therapy Education, the University of Kansas Medical Center in Kansas City, Missouri. She has 14 years of pediatric experience in educating students and in serving children and their families in a variety of settings.

Robin P. Glass, MS, OTR, is a pediatric occupational therapist and clinical infant specialist at Children's Hospital and Medical Center in Seattle, Washington. She received her bachelor of science degree in occupational therapy from Columbia University and her master of science degree in occupational therapy from the University of Washington. In addition to her clinical responsibilities, she is a Clinical Assistant Professor in the Department of Occupational Therapy in the Division of Rehabilitation Medicine at the University of Washington.

Jodie Redditi Hanzlik, PhD, OTR, is an Associate Professor in the Department of Occupational Therapy at Colorado State University where she teaches pediatrics in both the graduate and undergraduate programs. Dr. Hanzlik directed the development of the Pediatric Specialty Certification Program and currently serves on a variety of committees and boards on local and national levels that advocate for best practice in all aspects of pediatric health care.

Elise Holloway, MPH, OTR, is the Occupational Therapy Clinical Specialist, Department of Neonatology, at Huntington Memorial Hospital in Pasadena, California, and has worked in early intervention with children and their families for over 15 years. She has published, lectured, and consulted nationally in the area of occupational therapy in early intervention.

Susan Stallings-Sahler, MS, OTR, has over 16 years of experience as a pediatric occupational therapy clinician and educator. She is currently a doctoral student at the University of Illinois at Chicago and a developmental specialist at the National Association for Perinatal Addiction Research and Education in Chicago, Illinois.

Yvonne Swinth, MS, OTR, is an occupational therapist for the University Place School District, Tacoma, Washington. She is a doctoral student in the Department of Special Education and Rehabilitation at the University of Washington, Seattle, where she also earned her MS in Rehabilitative Medicine, Occupational Therapy Tract.

Barbara Burris Wavrek, MHS, OTR, is Director of Occupational Therapy at Children's Hospital in Columbus, Ohio. She has participated in a number of professional activities, including serving as editor for the *Developmental Disabilities Special Interest Section* newsletter and as an instructor for Sensory Integration International.

Lynn S. Wolf, MOT, OTR, is a pediatric occupational therapist and an infant clinical specialist at Children's Hospital and Medical Center in Seattle, Washington. She is also a research associate in the Department of Pediatrics at the University of Washington, which includes responsibilities such as research and clinical training.

□ □ □
□ □ □
□ □ □

Preface

The intent of *Pediatric Occupational Therapy and Early Intervention* is to provide guidelines and strategies for occupational therapists who work with both young children and their families. In the 1980s, major legislation and efficacy research resulted in dramatic changes in early intervention practice. As a result of these system changes, services to infants and their families have been enhanced and the overall practice of pediatric occupational therapy has been influenced. This book is divided into two parts: Part I defines the early intervention process and Part II provides specific information about occupational therapy interventions related to the developmental problems incurred in young children.

The principles and foundations of early intervention, which are presented in Part I, are espoused by leaders in the occupational therapy field. These principles and foundations serve to guide evaluation and planning for intervention as exemplified by the Individualized Family Service Plan (IFSP). Part I also describes evaluation tools and assessment methods appropriate for identifying child strengths and limitations, and family concerns and priorities. In Chapter 5, the last chapter in the part, Dr. Jane Case-Smith and Barbara Burris Wavrek explain medical and community models of service delivery and team interaction. In addition, they define strategies for creating continuity in services as the child and family transition between medical and community early intervention programs.

Part II applies occupational therapy theories and recent research to current early intervention practice. In Chapter 6, Elise Holloway explains the importance of early social-emotional development, emphasizing how sensory integration dysfunction may interfere with this development. By drawing on the research of prominent psychologists, she develops strategies for the therapist to use in promoting the infant's social-emotional development. In Chapter 7, Janice Posatery Burke enlightens the reader on the importance of play. She explains how therapists can engage the child in play and promote play skills in the young child. Chapter 8, by Robin P. Glass and Lynn S. Wolf, provides in-depth information about the critical functional area of feeding and oral-motor skills. Based on a wealth of experience in therapy with neonates and young infants and on current research, the authors present effective methods for resolving feeding problems. In Chapter 9, Dr. Jodie Hanzlik synthesizes current literature and research on parent–infant interaction. She addresses critical interactional issues that have a tremendous effect on developmental outcomes and draws conclusions of specific relevance for occupational therapists. In Chapter 10, Susan Stallings-Sahler applies sensory integration assessment and intervention methods to early intervention. In addition, she describes evaluation methods for identifying sensory integration problems in the young infant (e.g., sensory defensiveness, dyspraxia), and then explicates best practice intervention approaches for infants who exhibit these problems. The final chapter describes assistive technology that can promote function and independence in young children. The authors, Yvonne Swinth and Dr. Case-Smith, emphasize an interdisciplinary team approach for the evaluation of technology needs and for the integration of technology into the lives of young children with disabilities.

The contributors to this text, each with recognized expertise in early intervention, provide specific information about effective therapy methods that exist within the context of family-centered care. From a broad definition of family-centered early intervention to various specific therapeutic techniques that impact the neurophysiological system of the young child, this book presents critical information to guide pediatric occupational therapists.

Occupational Therapy in Family-Centered Early Intervention

1

□ □ □
□ □ □
□ □ □

Foundations and Principles

Jane Case-Smith, EdD, OTR

A Rationale for Family-Centered Services

Three decades ago, a British pediatrician, D.W. Winnicott, proposed that "there is no such thing as a baby", only a baby and someone else (Winnicott, 1964). He pointed to the absolute dependency of infants on their caregivers, and the importance of such relationships. In order to understand developmental and maturational processes, infants must be viewed in the context of their environment and in the context of their relationship with caregivers. Enduring and responsive relationships are critical for the infant. Caregivers provide the safety, comfort, nourishment, and stimulation that enable infant development to progress. Therefore, families are the basic foundation of the young child, determining the child's ability to adapt to and function in the environment. This unique, total dependency implies that intervention should always involve examining the family context.

Based on the family system, interactions among the family members are not only influenced by the infant, but also influence interactions with the infant. For example, an infant or toddler with a disability affects all family members, their roles, their relationships, and their values. At the same time, the personalities, roles, interaction styles, and relationships of the family members likewise affect the infant and influence his development.

The bidirectional influence means that the family affects the child's behavior and the child has an equally powerful effect on the parents' behavior.

Preparation of this chapter was supported by grant #H029F00034 of the Office of Special Education and Rehabilitation Services, U.S. Department of Education.

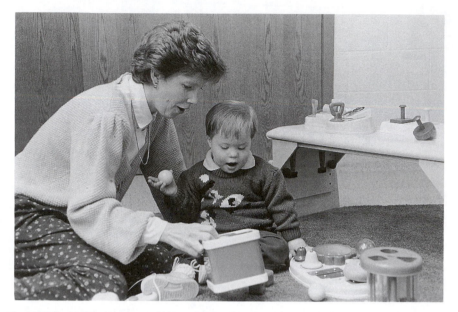

Figure 1-1 Mother and child

Sameroff and Chandler (1975), in their exhaustive review of the literature, provide strong evidence for the profound effect of parent–child interactions and relationships. They suggest that the interplay between children and their families is continual and progressive. The caregivers' interactions with the infant seem to have a major role in determining developmental outcome (Mahoney & Powell, 1988; Sameroff & Chandler, 1975). (See Figure 1-1.)

Occupational therapists have a major role in the provision of early intervention services for infants and preschoolers at risk for disabilities. More recently, the focus and the scope of intervention has expanded to include the family. This focus stresses that families are enduring and serve as the basic foundation in the young child's ability to adapt to and function in the environment (Sameroff & Fiese, 1990).

The family-centered approach in early intervention is promoted in Part H of Public Law (PL) 99-457, the Education of the Handicapped Act Amendments of 1986. The law contains numerous provisions to promote the family's participation in services as equal members of the early intervention team. One primary mechanism for building partnerships with parents is the Individualized Family Service Plan (IFSP). The plan is based on resources, concerns, and priorities of families, and results in the realization of goals for the family and the infant. Families are also assigned service coordinators who can assist them in obtaining and coordinating the appropriate services. Hence, the legislation validates the principle that infants and toddlers must be served within the family context.

The influence of the family on the child and that of the child on the family is illustrated in the Goodness-of-Fit model, a concept developed by Thomas and Chess (1977) and applied to early intervention by Bailey et al. (1986). The model proposes that the developmental outcome of children is significantly influenced by their environments and that this influence may be greater than that of physical endowment (Sameroff & Chandler, 1975). In particular, the infant's caregivers mediate his world. Through the child's physical environment and the experience that caregivers provide, growth within and across all developmental areas is nourished and impeded. Developmental outcome is related to the match, or fit, between the unique characteristics of the child and family as they interact. The focus of intervention is shifted from child variables or family variables to the relationship of the child and family members by using this concept to guide early intervention principles. The consonance, or fit, between the characteristics of children and families determines how well children cope with and adapt to their daily environment and experiences. Therefore, intervention considers child variables, family variables and resources, and perhaps most importantly, the family's perception of and relationship with the child (Simeonsson, Bailey, Huntington, & Comfort, 1986). The consonance of family interaction affects outcomes for the child and family (Turnbull, Summers, & Brotherson, 1986).

Principles in Family-Centered Early Intervention

Through the impetus of PL 99-457 (PL 102-119 and its regulations) and a growing body of research (Bailey et al., 1986; McGonigel, Kaufmann, & Johnson, 1991; Meisels & Shonkoff, 1990; Sameroff & Chandler, 1975; Shelton, Jeppson, & Johnson, 1987; Summers et al., 1990), an increasing understanding and appreciation of the meaning of family-centered care can be realized. This chapter discusses the following themes and principles as they relate to family-centered early intervention and occupational therapy:

- understanding family structures and family systems
- meeting the family's concerns
- building on family strengths
- respecting family diversity and cultural backgrounds
- acknowledging personal characteristics
- sharing information

- promoting partnerships and collaboration
- providing individualized, flexible, and accessible services
- accessing services that promote integration of the child and family into the community
- encouraging social support, recreation, and respite
- establishing interdisciplinary team collaboration
- facilitating interagency collaboration

Understanding Family Structures

The characteristics and structures of families shape their response to a child with a disability. Family structures are quite variable in present day society; in fact, a substantial proportion of families today are made up of single or divorced parents (Vincent, Salisbury, Strain, McCormick, & Tessier, 1990). The stress of raising a child with a disability as a single parent requires that emotional and social support have priority. In addition, a majority of mothers are now in the work force (Vincent & Salisbury, 1988). As a result, caregiving by family members is often shared with professional caregivers in homes or day-care centers. Although many parents are adolescents, first parents are often older than 35 years. These structural elements affect the goals and plans that are selected and the nature of therapy provided.

The family's structure also encompasses extended family. Grandparent involvement may be intense or there may be no involvement. Their role with the family and the child with a disability depends on their sense of investment and physical proximity. Grandparents can be an enormous source of support, providing respite for the parents, or they may create additional stress when they make assumptions about the child and the nuclear family (Fewell & Vadasy, 1986). The members who are included in the functional family unit and involved in the child's therapy may change over time as the family's circumstances change (e.g., if the mother develops health problems).

An open-ended definition of families, which includes a nuclear unit (e.g., a single parent and a child) or extended family members, is needed. Defining the functional family unit and the significant members of that unit is important in developing intervention plans and activities. The needs and resources of all the members who have primary involvement with the child need to be considered.

When the single mother of a young infant has the strong support of her mother, the therapist can build on that support. For example, therapy can be scheduled when both mother and grandmother are able to be present. Feeding methods could be discussed with both and techniques that would match their interaction styles could be suggested. By considering family configurations and structure, therapists can develop collaborative intervention activities that effectively match the needs of the child and family.

Understanding Family Systems

Family structure is only one aspect of the family system. Many interdependent parts make up a family, and the interaction of the parts creates properties not contained in any of the separate entities. Therefore, to understand and to work successfully with families, the relationships and interactions of the members must be understood and appreciated.

Within the family system, changes in an individual or in a relationship influence change throughout the entire system. Each member is affected by every other member. For example, a child with a disability affects all family systems, including the relationships between husband and wife, siblings, parent and child, and nuclear and extended family members. Furthermore, an intervention targeted toward one system will affect the others (Turnbull, Summers, & Brotherson, 1986). When therapy programs require that the mother devote additional time to the child with a disability, less time is available for other family members.

The various ways that family systems function can be described on a continuum (Barber, Turnbull, Behr, & Kerns, 1988). The continuum measures cohesion or strength of family members' emotional bonds versus their individual autonomy. Families with extreme dependency on each other are examples of *enmeshment* (Turnbull & Turnbull, 1991). A mother who is enmeshed with her child with a disability may become overly anxious about his progress. As a result, she may focus on the child's therapy to such an extent that her physical and mental health are affected, as well as her level of interactions and involvement with her other children. Important family functions, such as socialization and recreation, may become very low priorities due to time spent in caregiving and in therapy with the child who has special needs.

When family members are *disengaged*, the support needed to cope with crises and setbacks may not be available (Barber, Turnbull, Behr, & Kerns, 1988). Family members do not rally in support of each other. They may pursue individual interests, seldom communicate, and exhibit a lack of sensitivity to the needs of each other. Healthy family cohesion is characterized by a balance of unity and individualization in relationships (Simeonsson, 1988).

The family's adaptability also affects their response to a child with a disability and to intervention (Turnbull & Turnbull, 1991). Family adaptability enables the family to change in response to situational and developmental stress (Olson, Russell, & Sprenkle, 1980). Adaptable families easily and successfully meet with crises as well as with changes in routines and plans.

Families who are rigid are unable or unwilling to change in response to new situations and demonstrate a high degree of control and structure. Roles and rules change very little over time and change is stressful. The father who has the role of bread winner may not adjust to caregiving and housekeeping roles when the mother is overwhelmed with the caregiving needs of their child with a disability. Hinojosa (1990) provides a mother's description of the father's role:

> I do the majority of the hospitals and stuff with the twins because he has to work. But when I can't, he's there. And he helps in a million other ways. (p. 152)

Another mother reports the following:

> I say that Martin likes [my husband] more than he like me, because I have to do all the things that he doesn't like. . . . I have to put him on the bus in the morning, and um, make him take that bath that he doesn't want to take, and when daddy comes home his savior has arrived. [My husband] is real good around the house, usually I get out on the weekends while he takes over in the care of Martin. (Nastro, 1992, p. 43)

Many families have organized roles in which mothers perform the majority of caregiving and fathers provide for the family in other ways (e.g., care of house, financial support). On the opposite end of the continuum are families who are chaotic, in which membership or relationships may change dramatically in response to crises. Chaotic families demonstrate a low degree of control and structure. Rules are seldom enforced and often changing. The parents may ultimately separate or the responsibility of the children may be given to extended family members.

A balance between the two extremes of rigidity and chaos characterize well functioning families (Barber, Turnbull, Behr, & Kerns, 1988; Turnbull & Turnbull, 1991). However, more adaptability may be observed regarding some issues rather than others. When families have minimal adaptability, there should be additional preparation made to facilitate changes in intervention or transitions in services (Simeonsson, 1988).

A third element of family interaction is communication (Turnbull & Turnbull, 1991). Communication among family members may also be viewed on a continuum. At one extreme is the family with closed communication, where members seldom engage in meaningful discussion. The early intervention team may have difficulty in communicating with this family; for example, information communicated with one parent might not be shared with the other. Issues that are important to the parents may become buried because they are not expressed. In contrast, there is the family that discusses all topics openly, even those with high emotional charge that may cause distress in family members. Sensitivity to communication issues among family members enables the family to function as a whole. Optimal communication is open and honest with discretion used when sharing information among family members that involves sensitive issues. The communication skills of the family influence the therapist–family relationship and often create open pathways for communication or may create difficult, awkward, or infrequent communication that the therapists and team must work to positively influence (Case-Smith, 1991).

Meeting the Family's Concerns

Families of young children with disabilities have unique concerns and priorities that must be considered in the delivery of occupational therapy services. Although generalizations should not be made, some families have concerns about their ability to provide optimal care for their child. If the child has recently been diagnosed, the parents may be grieving, in denial, in shock, or angry. They may be anxious about the impact that a child with a disability will have on their family. Most parents in this situation want information, a listening ear, and the support of friends and extended family.

First-time, young parents may feel insecure about their ability to raise a child with a disability and, therefore, need assistance in developing caregiving skills and reassurance about their existing skills. Parents have many other needs related to their daily lives; these needs affect the child, the family, and the interactions between them. Examples of stressors are financial problems, need for respite care, need for acceptance by other families, and unstable relationships within the extended family (Bailey, 1988). These needs ultimately affect family function and parent–infant interaction and may become primary considerations of the occupational therapist. One mother reports:

> it all depends on insurance coverage. We went from a good insurance to not-so-great insurance. Under our current coverage, they pay fifteen OT approved visits for your lifetime. And so we pay for Martin's therapy ourselves. What we did was take out a home equity loan to pay for it because it's so expensive. It's very expensive but it's necessary. So we just give up other things, nobody is suffering for it . . . . (Nastro, 1992, p. 52)

Another mother explains:

> I went back to work while he was still in the hospital when he was like a month old. His insurance was through my employer so I had to

keep up with that, I went from working 40 hours to 30 hours and then to 25 and even at that point it felt totally stressed out, then last March, this company, I had worked for them for 10 years, they said either you take a 45 hour position each week or we don't need you . . . . (Nastro, 1992, p. 54)

Dunst, Trivette, and Deal (1988) refer to the needs defined by Maslow as a framework for understanding how families perceive and relate to their children with disabilities. According to Maslow's theory, unmet basic needs dominate behavior and interfere with higher level needs. When the family has basic needs for nutrition, shelter, and safety, their well-being is affected, and it is unlikely that they will become involved in intervention or be able to carry out occupational therapy home programs. When parents are concerned with providing for the basic needs of the family, they do not have the time or the energy to implement home programs. The family's concerns and resources related to everyday function influence well-being and family function in a broad sense, which in turn influence commitment to and involvement in therapy for their child.

Building on Family Strengths

To successfully meet the needs of families, the therapist builds on the family's strengths. Occupational therapy goals and plans emphasize existing family resources and respect the family's functioning style. Table 1-1 provides a list of possible family strengths (Dunst, Trivette, & Deal, 1988).

Compared to the enduring and intensive relationship of the child and nuclear family, the early intervention program influences the child and family for a brief period of their lives. Important supports come from the parents' social networks and extended families, and accessing these should be emphasized in therapy (Barber, Turnbull, Behr, & Kerns, 1988; Sameroff & Fiese, 1990). It is suggested that service providers encourage rather than interfere with family time and social-recreational events (Turnbull & Turnbull, 1991); therefore, the importance placed on therapeutic regimes is balanced with the need for time with friends and family.

While parents are encouraged to build skills that directly facilitate the child's development, it is equally important to encourage and enable parents to mobilize resources and services for their child. Effective intervention assists the family's use of natural support networks and neither supplants nor replaces them with professional networks (Dunst, Trivette, & Deal, 1988). Therapy programs that build on family strengths and capabilities enable families to

Table 1-1 Family Strengths

A combination of qualities appears to define strong familes, and define the unique family functioning style.

—Dunst, Trivette & Deal, 1988

Following are qualities of strong families.

1. A belief in and sense of **commitment** toward promoting the well-being and growth of individual family members as well as that of the family unit.
2. **Appreciation** for the small and large things that individual family members do well, and encouragement to do better.
3. Concentrated effort to spend **time** and do things together, no matter how formal or informal the activity or event.
4. A sense of **purpose** that permeates the reasons and basis for "going on" in both bad and good times.
5. A sense of **congruence** among family members regarding the value and importance of assigning time and energy to what the family considers its goals, needs, projects, and functions.
6. The ability to **communicate** with one another in a way that emphasizes positive interactions among family members.
7. A clear set of family **rules, values,** and **beliefs** that establishes expectations about acceptable and desired behavior.
8. A varied repertoire of **coping strategies** that encourage positive functioning in dealing with both normative and non-normative life events.
9. The ability to engage in **problem-solving** activities designed to evaluate options for meeting needs and procuring resources.
10. The ability to be **positive** and see the positive in almost all aspects of their lives, including the ability to see crises and problems as an opportunity to learn and grow.
11. **Flexibility** and **adaptability** in the roles necessary to procure resources to meet needs.
12. A **balance** between the use of internal and external family resources for coping and adapting to life events and planning for the future.

Source: Reprinted from Dunst CJ, Trivette CM, Deal AG: *Enabling and empowering families: Principles and guidelines for practice.* Cambridge, MA, Brookline Books, 1988, pp 25–26, reproduced with permission of the publisher.

meet their own needs and to cope with and adapt to their child's disability. One mother explains how important her informal support system has been to her:

My parents have always been a big help when Martin was first born, and in the hospital a lot. My parents came over and stayed with the other kids because my husband, of course, stayed around as often as he could, but eventually you have to get on and work, so my parents would come and then I could stay at the hospital with Martin. And then one of them would come down to stay with Martin so that I could come home and see the other kids. . . . What would we do if my parents weren't around? (Nastro, 1992, p. 46)

When the mother is the primary caregiver, husbands can be an important source of support and strength. (See Figure 1-2.) One mother reports the following:

I've had a lot of support from my husband, he's self-employed so he's home a lot with Peter and um, gives a lot of extra help. . . .

Another mother explains:

See, during the day, James [my son] gets all of my attention, it's my thing, but as soon as dad gets home, he's daddy's boy. James wants nothing to do with me, and I'll feel 'whew, thanks.' So I'll go cook dinner, and they will play and I try not to intervene. (Nastro, 1992, p. 44)

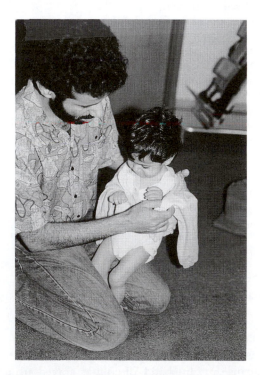

Figure 1-2 Many fathers, such as this one, share in everyday caregiving activities

Respecting Family Diversity and Cultural Backgrounds

Sensitivity to family diversity includes the acknowledgment that American society is flavored by people of many cultures, ethnic origins, and religions. In recent years, the changing demographics of the United States have underscored the need to consider the impact of culture and language. In 1984, 36% of the infants born in the United States were born to ethnolinguistically diverse families (Research and Policy Committee for Economic Development, 1987). By the year 2000, one-third of the projected U.S. population will consist of African Americans, American Indians, Asian Pacifics, Latinos, and other people of color (Chen, 1990). In the coming years, nearly 50% of all young children in many areas of the country will be from cultural and linguistic groups that are different from those of most early intervention professionals (Hanson, Lynch, & Wayman, 1990). A greater proportion of young children from these groups may need early intervention services due to lack of prenatal care and impoverished environments. As occupational therapists in early intervention work with these families, they need to understand their values, caregiving methods, and relationships (McCormack, 1987).

The structure of families from nonwhite ethnic origins often includes extended family members. The boundaries of the family may be undefined or family membership may change frequently, creating chaotic relationships among its members. Grandparents, aunts, and uncles may reside in the same household as the nuclear family. Grandparents often serve as the primary caregivers. The occupational therapist may find that she works with different family members at different times, requiring instructions and therapy to be constantly adjusted to the needs and desires of the various caregivers involved with the child.

Early intervention occupational therapists need to understand the specific impact of multiculturalism in the community in which they work. Knowledge of specific cultures, values, customs, and practices enables the therapist to make appropriate recommendations and suggestions that the family can understand and implement. While some commonalities exist among cultural groups, generalizations about families from certain cultures must always be viewed with caution, as each family has unique values and characteristics.

In particular, cultural beliefs and values about health, disease, and disability affect the way in which families respond to professionals. For example, Asian Americans often believe that disability is a punishment for sins committed by the parents. To hide this evidence of their wrongdoing, the child may be isolated from society and considered an object of shame for the family. To Hispanic Americans, the fastest growing minority group in the United States (McCormack, 1987), vitality and health are greatly valued; therefore, a child with a disability is often not seen as being in need of services or is hidden. Most Hispanic families are patriarchal; the husband seldom assists in the housework or in child care. As a result, the mother may receive minimal assistance from her husband in caring for the child with a disability (Anderson & Fenichel, 1989). However, grandparents and extended family may reside in the household and can implement therapeutic activities for the child or provide respite for the mother.

Some Hispanic Americans also hold beliefs in magical disorders believed to be brought on by a hex or witchcraft. Treatment for such disorders is often a ritual that has no medical base, such as holding the child over a pail of hot water to remove a virus. When such beliefs are strong, recommendations that conflict with these cultural rituals would be ignored. By acknowledging and respecting specific cultural values and beliefs, the occupational therapist can form partnerships with families of diverse cultures.

Another area in which cultural background strongly influences relationships is family and professional communication. When English is not the family's primary language, the professional jargon of the early intervention professionals is especially confusing and can be harmful rather than helpful. The concept of early intervention is difficult to understand when the family and professionals speak the same language. Ideally, one or more persons in the early intervention program knows the family's language. Interpreters may be used to assist team and family members understand nonverbal as well as verbal communication. Persons from other community agencies who work exclusively with one ethnic group can be instrumental in helping the early intervention team understand the cultural background of families and can be a liaison in communicating with families.

Respect for family diversity ensures that the intervention process is supportive of each family's efforts to enhance the development of the child's special needs, while attending to the needs of the entire family (McGonigel, Kaufmann, & Johnson, 1991). (See Figure 1-3.) Although each family's cultural values and norms are not always understood by the therapist, an effective relationship can be established when the identified concerns, resources, and priorities of each family are used as the basis for intervention programs.

Acknowledging Personal Characteristics

Personal characteristics of individual family members affect the way that the family functions. These characteristics serve as strengths or limitations to the family's ability to function as a whole. For example, a parent in poor physical health is less able to cope with stressful situations (Barber, Turnbull, Behr, & Kerns, 1988; Turnbull & Turnbull, 1991). Parents with mental illness or developmental disabilities may require special considerations; additional support systems may be needed. Occupational therapy

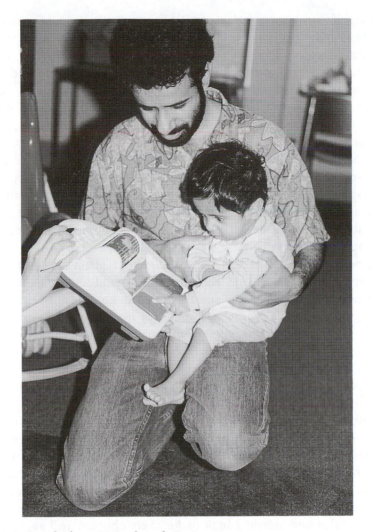

Figure 1-3 Family from United Arab Emirates

strategies should reflect activities that are realistic, appropriate, and consider the support needed to accomplish priority goals. The risks to children with parents who are mentally ill or who have mental retardation should be acknowledged and appropriate programming should be selected (Espe-Sherwindt, Kerlin, Beatty, & Crable, 1990). When the parent has a disability, the family's wellness receives more emphasis than the child's achievement of specific developmental skills.

Personality characteristics may influence both parents' involvement in therapy and their relationship to the child. Three aspects that seem to be associated with the parent's ability to cope are self-esteem, locus of control, and mastery (Dunst & Trivette, 1990; Turnbull & Turnbull, 1991). Parents with low self-esteem may feel inadequate in caring for a child with special needs. They may feel rejected by the child's inability to respond to them. Sense of mastery and locus of control describe the extent to which people believe that the events of their lives are under their own control rather than the control of someone else or fate. These factors determine the degree of initiative in the parent, the ability of the parent to participate in decision making, and the level of independence assumed in teaching the child and managing services.

The parents' history also influences their parenting style. The values and practices of their families form the basis for the values and practices that they practice when involved in early intervention. In families where deviations are not tolerated and achievement is emphasized, a child with delayed development or disabilities may be difficult for the parents to accept and be a source of continual stress.

The parents' educational levels and backgrounds affect their participation in therapy. Parents with knowledge in the areas of child development, atypical development, social systems, or social policy can more readily embrace the rationale and basis of early intervention. They may require less information about the early intervention program and may participate more than other parents due to a greater understanding of the purpose of the therapeutic activities. The parents' education level may affect the value that is placed on therapeutic services and the child goals that are priorities for the parents (Humphry, 1989).

Finally, the parents' personalities determine, to an extent, the match or fit achieved with the child. Parents who are warm, loving, and get great satisfaction from parenting may achieve a better fit with a child who has many parenting demands. Personalities influence the types of interactions that occur between parent and child. For example, some parents seem to automatically know how to handle children with postural insecurity; their own calm and steady hands make their children feel more secure. When children feel secure, higher levels of adaptation are elicited. A parent's sensitivity and responsiveness to others may also assist in accommodating a young child whose cues and efforts at communication are difficult to read.

Sharing Information

The information shared with parents should be complete and unbiased (McGonigel, 1991). Parents need information about programs, services, and community resources, in addition to information specific to their child. General information about the diagnosis and child development, as well as specific assessment results enable parents to problem solve and make decisions regarding their child. Gaining knowledge and understanding is one way parents become independent, competent caregivers. In particular, information about the community's special education and early intervention systems can empower parents to effectively move through bureaucracies and to gain access to services that will benefit their child.

Information sharing is an important part of therapy. Therapists should consider the manner in which information is shared. The professional who is sensitive and respectful of parents will communicate with warmth and empathy. Timing of information sharing is important. Parents should not be kept from learning their child's diagnosis, as a state of *non-knowing* often provokes greater anxiety than being told that their child has a specific diagnosis (Akerly, 1985; Ziskin, 1985). However, parents are not always ready to assimilate comprehensive information. They may need to discuss an issue repeatedly. This need should be respected.

The environment selected for information sharing is also an important consideration. The home may be the most comfortable environment for the family; however, homes with other children are often noisy and chaotic and may not be conducive to communication concerning important issues (Bailey & Simeonsson, 1988). Due to the time demands on therapists and parents, communication is not always ideal. Yet, when communication is not a priority, relationships deteriorate, misunderstandings easily develop, and, ultimately, effectiveness of intervention is affected. Positive interaction and communication are unstated goals of therapy.

Effective communication has been achieved when parents and professionals engage in a balanced give-and-take in which the views and perceptions of both are valued. Although parents know the most about their child, the therapist often assumes the role of information giver. Parents have a wealth of insights and knowledge about their child to share with therapists, and the parents' perspectives should always be solicited and explored. When providing information to parents, therapists should use jargon-free language and explanations that can be easily understood. Written communication and handouts are appreciated by parents (Nastro & Case-Smith, in press), especially to reinforce verbal communication that occurs in noisy, busy clinics. Therapists are sensitive to the parents' levels of knowledge and understanding, while at the same time they are concerned about increasing the parents' knowledge. The cultural background, education, and readiness of the parent should always be considered (Halpern, 1990; Wayman, Lynch, & Hanson, 1991).

Promoting Partnerships and Collaboration

Positive and sensitive communication is one aspect of parent–professional partnership. Collaboration is accomplished when professionals recognize and build on family competence and resourcefulness. Partnership does not imply that therapists and parents have the same roles in evaluation and intervention. Each brings his own perspective and expertise to the planning and implementation of therapy (Kjerland & Kovach, 1990; Winton; 1988).

Although parents have primary responsibility for their children, they also rely on therapists to contribute expertise and assistance. The relationships between parents and therapists are built on respect and cooperation, with a focus on the concerns and goals of the child (Healy, Keesee, & Smith, 1989). In a truly collaborative approach, the right of families to make decisions for their children and themselves exists in harmony with the reponsibility of therapists to share their knowledge, expertise, and concerns.

Two issues of parent–professional collaboration deserve consideration. First, partnerships are developmental and grow over time. Often the therapist initially provides instruction and direction, then she shifts roles from one of providing advice and recommendations to one of facilitating the parents' own problem solving; therefore, responsibilities for intervention goals may shift. Second, partnerships can be influenced by past experiences, family history, cultural values, and personalities. Therapists should recognize and attempt to understand these issues. Issues that affect the development of a positive parent–therapist relationship should be acknowledged and discussed as needed.

Collaboration is a skill. Often it is easier to collaborate with colleagues who have similar backgrounds and use the same language than with parents. Project Dakota has developed an exemplary model of parent–professional collaboration (Kjerland, 1986). In this project, the concept of parent involvement in services is replaced with the therapist's involvement with families. Parents' priorities and concerns are the basis of therapy and parents select the kinds of services that meet their needs and match their resources. One role of the therapist in the partnership is to consider the stress of raising a child with a disability and to demonstrate understanding by actively listening and offering support to the family.

Anderson and Hinojosa (1984) explain that occupational therapists frequently enter the parent–therapist relationship from a child advocacy position, as one who is committed to the child's developmental needs. Understanding of neurophysiological concepts and the interrelationships of sensory and motor systems enables the therapist to select activities and environments that promote development; therefore, therapists bring a new understanding of the child's function to the partnership. While the therapist's knowledge can and does promote the child's development, this knowledge cannot be effectively applied unless therapists first consider the parents' priorities and perspectives.

Establishing Individualized, Flexible, and Accessible Services

When personal characteristics, values, culture, structure, interactions, and levels of education and experience are considered, the complex nature of family systems underscores the need for individualized, flexible, and accessible services. The IFSP establishes the groundwork for services that are responsive to individual family needs. Services should be tailor-made to suit the specific strengths, needs, and resources of each child and family (Bailey et al., 1986; Kjerland & Kovach, 1990). Figure 1-4 provides a menu of services that might be offered to families as options.

Occupational therapists are also required to be responsive to individual needs. Several barriers have been identified that interfere with providing tailor-made therapy. Offering families flexibility in locations where services are delivered (e.g., in the home, clinic, or other community setting) may be desirable, but it is not always feasible. Costs are a limiting factor to flexible services; the expense of staff may limit the amount, time, and location of therapy. While center-based services tend to be more costly in terms of parents' time, home-based services may be more costly in terms of the therapist's time. The costs and benefits of the location of service delivery should be carefully evaluated; compromises on the part of therapists and parents are to be expected. The time for therapy should be flexible, but usually a number of factors limit the possible therapy times. While evening therapy may be ideal for some families; it may interfere with the therapist's family time.

Working through these issues should exemplify the collaborative relationship of the therapist, the team, and the parents. Reasonable solutions can be found if explored creatively and with an open mind. Rigid or highly structured programs may restrict the development of individualized, flexible, and accessible services for families. Hospitals, due to their size and the complexity of their organizational structure, may deter the provision of individualized services. This is particularly the case in hospitals that primarily provide acute care (see Case-Smith & Burris Wavrek, Chapter 5). When agencies and programs are highly structured, therapists may advocate for individualized services. Flexibility and responsiveness from the therapist, even within a system that lacks flexibility, facilitates the development of parent–professional partnerships.

Promoting Integration of the Child and Family into the Community

Parents of young children with disabilities often feel isolated from normal community life. The first step in the normalization process is to provide assistance that is normative and does not imply deviance or undue

SERVICE MENU

This menu is designed to stimulate thinking about the many ways services can be made available to families. Please don't let choices be limited to these! Families and staff may draw from all three categories in any combination. Subsidies and transportation assistance are available for community group settings. Preference is given to settings with non-delayed peers.

In the Child's Home:
With:
_____ one parent
_____ both parents
_____ and siblings
_____ and other family members

Where:
_____ family home
_____ EI center
_____ other locations
_____ requested by family via telephone

Time of Day:
_____ am   _____ pm   _____ eve

Day of Week:
_____ (Monday-Friday)

Frequency:
_____ 1x month
_____ 2x month
_____ 1x week
_____ 2x week
_____ 3x week

In the Community:
Locations:
_____ parent-child group
_____ family daycare
_____ neighborhood playmates
       with staff help
_____ church group/program
_____ recreation program
_____ group lessons such as
       tumbling, dance, swim
_____ nursery school, daycare
_____ other:

Facilitator Role:
_____ full assistance with child
_____ partial assistance with child
_____ consultation to group
       teacher
_____ consultation with family
       who carries out assistance
       or consultation with group
       teacher

At the Center:
Parent-Child Play Groups:
_____ am   _____ pm   _____ early evening
_____ 1x month   _____ 2x month   _____ 1x week   _____ 2x week

Child Groups:
_____ small, non-integrated group
_____ peer tutors (non-delayed older peers)
_____ one to one
_____ 1x week   _____ 2x week

Family Events:
_____ siblings
_____ grandparents
_____ support or coffee groups
_____ family retreats
_____ parent discussions

Figure 1-4 Service menu [Reprinted from Kjerland L: Early intervention tailor made. Eagan, MN: Project Dakota, Inc., 1986, reproduced with permission of the publisher.]

variations (McGonigel, 1991). Services provided in the home or day-care center are more normative than those provided in the hospital. The therapy environment should be comfortable and should contain toys and child-related equipment.

Therapy in an integrated environment, such as a day-care center, has a number of advantages. First, the center's personnel benefit from observing the therapist and discussing goals and activities for the child. Second, the child benefits from being around peer models who do not have disabilities. Dunst (1991) suggests that intervention is most effective if it does not imply deviance or undue variation when compared to the function and social activities of family friends and neighbors.

In addition to service delivery in normative settings, parents should be encouraged to engage in activities with families who do not have children with disabilities. Often parents of children with disabilities, due to the extra demands on their time and the perceived stigma of having a child with a disability, become isolated from the community. Mothers reported that having a child with a disability restricted their participation in community events, primarily as a result of the difficulty of finding someone to stay with the child. Even when a babysitter has had training in working with children with special needs, the parents often must provide explicit and detailed instructions about care of their child. As a result, the parents often find it easier to stay at home. Since experiences in community groups, church, and informal gatherings of friends help to support and revitalize the family, they should be encouraged to allocate the time and resources to become involved in local events.

Encouraging Social Support, Recreation, and Respite

While community involvement is desirable and parents of children with disabilities may benefit from active support systems, they often lack the support of friends and extended family. One parent describes this social phenomena, "a special loneliness is the most pervasive theme in the stories told by parents with disabled children. This loneliness is nourished from within and without. . . The two most prominent ingredients of a parent's loneliness are differences—his own and the child's and isolation" (Featherstone, 1980, p. 50).

Social isolation may occur because the family withdraws from the community. The time and energy required to care for a child with a disability may drain the parents' time, resources, and energy. In order to ensure the availability and adequacy of resources for supporting the family in times of crisis and need, the family's personal, social network should be strengthened and use of untapped sources of assistance should be promoted. The benefits of support are best realized if aid and assistance come primarily from informal sources (Dunst & Trivette, 1990).

Obviously, the family is greatly influenced by their social network. Extended family may be a major source of assistance in meeting individualized family needs. (See Figure 1-5 for a schematic diagram of the family's social support systems.) As previously mentioned, grandparents often help with child care, and provide material, psychological, and emotional support. Relatives who live in proximity to the family can assist in child care and be a resource when crises arise. Resource exchanges (i.e., gifts or household items), shared social and recreational activities, and frequent communication strengthen the bond among extended family members and bolster the family.

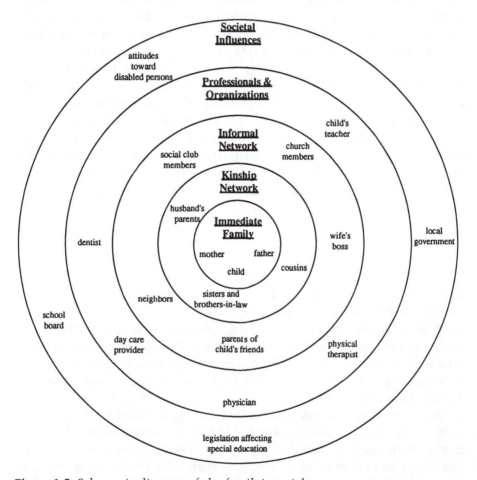

Figure 1-5 Schematic diagram of the family's social support systems

Friends and neighbors may also be an important source of support (Stagg & Catron, 1986), assisting in child care or meal preparation if the child with a disability is hospitalized. They can also provide a sense of renewal and reassurance. Assistance from others can be as simple as listening or can involve sharing of resources. Parents of children with disabilities often provide tremendous support to each other. In fact, networks of families who share similar experiences can help in many ways. First, other parents who have children with special needs help each other realize that they are not alone or unique in the problems they experience (Stagg & Catron, 1986). Parent-to-parent networks that connect parents of similar backgrounds or parents with similar children can help relieve the sense of isolation and can provide newer parents with the guidance of more experienced parents who will understand their feelings. Parent networks, both formal and informal, can give parents the opportunity to express their feelings to others who will listen and understand. As one parent expresses

> The challenge for us, as parents, is to allow ourselves feelings. The negative should not overwhelm the positive, but neither should parents be overwhelmed by guilt when they do experience negative feelings about their child. (Turnbull & Turnbull, 1991)

Parent-to-parent networks also offer parents a mechanism for sharing information (Bruder & Cole, 1991). Parents can help each other solve practical issues; for example, how to make adapted toys or how to find time to make dinner for other family members. Such inside information can reduce the daily stress and frustration that often accompanies having a child with extraordinary caregiving needs (Ackerman, 1985; Dunst, 1985).

Parents may also share information about negotiating the system and accessing resources. Often parents give each other related books or articles, sources for reliable respite care, or a preferred list of helpful community organizations. Parents offer each other a sense of connection with the larger community and a source of ongoing aid and friendship. Helping to develop this network may be of greater long-term value to families than the services that the early intervention programs provide for only a short period of their lives (Bennett, 1985; Dunst, Trivette, & Deal, 1988).

Establishing Interdisciplinary Team Collaboration

Teamwork in a variety of disciplines is part of quality service delivery. The types of interactions and relationships among team members influence the kind of care and service received. An interdisciplinary team approach is necessary to reduce the fragmentation and confusion that results when a number of professionals are advising a family. To be effective in serving young children with disabilities and their families, professional teams must be more than collections of persons pursuing their own interests.

Teams that are cohesive recognize their interdependence and choose to collaborate rather than act independently. Teams that effectively interact with families, effectively interact with each other and include the family on the team. Both informal (conversations at lunch) and formal (written reports and team meetings) modes of communication are essential to team function.

Teamwork evolves through a developmental process (see Case-Smith & Burris Wavrek, Chapter 5). Initially, when first formed, team members identify their skills, expertise, and resources. In this first stage, team roles, tasks, and values are defined. In the second phase, relationships among team members are formed, roles are clarified, and the team begins to develop strategies to manage conflict, make decisions, and solve problems. In the third stage, the team becomes cohesive, working together effectively and productively. Conflicts and problems are resolved through open discussions, and team members have a sense of mastery concerning their roles. In the fourth stage, the team achieves interdependence among its members; that is, members support, value, and depend on each other. At this stage, the team is highly productive and enjoys working together (Handley & Spencer, 1986).

The ability of the early intervention team to effectively function is determined by internal and external factors. The composition of the team and the structure of the home organization or agency will greatly influence how the team functions. Different models of team interaction have been identified and are discussed in Chapter 5. Most early intervention teams are dynamic structures that are eclectic in their approach and that change in response to team membership, client needs, and agency requirements. Values and beliefs also affect communication and interaction among team members (Blechert, Christiansen, & Kari, 1987).

Teams that work together to establish a philosophy and a mission statement find that they have a guide to assist them in decision making and problem solving. Cohesive teams that communicate openly help parents articulate their preference for involvement and identify their roles on the team. Such teams have well-established relationships, allowing them to be flexible with parents regarding their desired team role and style of interaction. Parents have a unique and central role on the team; they are both participants and recipients of services. Their needs and desires should guide the team's actions. When the parents' strengths and resources are emphasized, their roles as decision makers and as advocates for their child are strengthened (Dunst, Trivette, & Deal, 1988).

Facilitating Interagency Collaboration

Teams within agencies can be cohesive units with common missions and goals. However, in early intervention, the team that works with the family is likely to include members from other agencies. Multi-agency teams are a critical aspect of comprehensive early intervention services (McGonigel, Kaufmann, & Johnson, 1991). While multi-agency teams may not have singular missions and goals, they can collaborate, providing mutually beneficial and integral services, to meet family needs. The need for interagency collaboration is especially apparent when the family makes the transition from one agency to another. A primary example occurs when the child is discharged from the hospital. Communication between the hospital team and the agency, which provides community-based services, results in a smooth transition for the family and facilitates continuity of the child/family goals and maintenance of child progress. Often children with disabilities receive ongoing medical and educational services; therefore, linkage between the medical facility team and the early intervention program team can promote continuity for the family as they move in and out of these systems (Gilkerson, Gorski, & Panitz, 1990).

Due to time and resource constraints, interagency collaboration may not always be ideal. Therapists should routinely share written information and make phone contacts with other therapists or early intervention personnel who are involved with the family. Conflicts and confusion for the parents can be avoided if therapy goals and plans are shared. When possible, collaborative efforts should be made on behalf of the family. For example, interagency collaboration is needed when a child simultaneously receives occupational therapy in a preschool setting, from a private practice agency, and in a follow-up clinic of the hospital. Communication becomes critical among these therapists, particularly concerning the goals of therapy and the information shared with the family. The interests and perspectives of the therapists are quite different and the potential for duplication and conflict are great. Communication among service providers may be informal communication, such as a phone call, or may become more formalized when needed, such as an inter-agency meeting.

Summary

The principles and issues discussed in this chapter provide a general framework for occupational therapists who work in early intervention. From these principles and guidelines, a process of family-centered services evolves. This process is described in the following chapter and is illustrated in the other chapters of this book.

References

Ackerman, J. (1985). Preparing for separation. In H.R. Turnbull & A.P. Turnbull (Eds.), *Parents speak out: Then and now.* (pp. 149–158). Columbus, OH: Charles E. Merrill.

Akerly, M.S. (1985). False gods and angry prophets. In H.R. Turnbull & A.P. Turnbull (Eds.), *Parents speak out: Then and now.* (pp. 33–38). Columbus, OH: Charles E. Merrill.

Anderson, J., & Hinojosa, J. (1984). Parents and therapists in a professional partnership . . . occupational therapy in intervention with parents of handicapped children. *American Journal of Occupational Therapy, 38,* 452–461.

Anderson, P.P., & Fenichel, E.S. (1989). *Serving culturally diverse families of infants and toddlers with disabilities.* Washington, DC: National Center for Clinical Infant Programs.

Bailey, D.B. (1988). Considerations in developing family goals. In D.B. Bailey & R.J. Simeonsson (Eds.), *Family assessment in early intervention* (pp. 229–249). Columbus, OH: Charles E. Merrill.

Bailey, D.B., & Simeonsson, R.J. (1988). Home-based early intervention. In S.L. Odom & M.B. Karnes (Eds.), *Research in early childhood special education* (pp. 199–215). Baltimore: Paul H. Brookes Publishing Co.

Bailey, D.B., Simeonsson, R.J., Winton, P.J., Huntington, G.S., Comfort, M., Isbell, P., O'Donnell, K.J., & Helm, J. (1986). Family-focused intervention: A functional model for planning, implementing, and evaluating individualized family services in early intervention. *Journal of the Division for Early Childhood, 10,* 156–171.

Barber, P.A., Turnbull, A.P., Behr, S.K., & Kerns, G.M. (1988). A family systems perspective on early childhood special education. In A.L. Odom & M.B. Karnes (Eds.), *Early intervention for infants and children with handicaps.* Baltimore: Paul H. Brookes Publishing Co.

Bennett, J.M. (1985). A ten o'clock scholar. In H.R. Turnbull & A.P. Turnbull (Eds.), *Parents speak out: Then and now.* (pp. 175–184). Columbus, OH: Charles E. Merrill.

Blechert, T., Christiansen, M., & Kari, N. (1987). Intraprofessional team building. *American Journal of Occupational Therapy, 41*(9), 576–582.

Bruder, M., & Cole, M. (1991). Critical elements of transition from NICU to home and follow-up. *Children's Health Care, 20*(1), 40–49.

Case-Smith, J. (1991). The family perspective. In W. Dunn (Ed.), *Pediatric occupational therapy: Facilitating effective service delivery.* Thorofare, NJ: Slack.

Chen, S. (1990). Early intervention with culturally diverse families of infants and toddlers with disabilities. *Infants and Young Children, 3*(2), 78–87.

Dunst, C.J. (1985). Rethinking early intervention. *Analysis and Intervention in Developmental Disabilities, 5,* 165–201.

Dunst, C.J. (1991). Implementation of the Individualized Family Service Plan. In M.J. McGonigel, R.K. Kaufmann, & B.H. Johnson (Eds.), *Guidelines and recommended practices for the Individualized Family Service Plan.* 2nd ed. Bethesda, MD: Association for the Care of Children's Health.

Dunst, C.J., & Trivette, C.M. (1990). Assessment of social support in early intervention programs. In S.J. Meisels & J.P. Shonkoff (Eds.), *Handbook of early childhood intervention.* Cambridge, MA: University of Cambridge Press.

Dunst, C.J., Trivette, C., & Deal, A. (1988). *Enabling and empowering families: Principles and guidelines for practice.* Cambridge, MA: Brookline Books.

Early Intervention Program for Infants and Toddlers with Handicaps: Final Regulations, 34 CFR 303. (1989, June 22). *Federal Register, 54*(119), 26306–26348.

Education of the Handicapped Act Amendments of 1986 (PL 99-457), 20 U.S.C. Secs. 1400–1485. (1986).

Espe-Sherwindt, M., Kerlin, S., Beatty, C.L., & Crable, S. (1990). *Parents with special needs/mental retardation: A handbook for early intervention.* Cincinnati, OH: University Affiliated Cincinnati Center for Developmental Disorders.

Featherstone, H. (1980). *A difference in the family: Living with a disabled child.* New York: Basic Books.

Fewell, R.R., & Vadasy, P.F., Eds. (1986). *Families of handicapped children: Needs and support across the lifespan.* Austin, TX: PRO-ED.

Gilkerson, L., Gorski, P., & Panitz, P. (1990). Hospital-based intervention for preterm infants and their families. In S.J. Meisels & J.P. Shonkoff (Eds.), *Handbook of early childhood intervention* (pp. 445–468). Cambridge, MA: University of Cambridge.

Halpern, R. (1990). Community-based early intervention. In S.J. Meisels & J.P. Shonkoff (Eds.), *Handbook of early childhood intervention* (pp. 469–498). Cambridge, MA: University of Cambridge Press.

Handley, E.E., & Spencer, P. (1986). *Project Bridge: Decision-making for early intervention: A team approach.* Elk Grove Village, IL: American Academy of Pediatrics.

Hanson, M.J., Lynch, E.W., & Wayman, I.I. (1990). Honoring the cultural diversity of families when gathering data. *Topics in Early Childhood Special Education, 10*(1), 112–131.

Healy, A., Keesee, P.D., & Smith, B.S. (1989). *Early services for children with special needs: Transactions for family support.* Baltimore: Paul H. Brookes Publishing Co.

Hinojosa, J. (1990). How mothers of preschool children with cerebral palsy perceive occupational and physical therapists and their influence on family life. *Occupational Therapy Journal of Research, 10,* 144–162.

Humphry, R. (1989). Early intervention and the influence of the occupational therapist on the parent–child relationship. *American Journal of Occupational Therapy, 43*(11), 738–744.

Individuals with Disabilities Education Act (PL 100-476), 20 U.S.C. Secs. 1400–1485. (1990).

Kjerland, L. (1986). *Early intervention tailor made.* Eagan, MN: Project Dakota, Inc.

Kjerland, L., & Kovach, J. (1990). Family-staff collaboration for tailored infant assessment. In E.D. Gibbs & D.M. Teti (Eds.), *Interdisciplinary assessment of infants: A guide for early intervention professionals.* Baltimore: Paul H. Brookes Publishing Co.

Mahoney, G., & Powell, A. (1988). Modifying parent–child interaction: Enhancing the development of handicapped children. *Journal of Special Education, 22,* 82–96.

McCormack, G.L. (1987). Culture and communication in the treatment planning for occupational therapy with minority patients. *Occupational Therapy in Health Care, 4*(1), 17–36.

McGonigel, M. (1991). Philosophy and conceptual framework. In M. McGonigel, R.K. Kaufmann, & B.H. Johnson (Eds.), *Guidelines and recommended practices for the Individualized Family Service Plan.* 2nd ed. Bethesda, MD: Association for the Care of Children's Health.

McGonigel, M., Kaufmann, R.K., & Johnson, B.H. (1991). *Guidelines and recommended practices for the Individualized Family Service Plan.* 2nd ed. Bethesda, MD: Association for the Care of Children's Health.

Meisels, S.J., & Shonkoff, J.P., Eds. (1990). *Handbook of early childhood intervention.* Cambridge, MA: University of Cambridge Press.

Nastro, M. (1992). An ethnographic study of mothers of children with cerebral palsy and the effect of occupational therapy intervention on their lives. Master's thesis, The Ohio State University, Columbus.

Nastro, M., & Case-Smith, J. (in press). The effect of occupational therapy intervention on mothers of children with cerebral palsy. *American Journal of Occupational Therapy.*

Olson, D.H., Russell, C.S., & Sprenkle, D.H. (1980). Circumplex model of marital and family systems II: Empirical studies and clinical intervention. In J.P. Vincent (Ed.), *Advances in family intervention assessment and theory* (Vol. 1, pp. 129–179). Greenwich, CT: JAI Press.

Research and Policy Committee for Economic Development. (1987). *Children in need—Investment strategies for the educationally disadvantaged.* New York: Author.

Sameroff, A.J., & Chandler, M.J. (1975). Reproductive risk and the continuum of caretaking casualty. In F.D. Horowitz, M. Hetherington, S. Scarr-Salapatek, & G. Siegel (Eds.), *Review of child development research* (Vol. 4, pp. 187–244). Chicago: University of Chicago Press.

Sameroff, A.J., & Fiese, B.H. (1990). Transactional regulation and early intervention. In S.J. Meisels & J.P. Shonkoff (Eds.), *Handbook of early childhood intervention.* Cambridge, MA: University of Cambridge Press.

Shelton, T., Jeppson, E., & Johnson, B. (1987). *Family-centered care for children with special health care needs.* Washington, DC: Association for the Care of Children's Health.

Simeonsson, R. (1988). Unique characteristics of family with young handicapped children. In D.B. Bailey & R. Simeonsson (Eds.), *Family assessment in early intervention.* Columbus, OH: Charles E. Merrill.

Simeonsson, R.J., Bailey, D.B., Huntington, G.S., & Comfort, M. (1986). Testing the concept of goodness of fit in early intervention. *Infant Mental Health Journal, 7,* 81–94.

Stagg, V., & Catron, T. (1986). Networks of social supports for parents of handicapped children. In R.R. Fewell & P.F. Vadasy (Eds.), *Families of handicapped children* (pp. 279–316). Austin, TX: PRO-ED.

Summers, J.A., Dell'Oliver, C., Turnbull, A.P., Benson, H., Santelli, E., Campbell, M., & Siegel-Causey, E. (1990). Examining the Individualized Family Service Plan process: What are family and practitioner preferences? *Topics in Early Childhood Special Education, 10*(1), 78–99.

Thomas, A., & Chess, S. (1977). *Temperament and development.* New York: Brunner/Mazel.

Turnbull, A.P., Summers, J.A., & Brotherson, M.J. (1986). Family life cycle: Theoretical and empirical implications and future directions for families with mentally retarded members. In J.J. Gallagher & P.M. Vietze (Eds.), *Families of handicapped persons: Research, programs, and policy issues* (pp. 45–66). Baltimore: Paul H. Brookes Publishing Co.

Turnbull, A., & Turnbull, H.R. (1991). *Families, professionals, and exceptionalities: A special partnership.* 2nd ed. Columbus, OH: Charles E. Merrill.

Vincent, L.J., & Salisbury, C.L. (1988). Changing economic and social influences on family involvement. *Topics in Early Childhood Special Education, 8*(1), 48–59.

Vincent, L.J., Salisbury, C.L., Strain, P., McCormick, C., & Tessier, A. (1990). A behavioral-ecological approach to early intervention: Focus on cultural diversity. In S.M. Meisels & J.P. Shonkoff (Eds.), *Handbook of early childhood intervention.* Cambridge, MA: University of Cambridge Press.

Wayman, K.I., Lynch, E.W., & Hanson, M.J. (1991). Home-based early childhood services: Cultural sensitivity in a family systems approach. *Topics in Early Childhood Special Education, 10*(4), 56–75.

Winnicott, D.W. (1964). *The child, the family, and the outside world.* London: Penguin Press.

Winton, P.J. (1988). Effective communication between parents and professionals. In D.B. Bailey & R.J. Simeonsson (Eds.), *Family assessment in early intervention* (pp. 207–228). Columbus, OH: Charles E. Merrill.

Ziskin, L. (1985). The story of Jennie. In H.R. Turnbull & A.P. Turnbull (Eds.), *Parents speak out: Then and now.* Columbus, OH: Charles E. Merrill.

2

□ □ □
□ □ □
□ □ □

Defining the Early Intervention Process

Jane Case-Smith, EdD, OTR

Occupational therapy involves assessment, planning, intervention, and evaluation. These four interrelated processes are ongoing throughout the therapy. This chapter describes how they are implemented in family-centered occupational therapy with infants and young children. Occupational therapy is part of a comprehensive interdisciplinary team process that is both defined and exemplified by the development of an Individualized Family Service Plan (IFSP).

The events that transpire in developing the IFSP are more important than the written document that results. This process involves negotiation and collaboration between families and professionals (McGonigel, 1991) and represents the true spirit of the Education of the Handicapped Act Amendments of 1986, Public Law (PL) 99-457, and the Individuals with Disabilities Education Act, PL 102-119. Figure 2-1 illustrates the IFSP process.

Comprehensive Assessment

In family-centered early intervention, the infant is assessed in the context of the family. Assessment has multiple steps that require the time and input of family members and other professionals.

Screening

The family's entry into the early intervention system often begins with a screening or formal identification process that may focus on the child, the parents, or both. Screening identifies delays in the child's

Preparation of this chapter was supported by grant #H029F00034 of the Office of Special Education and Rehabilitation Services, U.S. Department of Education.

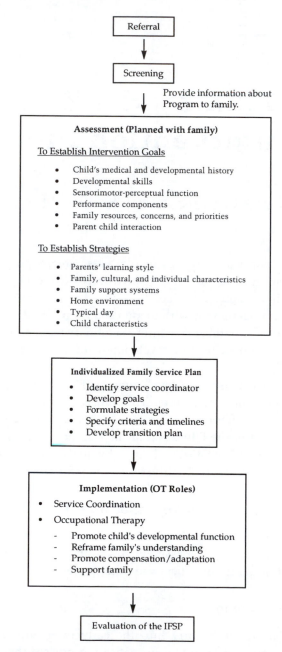

Figure 2-1 The IFSP process

developmental skills, areas of dysfunction, and risk factors that potentiate delays in development. Risk factors may be either biological or environmental. The infant is considered most at risk when biological risk factors combine with a caregiving environment that is not conducive to developmental growth. In medical diagnostic clinics, children who are considered to be high-risk are often evaluated by occupational therapists. In community child find, screening may or may not involve occupational therapists. While an essential part of the initial assessment, screening often occurs in an agency or a center that does not house an early intervention program, and a referral is made if testing indicates delays or high risk for developmental problems. Team members of the early intervention program undertake a comprehensive assessment in order to develop a plan for individualized services. Therefore, screening and assessment are often separate processes, serve different purposes, and use different evaluation methods. Chapter 3 provides an in-depth discussion of screening.

Assessment to Establish Goals

Assessment occurs across time and is accomplished in a series of steps. Figure 2-1, The IFSP Process, includes the major types of assessments performed by occupational therapists in family-centered early intervention. A comprehensive assessment should be guided by the family and involves both the family and multiple team members. As much as possible, families are to be given choices regarding what assessments should be used and when, as well as where and how assessment should occur. The essential components of the therapist's evaluation are family concerns, resources, and priorities; child's developmental levels and skills; performance components; and family interactions. Support systems, the parents' learning style, roles and values, cultural background, a typical day, and the home (day-care) environment are assessed to establish intervention strategies. Assessment begins when the child is identified as an appropriate candidate for early intervention services. Based on the results of the initial contacts, the family can be referred to another agency or it can be decided that the child and family do not need services at the time.

Logically, family resources, concerns, and priorities are assessed after the child is evaluated and is determined to be appropriate for services. This information, elicited using formal and informal methods, guides the planning process and is essential to the development of intervention goals and strategies.

Most often therapy and educational services begin during the assessment process. As child and family are assessed, information is provided about the scope of early intervention services, about child development, and, specifically, about the child's diagnosis. The assessment period also allows the team to view the child and family in different contexts. The occupational therapist observes the child's responses in a variety of situations with and without the parents. These observations result in an understanding of parent–child interaction patterns and the child's ability to cope with and master her environment. Therapy techniques are tried and the child's adaptive responses provide helpful information for establishing therapy goals and plans. During this time, the therapist develops an appreciation of the parents' perceptions, hopes, desires, and concerns for the child. Information given to the parents about developmental skills, the nature of the child's problem, and the service delivery system enables the family to fully participate in the assessment process. The parameters of assessment are described in the following section. Chapter 4 discusses specific evaluation methods, procedures, and instruments.

Medical and Developmental History

The child's history is gathered from an interview with the parents and from records, when available. A *medical history,* including events that occurred during the mother's pregnancy and during the birth of the infant, is collected. Records of therapy or intervention services provided by the hospital or other community agencies are reviewed. A *developmental history* provides the therapist with information about the child's developmental course and the parents' perception of the child's progress. A *sensory history* of the child's responses to the environment is critical for infants who seem to have sensory modulation or sensory integration problems. (See Chapter 4.) Queries about the infant's *sleep–wake cycle* provide information on the sleep patterns of the infant. Continually disrupted sleep can create a state of exhaustion in family members that compounds the perceived stress of daily events.

Child's Developmental Skills

Developmental skills are evaluated through informal observations, standardized scales, and parental reports. Reports from parents are valuable elements in confirming the therapist's impressions and in verifying or qualifying the behavior of the child. The occupational therapist's role in evaluating developmental function depends on the staffing and structure of the program. The therapist may be responsible for assessing all domains of development or may focus on specific domains (e.g., fine motor, perceptual motor, sensory integration, and self-care). When the concerns of the occupational therapist are limited, assessment is not given prior to integrating the results of performance in one domain with the results of a child's performance in other domains. Development is also interpreted in light of neurophysiological, medical, and environmental factors. For example, delays in motor development may be attributed to deficits in strength, atypical muscle tone, poor endurance, orthopedic problems, and environmental factors. The results of the developmental assessment cite the strengths of the child and describe areas of delay and of atypical performance.

Performance Components

Assessment of performance components in the areas of sensori-motor-perceptual function and daily living skills is essential to the development of specific goals for the child. Neurophysiological theories provide an essential framework for making the critical observations that enable the occupational therapist to analyze the basis of an infant's skills. Through in-depth analysis of the quality of skill, the therapist formulates goals and methods to be implemented and reframes the parents' perception of the child's behaviors based on the child's underlying sensorimotor capabilities. Instruments and methods used to analyze the neuromotor and sensory components of the infant's developmental skills are described in Chapter 4.

Occupational therapists often focus on sensory, motor, and perceptual functions of the child (Gilfoyle, Grady, & Moore, 1991). The therapist assesses these areas by observing the child in naturalistic interaction with the parents or others. Evaluation information is also gathered from the child's responses to specific stimuli. The environmental context is considered, since factors such as familiarity with persons in the environment, presence or absence of parents, and level of sensory stimulation impose strong influences on the child's responses. By observing the infant's response to specific handling and sensory input, the therapist judges the skills that seem to be amenable to change, that can be targeted in the therapy plan.

Daily Living Skills

In the case of infants, *daily living skills* refers to self-sustaining skills, such as feeding patterns and sleep patterns. In Chapter 8, Glass and Wolf describe assessment of feeding in detail. Sleep patterns may be evaluated from the parents' description of a typical day (discussed later in this chapter) or the parents may be asked to maintain a week-long record of the infant's sleep and wakeful periods in each 24-hour day.

The daily living skills of the infant also refer to bathing and dressing, which involve the parent. Occupational therapists can observe the parents during these activities and then offer suggestions for making the activities easier or more therapeutic for the child. When observation is not possible or is not a priority of the parent, the therapist may discuss daily caregiving activities with the parent to assess the parent's sense of enjoyment or frustration during routine caregiving. As a result, the therapist may suggest alternative handling methods, adaptive equipment, or adaptations to the environment that can facilitate the activity or conserve the parent's energy during the activity. Because the caregiving activities of bathing, diapering, and dressing are interactional situations for both parent and child, therapy goals may also be addressed during these times.

Family Concerns, Resources, and Priorities

Family concerns, resources, and priorities are evaluated during ongoing contacts with the family and may be formally evaluated in an interview, which may or may not include completion of a written form (Kaufmann & McGonigel, 1991). When the primary needs and desires of the family are identified, the assessment and planning process can focus on those family priorities. Deal, Dunst, and Trivette (1989) propose that families are more receptive to and willing to participate when assessment and intervention are based on family needs and aspirations. Intervention becomes most effective when the assistance offered is congruent with the family's appraisal of the problem and need (Dunst, 1991). Comprehensive evaluation of concerns and resources provides the therapist with the information needed to guide the family toward resources that will strengthen the family unit and improve their ability to cope (Zeitlin & Williamson, 1989). Goals and plans that build on family strengths and resources are more likely to be accomplished than those that arise from the therapist's priorities.

Assessments to Determine Intervention Strategies and Plans

Multiple family variables influence intervention strategies and methods. Many times characteristics of the mother or father determine the intervention strategies and plans selected. The presence of a disability in either or both parents (e.g., deafness, mental retardation, or mental illness) will greatly influence the role of the early intervention team and the goals and plan determined.

Parents' Learning Styles

One variable that seems particularly important to the occupational therapist is the parents' learning style. Therapy often involves instruction to the parent(s) regarding methods for facilitating the child's developmental skills through play activities and daily interactions. The parents may prefer written instructions or illustrations, videotapes, or the opportunity to observe the child's interaction with the therapist. The preferred learning methods of parents in a qualitative study by Hinojosa (1990) was observation of the therapist with the child. Other parents benefit from performing the activity (e.g., facilitating head control during dressing) with the therapist's guidance and feedback. It is important that the parents' preferred activities guide the therapist's selection of strategies.

Family Support Systems

Support systems and resources are other variables that may not be directly assessed by the occupational therapist, but are important in establishing intervention plans. The family's support systems are closely tied to their ability to cope with stress (Dunst, Trivette, & Deal, 1988). The family's social support systems may be formal (e.g., church) or informal (e.g., friends in the neighborhood). Extended family can be an important source of support. An assessment of support systems includes not only identifying friends and extended family, but also assessing the parents' perception of their support systems. Often, support systems change when a child with a disability enters the family system, and shift according to the family's developmental stage.

Home Environment

Assessment of the home environment gives the therapist a picture of the child's learning environment. Aspects of the home environment that influence the selection of strategies are: (1) safety, (2) space, (3) toys available, (4) amount of general sensory stimulation (visual and auditory), (5) roles of nuclear and extended family members who reside in the home, and (6) equipment available (e.g., strollers, playpen, swing, high chair).

By identifying the resources available in the home, the therapist can provide the most appropriate suggestions for activities to be undertaken with the child. The activities can be individualized to the equipment and toys already present in the home. In addition, the equipment that is already present may need to be modified to meet the child's needs. For example, if the parents have purchased a high chair that does not provide the support and stability needed for feeding, adaptations can be made. The therapist may discourage use of Johnny-Jump-Ups™ and certain types of walkers. Evaluation of the child while he is using the equipment helps the therapist determine if its use is inappropriate and, if so, how to adapt the equipment to promote the child's function. A visit to the home provides the therapist with a visual image so that recommendations and suggestions match the resources available and take into consideration the child's natural environment. When services are clinically based, arrangements should be made so that the therapist has the opportunity for occasional home visitation.

A Typical Day

Another assessment that provides essential information for planning intervention activities and strategies is the parents' description of *a typical day*. The therapist guides this description, using open-ended questions (e.g., "Tell me about a typical day.", "Beginning with when you first awaken, describe all of your activities in a typical day."). A description of the typical day serves three purposes. These purposes are as follows:

1. The therapist gains an understanding of the amount of caregiving that the child requires in a typical day and of the amount of daily attention and energy that the parents devote to the child.
2. The therapist learns the structure of the family's day so that the recommended activities fit into their schedule. Suggestions are also made for optimal times to perform certain activities.
3. The therapist learns about difficult times in the family's day. The parents may explain that feeding each meal requires an hour and a half or that baths are given only twice a week by the father, because the child is too difficult for the mother to handle in the bathtub. Therefore, requesting a description of the typical day may uncover daily problems that the family may not have included in their original problem list (Rainforth & Salisbury, 1988).

Child Characteristics

Child assessment influences both the goals established by the team and the strategies and activities that are planned. Assessment of the child must occur in the presence of the parent(s) so that observations can be verified with the parents and reports about typical responses can be obtained. The parent can assist in administering test items or in engaging the child in play if the child appears anxious or fearful of the therapist. Certain child characteristics generally create stress for family members and tend to interfere with the family's daily routine. Three variables that seem to have a strong influence on the family's function are the severity of the disability, behavioral problems, and whether the child has a difficult temperament.

Assessment of the effects of the child's disability (and required care) on the family is particularly relevant when the child has severe or multiple disabilities. Some children with ongoing medical problems need almost continual care. The amount of time in direct care can be assessed through the parents' description of a typical day. Children with feeding tubes do not necessarily require more time to feed; in fact, they often require less time and effort to feed. Children on cardiorespiratory monitors may not require more time, but may create a sense of anxiety in the family.

The time and effort required of the parents in daily care and the amount of progress made by the child are the critical family function issues that are relevant to occupational therapy evaluation. The developmental progress of the child often determines the parents' sense of competence. While rapid progress can create parental satisfaction, lack of progress can be frustrating or disappointing for parents. A child who makes slow, steady progress seems to be less a source of stress than a child who makes progress and then loses ground (e.g., a child with severe seizures).

While therapists make informal observations about children's behaviors, in-depth assessment of behavior and temperament is usually accomplished by disciplines other than occupational therapy (e.g., psychology). Observation of general behavior and temperament is an important part of the comprehensive assessment. Behaviors that are particularly relevant to family function are listed in Table 2-1.

Table 2-1 Child Behaviors that Affect Family Function

Behaviors	*Relevance to Family*
Hyperactivity	• Is a source of disruption • Requires tremendous energy
Socially unresponsive behaviors	• Cause interactions between family members and child to be less frequent or one-way • Can interfere with the formation of positive relationships
Repetitive behaviors (can evolve into self-abusive behaviors)	• Are distracting to family • Can be a source of great anxiety for the parents
Lability Unpredictable or extreme mood swings	• Can be confusing for parents • Can decrease parents' sense of competence in caregiving
Poor adaptability to new environments or new situations	• Often requires comforting or other kinds of attention to adapt to change

Goodness-of-Fit between Parent and Child

Behaviors such as those listed in Table 2-1 have different effects on family function and interaction according to the goodness-of-fit model. Handling a child who is hyperactive may be less stressful for energetic, active parents than for less energetic, more sedentary parents. Easygoing parents may not be as affected by a child with lability and unpredictable moods. Therefore, while the listed child variables are an essential part of early intervention assessment, their impact on family function must be considered in light of the parents' characteristics.

McWilliams (1991) describes the relationship between a child and a single mother who suffered an emotional breakdown that resulted in her being hospitalized in a state institution for the mentally ill. Her description depicts the goodness-of-fit between parent and child that is essential not only to the child's development, but to their lives together.

> Carol feels that Joy [mother] is fairly capable of living on her own and caring for Bobby providing she has a reasonable level of support. Bobby obviously means the world to Joy. She loves him as much as any mother could love any child; handicapped or not. Joy talks to Bobby constantly, rocks him, and tries to play with him by showing him toys and books. In some ways, her low-key personality, patience, and lack of expectations for him provide a better environment than the fast pace environment of most homes and preschool centers. In short, she knows how to wait for a response from him and is capable of repeating an activity over and over again. . . . Carol remembers her astonishment at Joy's ability to wait for Bobby to respond. What amazed her more was the fact that Bobby only cooed when Joy stopped speaking and that he seemed so intent upon Joy's face. (McWilliams, 1991, p. 81)

Planning Intervention

The information gathered from the assessment administered by the occupational therapist and by other disciplines is shared among the team members, including the family. The occupational therapy assessment results are interpreted in light of the results of other disciplines and combined into a comprehensive picture of the child. Using the collective results, the team and family together develop an IFSP that will serve as the basis for the intervention program. The process of developing an IFSP is intended to be continually responsive to the child's and family's changes in priorities. As such, the intervention plan can be described as *fluid*, which implies that the plan is flexible and can change at any time as the child and/or the family needs change (Deal, Dunst, & Trivette, 1989).

The specific plan goals are derived from the assessment information. This information is based on the therapist's previous experience with similar children and the therapist's impressions about the potential of the involved child. Given a list of potential goals, the family decides which goals are priorities. Goals that specifically relate to the family's concerns about caring for their child are acknowledged and incorporated into the plan. When the occupational therapists or other team members have additional concerns, these should be explained to the family, who then decides whether they are to be included in the plan. Bailey (1988) suggests that when the family's high-priority goals are targeted first, family members are more likely to invest in their attainment and to work harder to achieve them. Successful attainment of the priority goals may give the family the energy and confidence to work on other goals not initially viewed as important by family members.

With certain goals established, the team progresses and begins to formulate strategies. The strategies or plans are based on the assessment results as well as the interests and resources of the family. In the plan, the team identifies who should be involved in accomplishing each goal and how that goal might best be attained. The occupational therapist designs strategies based on her impressions as to what activities and environments seem to elicit the child's best responses and highest level of behavior. The plans are also based on the family's resources, their desire for level of involvement in intervention, and their values. Plans that involve the purchase of equipment or adapted toys clearly must consider the family's resources. The parent should be given a range of equipment choices, with specific information about the advantages and disadvantages of each choice. The parent may choose to be present during all intervention sessions or to request that therapy be provided at the child's day-care center, to assist those caregivers in working toward the intervention goals. The flexibility of the early intervention team will determine the variety of strategies that are planned. One mother expressed her appreciation of such flexibility:

> It has been nice to have Joan [occupational therapist] come to our house and she always works around our schedule and tries to come at the best times for Brian. One day, when my parents were visiting, she came early in the morning before the rest of the family was up and going. Because Joan is flexible, so are we. Adaptability is very important. It's a big key in how to get along and you have to get along with your therapists. (Nastro, 1992, p. 51)

Situations arise in which the parents' values or actions are clearly detrimental to the child. In some families, parents use physical punishment daily (e.g., spanking) to discipline the child. When such problems in parenting are identified, they should be directly addressed and support systems should be identified to assist the parents in remediating the problem and providing adequate and appropriate child care. A positive relationship between team members and the parents will help facilitate change in the parents' behavior (Bailey, 1987). In some instances, a referral to persons and agencies outside the early intervention agency may be necessary.

Intervention

Service Coordination

The occupational therapist often takes on the role of service coordinator for the family, when he is the primary interventionist for the family (Case-Smith, 1991a). As the service coordinator, the therapist has primary responsibility for coordinating the IFSP. Agencies, team members, and families are invited to participate in developing the IFSP and to attend the planning meeting. The service coordinator may also have the responsibility of gathering the assessment information from all team members and facilitating collaboration with the family. Even further, the role of service coordinator extends beyond development of the IFSP into implementation of the plan. While the occupational therapist/service coordinator may not carry full responsibility for implementing the IFSP, he often has continuing responsibility for assisting the family in procuring resources, in maintaining communication among the multiple agencies serving the family, and in monitoring progress relevant to the IFSP (Case-Smith, 1991a; Dunst & Trivette, 1989).

A Conceptual Framework for Occupational Therapy

The goals and plans that have been developed serve to guide intervention, and the results of intervention lead directly to changes in these same goals and plans. The circular relationship of intervention goals, strategies, and results is described in Figure 2-2. This model suggests that goals and strategies are continually evolving with child response and family input and that decisions to change intervention may be reached by the mutual agreement of parent and therapist. Therapy consists of turn taking between the child and therapist, parent and therapist, and parent and child. The therapist establishes an environment for play or performance in another domain (e.g., feeding).

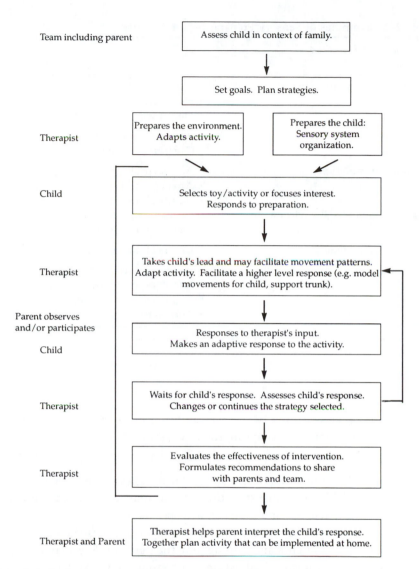

Figure 2-2 Early intervention therapeutic process

Sensory Preparation for Activity

The therapist sometimes prepares the child for activity by means of sensory input. This is accomplished through the following sources of stimulation. Table 2-2 lists some examples of sensory input and the expected effect that each example might have on the child. While preparing the

Table 2-2   Examples of Sensory Preparation for Activity

Description of Handling or Sensory Input	Effect on the Child
Deep pressure, proprioception	• Calms child • Helps organize responses • Decreases hypertonicity
Stroking	• Activates muscle groups • Organizes movement
Vestibular stimulation	• Alerts child • Arouses child • Calms child
Organization of visual environment	• Increases visual focus • Increases attention
Music/rhythmic voice	• Calms child, helps focus attention
Joint mobilization, weight-bearing	• Increases range of motion • Improves joint co-contraction • Improves joint stability • Activates muscles or inhibits muscle tone

child, the therapist continually observes and interprets the infant's response for adjusting the input and adapting the environment.

Creating an Environment of Turn Taking Interaction

Within the context of the environment that the therapist has created, the child selects an activity and responds both to handling and to choices for play in the environment. The therapist follows the child's lead and offers support and guidance throughout the activity. She may facilitate movement, assist in postural adjustment, or guide movement with tactile cues. The activity can also be adjusted so that a higher level of response is required. This adjustment is a natural evolution of the activity. For example, the toys are moved to facilitate crossing the midline or reaching over the head. The therapist's support of the upright position is gradually removed and is reapplied only as necessary. Whether the activity is adapted to increase or decrease difficulty, the appropriate challenge is created for the child. Environment, activities, and handling that offer the optimal amount of challenge engage the child's interest and facilitate the highest level of response. Interaction is easily sustained at this level.

After introducing a stimulus, the therapist waits for the child's response.

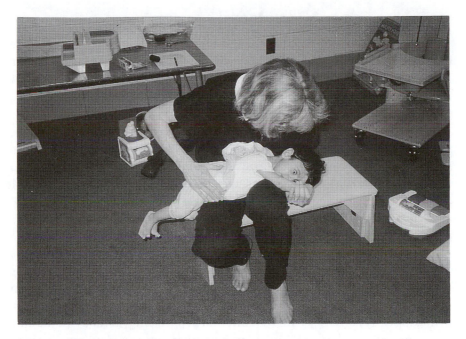

Figure 2-3 Therapist applies NDT techniques based on the infant's responses

Each input offered, is based on the child's response, whether it requires special-ized handling, adaptation of the environment, or simple repetition of the selected activity. With each response, the therapist decides whether to con-tinue or to change the activity. The reciprocal turn taking continues as the child responds to the environment and initiates activity. Meanwhile, the therapist formulates an overall impression of the effectiveness of the activity toward promoting function. Based on evaluation of the effectiveness of the activity, the therapist plans new strategies and formulates recommendations for the family and other team members. (See Figure 2-3.)

Parent Participation

The parent participating in the therapy can join the interaction at any point. The parent can choose to be involved in the turn taking as a third participant or to engage the child in reciprocal interaction as a dyad. The interaction should flow between the child and therapist, child and parent, and parent and therapist. Infants usually focus on a single stimulus at a time; therefore, interaction with one individual elicits the best response. The therapist can model handling for the parent to imitate; guide the parent's responses, either physically or verbally; and reinforce the parent's interaction with the child.

Goals of Occupational Therapy

The occupational therapist has four overriding goals that set the stage for interactions between the child and family. The first is to *promote change in the child's developmental function.* Emphasis of remediation is in the developmental areas that are delayed and are within the realm of occupational therapy. Changes in the child create changes in the family.

A second goal of occupational therapy intervention is to *reframe or redefine the child's behavior.* From the early days of the parent–infant relationship, the parents begin to categorize and interpret the infant's behaviors. For example, a child with sensory defensiveness may be viewed as a child unable or unwilling to attach to them. Therapists help parents understand the child's behaviors from a different perspective based on an understanding of neurophysiological, developmental, and sensory integration principles (Fisher & Murray, 1991).

A third goal of intervention is assisting the family and child to *compensate for and adapt to the disability.* Often the child's problems require adjustment in the family's life together. Occupational therapists assist the family in managing daily activities with the child and in providing methods for the child to compensate for the disability. Adaptive equipment or adaptive methods are suggested to the family to make care of the child easier and to improve the child's function.

A fourth goal of occupational therapy is to *support family members.* By offering ongoing, nonjudgmental support of the parents and other family members, the therapist promotes family–child relationships. Listening to, respecting, and demonstrating family concerns helps the family cope and strengthens their ability to manage stressful situations.

Therapy to Promote Child's Developmental Function

The intervention process that promotes function and skill building involves and affects the family in two general ways. First, the therapeutic model facilitates new skills in the child. A higher level of responses in the child often bolsters the parent–child relationship, since developmental progress is viewed positively by parents. A higher level of sensorimotor skills may enable the child to respond more effectively in interactions with family members. Change may also occur in the child's ability to initiate interaction and to be involved in turn taking with the parent. As sensorimotor skills improve, the child's cues and responses become easier for the parent to read, promoting communication in the dyad. Improved head control may facilitate improved oculomotor skills and better eye contact with the parent. Increased reaching enables the infant to touch the parent's face. Increased arousal and alertness results in improved attentiveness and more opportunities for interaction.

Second, progress in developmental skills also promotes the parents' sense of competence. While it is important that the parents understand that their child's developmental progress is not necessarily linked to their parenting skills, most parents take great joy in observing developmental changes in their child. They gain a sense of achievement and confidence from watching their child's growth. Overall, parents are empowered as competent caregivers when new skills are demonstrated by their child (Case-Smith, 1991b).

The occupational therapist becomes a primary source of information in the promotion of growth in a child. Information is shared throughout the intervention process in a variety of forms. One of the first bits of information shared is a description of child development. The family benefits most from understanding their child's present skills on the continuum of typical development. The next developmental steps are shared with the parents in order to guide their selection of toys, equipment, and activities for the child. The interaction of developmental domains is often helpful for family members in understanding how function in one area affects function in other areas.

The occupational therapist gives parents specific recommendations for activities that promote developmental function and the child's ability to interact with family members. The recommendations are based on the interpretation of a number of variables that influence the parent–child interactions and the daily environment of the child. These variables are as follows:

1. the priorities of the family
2. strengths and needs of the child
3. interpretation of the child's response to sensory stimulation
4. materials and resources available in the home
5. parents' level of involvement and interest in the early intervention program
6. parents' learning style and preference of type of information (visual, verbal, physical modeling)
7. input from other team members regarding goals, strategies and recommendations for the child
8. the daily routines of the family

Recommendations that are easy to apply and fit naturally into the parents' daily routines are most likely to be implemented. Some parents request specific, concrete suggestions for activities that promote the child's skill development. Other parents benefit most when the goals for the child are shared and a range of activities are given for accomplishing the goal(s). Through the parent's description of a typical day, the stressful, demanding times with the child are identified. Suggestions for strategies to help the parents manage these difficult times are given. The number of suggestions should be limited (one or two may be best) because long lists of recommendations can overwhelm parents and be abandoned immediately.

Mothers of children with cerebral palsy reported that they did not have the time, energy, or confidence to implement a therapist-directed home treatment program. Nevertheless, they did incorporate previously learned treatment strategies into daily interactions with their children (Hinojosa & Anderson, 1991). When the number of recommendations cannot possibly be implemented, the parents may feel guilty or feel that their caregiving is inadequate. Recommendations that can be accomplished in play with the child or in the family's natural daily routine will most likely promote the parents' sense of competence and positively affect the parent–child relationship. Studies have demonstrated that when parents become therapists of the child, their interactions tend to become negative (Kogan, Tyler, & Turner, 1974). Therapeutic exercises are an unnatural context for interaction and may be stressful for the parent and confusing for the child. Directed exercises may replace time that could be spent in play or more natural interactions.

A variety of methods are used by the therapist to help parents promote the child's development, including specific therapeutic techniques. Usually, a combination of methods proves to be most effective in remediating delays and problems. The visual image of feeding, handling, or interacting with the child, as shown in Figure 2-4, may be the best source of information for the parent who wishes to implement similar strategies at home. Through modeling and explanation, therapists have the opportunity to give examples of the types of activities that will promote developmental skills and of ways to promote positive interactions while implementing those activities. (See Figure 2-5.)

The therapist may also suggest adaptations to the home environment, which can enhance the child's development. These suggestions often relate to creating a sensory milieu that provides the best learning environment for the child. Infants with sensory defensiveness may benefit most from quiet, nonstimulating environments. Specific suggestions can be made to rearrange the position of the child's crib, to allow more play on the carpet, or to arrange furniture so that the child can easily pull himself to a standing position. An environment that allows exploration and is open, yet safe, enables the child to achieve a sense of mastery over the environment.

The therapist's responsiveness and sensitivity to the child often promotes those qualities in the parent–child relationship. In contrast, interactions that are therapist-directed and highly structured may reinforce excessive parent-directed interaction. The interaction style of parents who have children with special needs tends to be more directive and less responsive than that of other parents (Mahoney, Finger, & Powell, 1985). This directive, nonresponsive

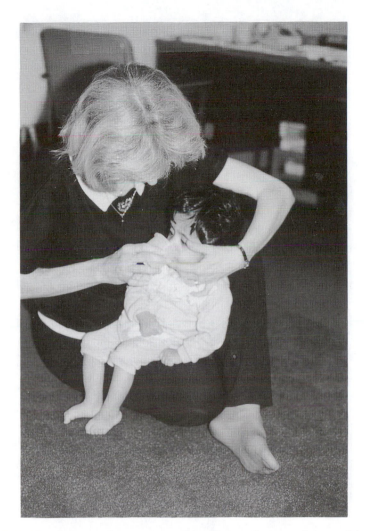

Figure 2-4 The therapist demonstrates handling techniques for cup drinking
that help the parents manage this activity and improve the child's jaw stability

style of interaction appears to be less effective in promoting development
than sensitive interactions that are responsive to child-initiated activities
(Hanzlik, Chapter 9; Mahoney & Powell, 1988).

The natural turn taking that occurs between parent and child is often
different when there is a child with a disability in the family. Children with
Down syndrome demonstrate slower responses and, therefore, the parent
must often patiently wait to allow the child ample opportunity to respond.
Children with poor motor control often require repeated attempts to respond
and assistance to successfully accomplish a response. The assistance provided

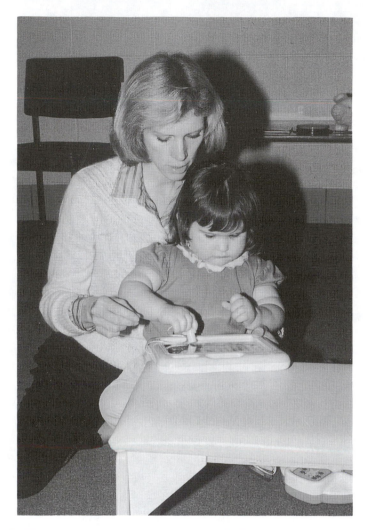

Figure 2-5 Therapist modeling turn taking with child

is clearly a supportive rather than a directive effort by the parent or therapist. By assisting parents in adapting their interaction style and patterns of reciprocal turn taking to the child's level of response, the goodness-of-fit between parent and child is promoted, which then fosters the child's development.

In addition to modeling interaction, specific handling methods, and adapting developmental activities, therapists also provide specific recommendations to parents regarding their selection of toys, equipment, and activities at home. Therapists may be a source of positive reinforcement or of consultation for parents when the parents are making decisions and plans for their child. It is important that, as a consultant, the therapist is aware of the recommendations made by other team members. Consultation may also be most effective when the therapist has observed the home environment and the family interaction in that environment. Service delivery that includes therapy at home increases the occupational therapist's ability to provide the most appropriate and effective consultation. Intervention within the home helps the therapist understand the family's style, routines, and resources within their natural environment and provides a more complete picture as the basis of the consultation.

Reframing: Increasing Understanding of the Child

Occupational therapists are instrumental in helping others to understand and appreciate a child who has a disability. This process of increasing or changing the family's understanding of the disability and of teaching the family to perceive a child's strengths has been termed *reframing* (Fisher & Murray, 1991). By reframing the situation, caregivers, teachers, and others can more easily comprehend the nature and the reasons for the child's behavior.

While some parents have a good understanding of child development (e.g., parents with several children), most parents have minimal knowledge of disability. Specific information about the child's disability helps parents form expectations, become more sensitive to certain areas of child development, access resources that may be beneficial to the child, and communicate with professionals and service providers.

When a child with delays is not given a specific diagnosis or when minimal information about the disability is available, many parents report anxiety, stress, and confusion connected to caregiving. One mother tells how lack of information affected her: "Our failure to obtain realistic data made our experience much worse than it had to be. Certainly, there is a dashing of hopes and expectancies as professionals are quick to point out. Stress and anxiety are relieved when a diagnosis is made" (Roos, 1985). The therapist should explain the disability in understandable terms and with the amount of detail and specifics desired by the parents. Understanding the basis of the disability helps parents understand the intervention; they begin to understand the rationale for specific activities with the child. Insight into the disability and appropriate intervention enables the parents to adapt and change the suggestions of the therapist to fit their daily family routines without losing the intended purpose. It enables them to begin to successfully problem solve through daily management of the child.

For parents, information about their child's disability helps them select appropriate services and monitor the effectiveness and benefit of those services. The therapist should gauge the amount and type of information shared according to the desires, needs, and learning styles of the parents. Explanations are most helpful when they specifically apply to the child; for example, general information about cerebral palsy is not as helpful to parents of a child with spastic athetosis as information about spastic athetosis. Parents may be informed about the types of materials available and then be given specific resources as they request. Often, they need to be ready to hear information in order for it to be meaningful or understood.

Occupational therapists offer explanations of the child's problem based on analysis of the sensory integrative and neurophysiological foundations of behavior. For example, the therapist teaches parents that skill mastery requires a balance of environmental demands and the child's ability to accommodate to the environment. The therapist further explains that when the child accurately perceives, attends to, and organizes sensory experiences, and adaptively responds, he is able to learn from the environment and to develop a high level of developmental skills. Critical to developmental growth is a match between the demands of the environment and the child's ability to adapt to those demands.

A mismatch of too much or too little stimulation in the environment creates disorganized or nonpurposeful behaviors in the child that do not foster developmental growth. By applying these principles to the individual strengths and needs of the child, therapy offers the parent insight into beneficial methods for enhancing the child's function. To help parents provide an environment that fits the child's sensory needs, the therapist first analyzes the child's ability to integrate and organize sensory experiences and then the types of sensory inputs provided by the parents and the environment. By explaining sources of mismatch, the occupational therapist can help parents understand their child's behavior. Recommendations for appropriate, growth-fostering environments result in increasing the child's adaptive responses. (See Stallings-Sahler, Chapter 10.)

Helping parents understand the disability also assists them in understanding their child's future and in making decisions regarding services and programs. By reframing the problem, parents can best strategize the experiences that will promote the child's development and mastery. A child with dyspraxia may have been perceived as having mental retardation. By reframing the child's problem, an emphasis can be placed on providing practice of motor skills and specific sensory input. A child with tactile defensiveness may be perceived as unaffectionate. By explaining to the parents that the child is uncomfortable with touch, the appropriate tactile stimulation can be given and modifications in the environment can be made. As the parents approach the child in ways that are more acceptable to her, her responses become more positive. Understanding the basis for problematic or unusual behavior helps the parents accept the disability and adjust to child behaviors or characteristics that they are unable to change. This understanding also helps them explain the behavior to friends and extended family. Increased understanding also enables others to respond to and interact with the child with increased competence and confidence. Explanations about the child's disability and the anticipated rate of development for that type of disability can help parents accept small goals and have realistic expectations for developmental changes.

Reframing the child's behavior improves the goodness-of-fit between caregivers, parents, family members, other professionals, and the child. When the sensory environment fits the needs of the child, it facilitates sustained and positive interactions that enable the child to increase skill mastery and to develop positive relationships with others.

Promoting Compensation and Adaptation to Disability

In children with disabilities, not all problems and behaviors can be changed. The child may never reach normal levels of developmental achievement. Many conditions require that the child and family learn to adapt to and compensate for the disability. Occupational therapists help families adjust to or adapt to their child's disability in a number of ways. They may recommend changes in the home to improve the child's quality of life and to compensate for functional limitations. For example, the therapist may recommend that an infant with reflux (i.e., vomitting after eating) be fed in an upright position and remain upright for 30 minutes after feeding. It may be suggested that the hyper-responsive infant be fed initially in a quiet, low-lit room, and gradually introduced to more intense sensory experiences. A small table and chair may be recommended for a toddler with spastic diplegia who frequently sits on the floor.

The strategies that help the infant compensate for a sensorimotor problem can also help the family compensate for the time and energy required in caring for a child with special needs (Case-Smith, 1993). Adaptive equipment, such as a modular wheelchair, helps support the child for play and for observation of the environment in an upright position. In fact, a wheelchair may offer a child his first form of mobility. Wheelchairs also help the family transport their child and assist the parents in positioning and managing the child during feeding and other daily activities. Therapists are familiar with the range of equipment available and provide information that assists the family in selecting equipment and adapting the home to best meet the needs of the infant. Compensation methods help normalize family function. Simple equipment may enable a child to feed himself so that the family can eat together at mealtime. A wheelchair with postural supports may enable the family to dine in a restaurant. A corner chair on wheels can enable the mother to take her infant with her from room to room as she cleans the house.

Practical suggestions for the daily care of a child with special needs are often the advice parents value most (Hinojosa, 1990). The therapist should particularly keep in mind the time involved in daily care of the child and should make suggestions that specifically decrease rather than increase the time any one activity requires. When the therapist suggests that extra time be spent in a particular activity (e.g., performing range of motion while bathing the infant), it should be to accomplish specific agreed-upon goals. Extra tasks with the child take away the parent's time with other family members. This imbalance of attention can occur gradually, without the parent's being aware of how they are devoting their time. The therapist may suggest a review of the typical day to help parents become aware of the areas of their lives that are being neglected.

Compensation strategies should help each parent conserve energy (Case-Smith, 1993; Stewart, 1990). To help parents in energy conservation, therapists suggest ways that parents can organize their home environment to reduce the time spent in daily caregiving. When children are fed by gastrostomy tubes, several feeding stations can be arranged in different areas of the house so that the parent can conveniently feed the child while attending to other children at the same time. Parents with children who have severe disabilities are particularly in need of energy conservation techniques. Therapists can suggest a number of ways to set up activities for independent play (e.g., mirrors on the side of the crib or overhead play gyms) that give the parent time to attend to others. Toys can be arranged to support the child's independent exploration so that she is more likely to engage in self-initiated play rather than parent-supported play. (See Figure 2-6.) By helping the parents establish safe environments for play, therapists can teach parents to accomplish other activities without keeping a constant eye on the child.

Energy conservation is also important for the parents of a demanding or irritable child. Therapists may suggest ways to relax during periods of crying and cope with, rather than anguish over, the child's irritability. It may be suggested that family members alternate in attending to the child so that the responsibility is shared rather than shouldered by a single caregiver. Assisting parents in energy conservation may involve adapting daily activities so that they are easier to perform; it may also involve activities that renew energy during a draining day of child care. The activities that renew energy are quite varied among individuals and often include walking through the park, reading a magazine, cooking a gourmet meal, or visiting with a neighbor. The occupational therapist may suggest ways for the caregiver to have the needed time-out, and should emphasize the importance of each parent's having some time for renewal of energy.

Supporting Families

Recommendations that help parents increase efficiency in daily tasks and organize their home environments are also ways to support family function. Support by professionals, friends, and extended family is essential

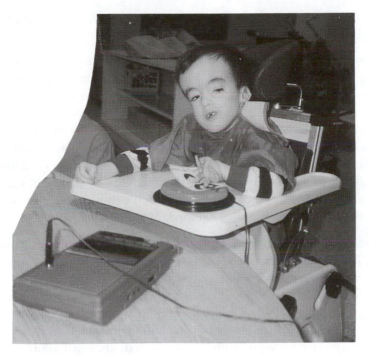

Figure 2-6 Child in Care Chair® using a press switch to operate a tape recorder

to the family's well-being and ability to cope with a child's disability. Deal, Dunst, and Trivette (1989) recommend that the major emphasis of early intervention be placed on strengthening families and their natural support networks, and not on supplanting their personal social support networks with professional services. They advocate that assistance first be sought from informal sources; for example, extended family should be trained to care for the child prior to accessing community agencies and respite care services. The support of family members is shown to be particularly important in adapting to a child with a disability (Simeonsson, Bailey, Huntington, & Comfort, 1986).

Other good resources are often those closest to the family unit. Encouraging families to develop a support network of friends within their neighborhood may lead to opportunities for the child to play with peers and for the parents to have a reliable source of respite care. Play with the other neighborhood children may facilitate social play skills, language, and mobility. Families that balance their day-to-day activities with family recreation and social occasions seem to be better able to cope with stress and to maintain family cohesion (Dunst, Trivette, & Deal, 1988). It is important for parents to keep in perspective that their child is a child first and that his most important growth occurs in natural play interactions. Diamond, a psychologist with a physical disability, explains:

> Something happens in a parent when relating to his disabled child; he forgets that they're a kid first. I used to think about that a lot when I was a kid. I would be off in a euphoric state, drawing or coloring or cutting out paper dolls, and as often as not the activity would be turned into an occupational therapy session. "You're not holding the scissors right." "Sit up straight so your curvature doesn't get worse." That era was ended when I finally let loose a long and exhaustive tirade. "I'm just a kid! You can't therapize me all the time! I get enough therapy in school every day! I don't think about my handicap all the time like you do!" (Diamond, 1981, p. 30)

Social activities may offer a time of family renewal and family unity that can heal some of the stress and separation created by hectic and demanding daily schedules. It has been demonstrated that social support enhances well-being and lessens the likelihood of distress. When parents successfully identify and mobilize resources and support, they gain confidence to solve future problems and to meet the needs of their child (Hunt et al., 1990).

Although family support often comes from informal sources, such as friends and extended family, the therapist can be a great support to the family. Parents have indicated that the most important aspect of their encounter with a professional is her sensitivity to them and the needs of their child (Beckman-Bell, 1981). Hinojosa (1990) interviewed mothers of young children with cerebral palsy and found that all of them thought that personal relationships with their therapists were important. The mothers reported that the therapist as a person was more important than the technical services offered. Some mothers and therapists developed relationships characterized by personal and intimate sharing. The mothers appreciated the opportunity to discuss issues with therapists as friends who appreciated and understood their children.

Actively listening to parents is an essential element of therapy that helps keep the therapist on a course that addresses family priorities. It also reinforces the parents' sense of worth as individuals whose opinions are valued and respected. Healy, Keesee, and Smith (1989) state that "early intervention as a service takes place in the relationship and interactions between families and professionals" (p. 120). This implies that the establishment of positive relationships between families and professionals is a worthy goal in and of itself (McGonigel, Kaufmann, & Johnson, 1991).

Communication skills are essential in developing this relationship and in establishing a collaborative partnership. Key skills are attending to the parent and demonstrating respect and empathy (Stewart, 1990). These simple methods of relating to parents help therapists understand the family's perspective and build the parents' sense of control and competence as caregivers.

Summary

Occupational therapists have adopted a family-centered approach for working with infants and their families. Specific intervention strategies are presented in this chapter as a framework for the topics discussed in the remaining chapters. Table 2-3 summarizes goals and activities of the occupational therapist in early intervention, and the following chapters offer specific examples of therapy with young children and their families.

Table 2-3   Family-Centered Early Intervention

Goals	Therapy Activities	Effects on Family
Promote change in child (remediation). Promote developmental skills.	• Provide information • Educate parent • Prepare child and environment • Model activities • Make recommendations in daily living activities, positioning, and equipment play • Provide feedback to parents • Suggest handling methods and home environment adaptations	• Promotes positive relationship between parent and child • Increases child's ability to interact with family members • Increases parents' sense of competence • Enhances goodness-of-fit • Makes daily activities and home management easier
Reframing. Promote understanding of child.	• Provide information and reading materials about disability • Interpret and explain basis for delays • Explain sensory integration and neuromotor development	• Promotes parents' understanding of child's behavior • Helps parents focus on positive aspects of child • Assists parents in providing appropriate environments and sensory input • Helps parents explain child's behavior to extended family and friends

(continued)

Table 2-3   *Continued*

Goals	Therapy Activities	Effects on Family
Promote compensation and adaptation to child's disability.	• Recommend adaptations at home • Recommend equipment for child • Teach child to compensate for the disability • Support family in adapting to the child's disability • Suggest methods for assisting parents in caring for children with unusual caregiving needs • Teach family energy conservation • Suggest methods to make daily living activities easier and less time-consuming	• Helps family adapt home environment and family activities • Helps family focus on child's strengths • Makes home management and daily activities easier • Helps family select activities, interventions, and resources that match the child's needs • Helps normalize family function • Helps family with time management and energy conservation
Support families.	• Listen to parents • Give positive reinforcement regarding parents' caregiving skills • Help families access community resources (case management) • Encourage social and recreational family activities	• Promotes positive family–child relationships • Helps parents cope, reduces stress • Enhances goodness-of-fit between family and child • Helps parents gain an ongoing social support system

References

Bailey, D.B. (1987). Collaborative goal setting with families: Resolving differences in values and priorities for services. *Topics in Early Childhood Special Education, 7*(2), 59–71.

Bailey, D.B. (1988). Considerations in developing family goals. In D.B. Bailey & R.J. Simeonsson (Eds.), *Family assessment in early intervention* (pp. 229–249). Columbus, OH: Charles E. Merrill.

Beckman-Bell, P. (1981). Child-related stress in families of handicapped children. *Topics in Early Childhood Special Education, 1*(3), 45–53.

Case-Smith, J. (1991a). Occupational and physical therapists as case managers in early intervention. *Physical and Occupational Therapy in Pediatrics, 11*(1), 53–70.

Case-Smith, J. (1991b). The family perspective. In W. Dunn (Ed.), *Pediatric occupational therapy: Facilitating effective service delivery.* Thorofare, NJ: Slack.

Case-Smith, J. (1993). Self care in children with developmental disabilities. In C. Christianson (Ed.), *Ways of living.* Rockville, MD: American Occupational Therapy Association, Inc.

Deal, A.G., Dunst, C.J., & Trivette, C.M. (1989). A flexible and functional approach to developing Individualized Family Support Plans. *Infants and Young Children, 1*(4), 32–43.

Diamond, S. (1981). Growing up with parents of a handicapped child: A handicapped person's perspective. In J.L. Paul (Ed.), *Understanding and working with parents of children with special needs* (pp. 23–50). New York: Holt, Rinehart, & Winston.

Dunst, C.J. (1991). Implementation of the Individualized Family Service Plan. In M.J. McGonigel, R.K. Kaufmann, & B.H. Johnson (Eds.), *Guidelines and recommended practices for the Individualized Family Service Plan.* 2nd ed. Bethesda, MD: Association for the Care of Children's Health.

Dunst, C.J., & Trivette, C.M. (1989). An enablement and empowerment perspective of case management. *Topics in Early Childhood Special Education, 8*(4), 87–102.

Dunst, C.J., Trivette, C., & Deal, A. (1988). *Enabling and empowering families: Principles and guidelines for practice.* Cambridge, MA: Brookline Books.

Early Intervention Program for Infants and Toddlers with Handicaps: Final Regulations, 34 CFR 303. (1989, June 22). *Federal Register, 54*(119), 26306–26348.

Education of the Handicapped Act Amendments of 1986 (PL 99-457), 20 U.S.C. Secs. 1400–1485.

Fisher, A., & Murray, E. (1991). Introduction to sensory integration theory. In A. Fisher, E. Murray, & A. Bundy (Eds.), *Sensory integration.* Philadelphia: F.A. Davis Co.

Gilfoyle, E., Grady, A., & Moore, J. (1991). *Children adapt.* 2nd ed. Thorofare, NJ: Slack.

Healy, A., Keesee, P.D., & Smith, B.S. (1989). *Early services for children with special needs: Transactions for family support.* Baltimore: Paul H. Brookes Publishing Co.

Hinojosa, J. (1990). How mothers of preschool children with cerebral palsy perceive occupational and physical therapists and their influence on family life. *Occupational Therapy Journal of Research, 10,* 144–162.

Hinojosa, J., & Anderson, J. (1991). Mother's perceptions of home treatment programs for their preschool children with cerebral palsy. *American Journal of Occupational Therapy, 45,* 273–279.

Hunt, M., Cornelius, P., Leventhal, P., Miller, P., Murray, T., & Stone, G. (1990). *Into our lives.* Akron, OH: Children's Hospital Medical Center.

Individuals with Disabilities Education Act of 1990 (PL 102-119), 20 U.S.C. Secs. 1400–1485.

Kaufmann, R.K., & McGonigel, M.J. (1991). Identifying family concerns, priorities, and resources. In M.J. McGonigel, R.K. Kaufmann, & B.H. Johnson (Eds.), *Guidelines and recommended practices for the Individualized Family Service Plan.* 2nd ed. (pp. 47–55). Bethesda, MD: Association for the Care of Children's Health.

Kogan, K.L., Tyler, N., & Turner, P. (1974). The process of interpersonal adaptation between mothers and their cerebral palsied children. *Developmental Medicine and Child Neurology, 16,* 518–527.

McGonigel, M. (1991). Philosophy and conceptual framework. In M. McGonigel, R.K. Kaufmann, & B.H. Johnson (Eds.), *Guidelines and recommended practices for the Individualized Family Service Plan.* 2nd ed. Bethesda, MD: Association for the Care of Children's Health.

McGonigel, M., Kaufmann, R.K., & Johnson, B.H. (1991). *Guidelines and recommended practices for the Individualized Family Service Plan.* 2nd ed. Bethesda, MD: Association for the Care of Children's Health.

McWilliams, P. (1991). *The families we serve: Case studies in early intervention.* Carolina Institute for Research on Infant Personnel Preparation, Frank Porter Graham Child Development Center, The University of North Carolina at Chapel Hill.

Mahoney, G., Finger, J., & Powell, A. (1985). The relationship of maternal behavior style to the developmental status of mentally retarded infants. *American Journal of Mental Deficiency, 90,* 296–302.

Mahoney, G., & Powell, A. (1988). Modifying parent–child interaction: Enhancing the development of handicapped children. *Journal of Special Education, 22,* 82–96.

Nastro, M. (1992). An ethnographic study of mothers of children with cerebral palsy and the effect of occupational therapy intervention on their lives. Thesis. The Ohio State University, Columbus.

Rainforth, B., & Salisbury, C.L. (1988). Functional home programs: A model for therapists. *Topics in Early Childhood Special Education, 7*(4), 33–45.

Roos, P. (1985). Parents of mentally retarded children—misunderstood and mistreated. In A.P. Turnbull & H.R. Turnbull (Eds.), *Parents speak out: Growing with a handicapped child.* Columbus, OH: Charles E. Merrill.

Simeonsson, R.J., Bailey, D.B., Huntington, G.S., & Comfort, M. (1986). Testing the concept of goodness of fit in early intervention. *Infant Mental Health Journal, 7*, 81–94.

Stewart, K. (1990). Collaborating with families: Reflections on empowerment. In B. Hanft (Ed.), *Family-centered care.* Rockville, MD: American Occupational Therapy Association, Inc.

Zeitlin, S., & Williamson, G. (1989). Enhancing the coping of families. *Developmental Disabilities Special Interest Section Newsletter, 12*(2), 1–3.

3

□ □ □
□ ■ □
□ □ □

Screening and Identification in Early Intervention

Debra Galvin Cook, MS, OTR

The identification and screening of high-risk infants, children, and their families is the first phase in the assessment–intervention cycle. Identification involves a three-step process that determines which infants and children are in need of intervention, due to either an existing disability, or to a physical/environmental status that strongly suggests the possibility for the development of a disability. The three steps of identification include location, screening, and diagnosis and evaluation (Scott & Hogan, 1982). *Location* involves finding children who qualify for developmental services and who are, therefore, potential candidates for screening. Infants and children are often initially located in hospital and community settings based on identified specific or general risk factors. Once a child with high risk for developmental problems is located, screening and diagnosis follow. These evaluation processes are the topics of this chapter and Chapter 4.

Identification of At-Risk Infants

The process of identification centers on correctly labeling biological and environmental risk factors. *Risk factors* are defined as those elements that, in the absence of any manifest evidence of a disability, suggest that a child is at greater-than-normal risk for developing a disabling condition. Risk factors can be described according to the categories of established risk, biological risk, and environmental risk.

Established Risk

Those infants with known chromosomal, structural, or metabolic defects can be classified as having an established risk. Prenatal diagnostic methods such as amniocentesis, chorionic villus biopsy, and restriction enzyme analysis can determine if the child has an established risk. Amniocentesis has been useful in identifying more than 250 genetic disorders (Batshaw & Perrett, 1988). Chorionic villus biopsy, in which fetal cells present in the chorion are microscopically analyzed, allows for measurement of the activity of specific enzymes present in certain chromosomal abnormalities. This technique is not as safe and readily available as amniocentesis. Restriction enzyme analysis, or gene splicing, is a technique geneticists use to diagnose a number of diseases that previously had no prenatal diagnostic test, such as phenylketonuria (PKU), sickle-cell anemia, and cystic fibrosis (Batshaw & Perrett, 1988). Methods of detecting other established risk factors, such as viral and bacterial insults and maternal exposure to toxins (drugs), include simple blood and urine screens. From these relatively simple exams of maternal blood and urine, toxins (i.e., cocaine and alcohol) and viruses such as the TORCH complex (toxoplasmosis, other, rubella, cytomegalovirus, and *herpes genitalis*) can be detected.

Specific examples of chromosomal defects include Down syndrome, Turner's syndrome, and cri du chat syndrome. Additionally, genetically linked disorders such as Tay-Sachs disease, an autosomal recessive disorder, and achondroplasia, an autosomal dominant disorder, are also considered established risks for developmental concerns. Neural tube defects, such as spina bifida, appear to have a multifactorial genetic basis. It appears not only that some women have a genetic predisposition toward bearing children with myelomeningocele, but that certain intrauterine factors are also associated with this disorder (Shonkoff & Marshall, 1990). Metabolic disorders such as PKU are caused by a single gene abnormality.

Biological Risk

Infants and children with a potential for neurodevelopmentally or educationally identifiable disorders, secondary to a history of prenatal, perinatal, or neonatal insult, are categorized as having a biological risk. Conditions such as apnea, respiratory distress syndrome, patent ductus arteriosus, and intraventricular hemorrhage are a few examples of complications that affect the health and developmental status of the infant. Cerebral palsy and mental retardation are more likely to occur in infants born with very low birth weight (VLBW) (<1500 g). Intraventricular hemorrhage (IVH) and periventricular leukomalacia (PVL) are both significantly associated with these two developmental disabilities. Medical testing of the infant while in the neonatal intensive care unit can reveal when these neurological insults have occurred (Mantovani & Powers, 1991).

These infants can be identified in the neonatal period by interdisciplinary team members, while actual disabilities can be detected from infancy through school age. For example, these children may be classified in the infancy period as being developmentally delayed, and later identified as having cerebral palsy or a learning disability.

Environmental Risk

This category describes infants and children with a potential for delayed development secondary to family and social stressors. The effect of the environment on the child's development is profound. Specific examples of family and social stressors include adolescent parenting, low socioeconomic status, and a history of drug abuse, child abuse, and neglect. Other factors that place the child at developmental risk are problems in the parents' mental health, family support, and mother–child or father–child interactions.

Environmental risk factors can be identified prenatally, as in the single, adolescent mother, or are not apparent until after birth, as in child abuse. Maternal drug addiction places the infant at biological and environmental risk. Since the child's environment changes as he develops, risk factors should be monitored throughout the early years. For example, parents may divorce or one parent may become seriously ill, creating stress in the family. Environmental factors generally associated with stress to the family support system (e.g., drug addiction of one or more members, abusive relationships) can interfere with parent–child attachment (Griffith, 1988). While occupational therapists should be aware of environmental factors and alert to environmental risks, it is not always their focus in the child screening (i.e., the social worker may assess environmental and interactional variables). However, when the therapist is the sole individual administering a screening, it is essential that major environmental risk factors be considered. In general, when the child has both environmental and biological risk factors, referral to a program is indicated. Table 3-1 summarizes the three previously discussed categories of risk factors (Tjossem, 1976).

Impact of Risk Factors

Numerous researchers (Meier, 1976; Scott & Hogan, 1982; Thoman & Becker, 1979) have reported that the conditions that denote risk in early infancy, which subsequently lead to developmental delay, are difficult to identify and, thus, to accurately assess. Difficulty in identification is due

Table 3-1 Three Categories of Risk Factors

Established Risk
Chromosomal defects
Neural tube defects
Genetically linked defects
Viral insults
Bacterial insults
Metabolic defects
Maternal exposure to toxins (drugs)
Maternal age
Maternal nutrition and anatomic variations
Sometimes detected in utero

Biological Risk
Initially biologically sound
History of prenatal insult
History of perinatal insult
History of neonatal insult
Absence of, or inadequate, prenatal care
Born prematurely (before 38 weeks)
Born postmaturely (after 42 weeks)
Low birth weight
Detected in neonatal period

Environmental Risk
Social stressors
Family stressors
Adolescent parenting
Low socioeconomic status
History of drug abuse
History of child abuse and neglect
Sometimes detected in neonatal/infancy period

in part to the following factors: transient infant delays, inconsistent tracking of infants, lack of professional expertise, and inadequate screening and assessment tools. The identification of risk levels is useful in determining which infants and families are in jeopardy (Ensher & Clark, 1986).

It is essential to identify both biological and environmental factors. The interplay of the child and environment across time is the key to accurate and effective identification. It is not sufficient to focus on a single or even a couple of factors when identifying at-risk infants and children. It is the number rather than the nature of risk factors that is the best determinant of outcome, except in the case of clearly identifiable biological dysfunction (Sameroff & Fiese, 1990). In infants with neurological difficulties, researchers have supported the number of risk factors secondary to numerous perinatal problems (Palmelee & Haber, 1973) in family difficulties for children with numerous psychological difficulties (Rutter, 1987), and in both biological and family difficulties in families considered to be multi-risk (Greenspan, 1981).

The Purpose of Screening

Screening is the process of quickly and economically testing children to identify those who have or are at risk for developmental delays. The child undergoes this review when she potentially qualifies for services. The purpose of screening is to gather as much data as possible in as little time as necessary so that a hypothesis on the needs of the child and family can be generated. Screening is performed to determine *if* there is a cause for concern. If a concern has already been identified, the next appropriate course is evaluation, rather than screening.

Screening also serves to determine the need for evaluation and treatment. The focus of screening in occupational therapy is to identify clients who may present problems in occupational performance (e.g., work, self-care, and play or leisure). Screening may be performed independently by occupational therapists or by a member of an interdisciplinary team. The methods used for screening should be appropriate to the child's age, medical status, cultural background, and functional ability and can include a review of medical records, an interview of family members, and an informal or structured observation of the child. The focus of screening should exemplify a family-centered approach, rather than a child-centered approach. Hanft (1989b) offers guidelines for determining whether screening services are truly family-centered. In family-centered screening, the family's concerns and resources are ascertained, in addition to assessing child performance. For example, the child's sensorimotor skills are observed in relation to the family's perceptions and priorities regarding the child's limitations and strengths. Additionally, the family's ability to cope and access resources for the child are included in the screening. Family risk factors (e.g., a single parent, adolescent parents, and history of drug abuse) are considerations in screening the child and in determining the most appropriate program for referral.

The setting, facility, or program often dictates the type and extent of identification and screening. Pursuant to Public Law (PL) 99-457, each state must define *at-risk* and *developmental delay*, thus emphasizing the vital role of identification and screening. The lead agency that directs implementation of the state plan tends to influence how early identification is addressed. The influence of the medical model might be more readily apparent in states where public health is the lead agency, while the influence of the education model is apparent in states where the education department functions as the lead agency. In states where local collaborative groups administer and manage the child find programs, an interagency model of screening is implemented.

In this model, identification is accomplished through a variety of agencies that can facilitate the family's access to the system. Established programs that offer early identification, screening, and intervention services typically have statements of the facility's mission for service provision that identify and define the biological and environmental risk factors necessary for qualification of services. Examples of levels of risk and recommended follow-up are highlighted in Table 3-2.

The screening process has its place not only in identifying children who are at risk, but in following or tracking them as well. Child find programs in the community and follow-up clinics in medical settings typically use the screening process for tracking and subsequent referrals for further evaluations. Child find programs in the community function differently than follow-up clinics in medical settings. Community programs typically consist of educators and nurses and tend to fit more closely with education models. In contrast, follow-up clinics in medical settings tend to fit more closely with medical models and are typically comprised of specialized physicians (e.g., neonatologists, developmental pediatricians), occupational and/or physical therapists, psychologists, and speech pathologists. The role of the occupational therapists in both types of settings varies according to the constellation of group members and the mission of the facility. Chapter 5 discusses the similarities and differences among professional roles in both community and medical settings.

The Role of the Occupational Therapist in Identification

As members of teams, occupational therapists are called on to contribute to the data collection process, which can result in identification. A therapist can independently administer screening instruments, eventually sharing the results with the team and family or contributing to interdisciplinary screening. Screening requires specific skills, such as making judgments and recommendations from limited information that is usually attained during a brief period of time. The average screening session can be completed in 20 to 30 minutes of interaction with the child and family. In order to make quick, accurate judgments and appropriate recommendations, adequate training in the medical conditions of infants and children, as well as advanced clinical reasoning skills grounded in neurobiology, social sciences, and current efficacy research, are required.

Therapists who provide screening services should have specialized training to meet the complex demands of early identification and intervention (Hanft, 1989a). Specifically, the therapist must be able to recognize subtle signs of sensorimotor-perceptual problems. He must be firmly grounded in

Table 3-2 Levels and Conditions of Risk in Undifferentiated Infant Populations and Recommended Follow-Up in the First 18 Months

Level	Conditions of Developmental Risk		Frequency and Mode of Follow-Up
	Infant	*Family*	
III Severe	*Presence of one or more conditions*	*Presence of two or more conditions*	*Further evaluation with positive findings*
	Persistent atypical patterns of neurological behavior	History of developmental disabilities	Direct screening every 3 months
	Severe respiratory distress requiring mechanical ventilation	History of drug addiction or alcoholism	
	Intracranial hemorrhage	Inadequate parenting of other children	
	Gestational age between 26 and 30 weeks	Evidence of emotional problems; self-destructive behavior; poor attitude toward pregnancy	
	Small for gestational age, with a birth weight of less than 1750 g	Teenage parents	
	Congenital infections	Limited education	
		Poor support system	
II Moderate	Birth weight of less than 1750 g	Poor history of parenting by own family	Follow-up by phone and/or mail every 6 months
	Hyperbilirubinemia	Inadequate housing and caregiving facilities; inadequate economic resources	
	Congenital heart disease	Poor utilization of medical care and other community resources	
	Respiratory distress without mechanical ventilation	Unrealistic and/or inappropriate expectations	
	Post-maturity		
	Metabolic disorders not associated with mental retardation		
I Mild	Birth weight of 1750–2500 g	Extended separation of parent and infant	Follow-up by mail every 12 months
Typical Growth and Development	Birth weight of 1750–2500 g, without complications		

Source: Reprinted from *Newborns at Risk: Medical CARe and Psychoeducational Intervention* by G. Ensher and D. Clark, p. 151, with permission of Aspen Publishers, Inc., © 1986.

normal development and its variation so that deviance that is suspect or abnormal is recognized. In addition, therapists must be able to understand how screening fits into the larger picture of identification and intervention and to use the limited time allowed for screening to the child's and family's full advantage.

Because screening is often the initial entry into the service provision process, the outcome is crucial to the subsequent processes of evaluation and intervention. The occupational therapist enters a screening process asking the following questions:

1. From the written records, what kinds of problems might be expected? For example, is the child at risk due to a history of premature retinopathy? Is the child at risk for feeding problems due to a history of bronchopulmonary dysplasia?
2. What are the parents' concerns? What are their priorities?
3. How do the parents perceive the child's development, including her ability to interact and to play?
4. What are some of the child care issues at home (feeding, dressing, sleep activity)?
5. How does the child respond to sensory input?
6. How does the child move? Quality of movement indicators include amount of movement, smoothness, and grading. Is postural stability and isolated movement appropriate for the child's age?
7. How does the child interact with her parents? With others?

Not only must the occupational therapist be an expert in how to screen, but he must also have a clear understanding of what others who are engaged in the screening process are doing. Skills in screening include the ability to make critical observations, to verify observations through the parents' report, and to quickly select appropriate screening methods. In order to be prepared to meet the complex challenges of quick and accurate decision making, therapists must critically analyze whether they are truly prepared and qualified to provide screening in the best-practice model. In addition to screening skills, the therapist needs to be knowledgeable about available community resources and referral options. Given a quick analysis of both family and child needs, the therapist should recommend that the family seek further assessment and intervention at their choice of appropriate services.

To be prepared to meet this challenge, occupational therapists interested in specializing in early intervention must secure advanced training and skills (Bajnok, 1988; Dunn & Rask, 1989; Hanft, 1989a). Specific training, education, and experience can prepare therapists to meet the necessary demands of screening. Opportunities for mentoring and self-study are methods to meet training and education objectives (Sweeney, 1986). It is important that therapists not only have the skills to identify developmental delays or problems, but also have knowledge of community services and systems so that family and child needs can be matched to services. When concerns about the child are identified, the family should receive information about the range of early intervention resources and services available to them.

The responsibility for early identification is shared across professional groups (Rossetti, 1990). Low-prevalence disabilities are most likely to be identified by physicians, while high-prevalence disabilities are most likely to be identified by other professionals, such as educators (Palfrey, Singer, Walker & Butler, 1987). Each team member's contribution to the screening is specialized and unique. Occupational therapists may offer expertise in identification of deficits or concerns, as well as of strengths in specific performance components of the child. The therapist also analyzes the hypothesized effects that other family members and life environments can have on the child's behavior. Ecological approaches to screening emphasize important contextual relevance of specific strengths and concerns. For example, the occupational therapist can provide specific information on delayed or abnormally developing sensorimotor skills, and predict their impact on the child's caregivers at home and in the day-care setting. Expanding on this example, the occupational therapist relates the child's chronic irritability and delayed acquisition of major motor milestones to sensory defensiveness and abnormally persistent primitive reflexes. The therapist explains the impact that multiple caregivers can have on the child's performance, including optimal environments that may reduce the level of arousal. The perceptions and resources of the family are an integral part of providing family-centered screening. The therapist explores and validates the impact that the child's performance has on other family members and makes recommendations for additional referrals to professional and community-based services that can address the family's evaluation and intervention concerns and needs.

Characteristics of Professionals

Since screening is often one of the first contacts that families have with professionals, the impressions left with the families are lasting and often facilitate or inhibit the family's ability to successfully access and interact with team members and, ultimately, acquire adequate, appropriate services. A parent describes her feelings about her encounters with early intervention professionals:

> Not being treated like an individual—not being listened to—is
> parents' greatest complaint about professionals. . . . I need them

because they hold the key to my child's future. . . . The power they exert over you is enormous. (Simons, 1987, p. 47)

Simons (1987) supports the importance of positive interactions with professionals. Respect, responsivity, and sensitivity by professionals seem to be as important as selecting an appropriate screening tool. Interactions among team members can promote or deter effective communication with families. Maple (1987) poses questions that can be addressed by teams to assist in their development of positive collaboration with each other and families. These questions include the following:

1. What kind of background does each individual bring to the team?
2. What does each member expect to contribute?
3. What does each member expect to gain?

Areas of potential conflict, which prevent the screening mission from being carried out, include power conflicts within the team, inadequate and ineffective communication skills, and unclear expectations from team members and parents. Specific characteristics of professionals that lead to good rapport with families include genuineness, warmth, respect, empathy, and a sense of humor (Sattler, 1988). There is no substitute for an attitude of acceptance, understanding, and respect for the integrity of the child and family (Cook, 1991). Again, the screening process may be the first time the family has come into contact with a group of professionals who are interested in their child's well-being. It is most important that professionals never forget the potential impact of the first impression.

Screening Tool Selection Criteria

Selection of specific tools is dependent on five desirable characteristics: validity, reliability, objectivity, efficiency, and freedom from bias (Smith, 1990). The sensitivity and specificity of the instrument are indications of the tool's validity (Chandler, 1990). The *sensitivity* of an instrument indicates its ability to accurately identify a problem or delay. The *specificity* of an instrument refers to its ability to accurately identify an infant who is without developmental delay. A tool that is highly sensitive and specific can offer a true, positive identification of the infant or child. A tool with inadequate sensitivity may fail to identify a child who has problems or delays and a tool with inadequate specificity may fail to identify a child who is without delays. For example, the Denver Developmental Screening Test, Revised, (Frankenburg, Fandal, Sciarillo, & Burgess, 1981) may not correctly identify a 6-month-old infant with mild spastic cerebral palsy with hemiplegic distribution because the tool is not a sensitive measure of muscle tone and postural asymmetries.

Stangler, Huber, and Routh (1980) state that desirable screening procedures include acceptability of the tool to all who will be affected by it, simplicity in training and administration, and consideration of the total cost of the test (including time in administration) in relation to the benefits of early detection. When professionals use screening tools that do not have a previous record of reliability and validity, potential errors will occur in the identification process (Collier, 1991). Other factors to consider in establishing screening programs and selecting tools include the domains to be screened, time constraints, availability of personnel, ease of administration and interpretation, and acceptability by the referral source.

Tools used for screening purposes typically fall into three categories: norm-referenced tests, criterion-referenced tests, and informal, structured observation scales. If any of the previously listed tools are used, adjustment of chronological age for prematurity is recommended until age 2 years. Use of a norm- or criterion-referenced tool should be combined with careful observations of the child and family. When structured observations are combined with norm- or criterion-referenced tools, the qualitative aspects of the child's and family's needs can be accurately identified and the basis for delays or failed items can be analyzed.

The mission of the facility or program often shapes the type of tool that is selected. The number of professionals participating in the screening process and the format of the screening are also factors that influence tool selection. For example, in interdisciplinary screening, several professionals may want to use the same tool, each administering or scoring particular portions. Screening tools, such as the Denver Developmental Screening Test, Revised, can be separated into domains that individual team members administer independently. Arena assessment is effective when the structure of the assessment is flexible and observation is informal. A standardized assessment is usually invalid when administered within an arena model.

Areas to Consider in Family-Centered Screening

The role and expertise of the occupational therapist, together with the mission of the team, influence what areas will be covered during a screening session. Infants and toddlers are typically served by different tools than preschoolers. Consideration and discussion of the areas to be screened are made by the team members, including the parents. Screenings are inherently brief in terms of the length of time allotted to gather data, and areas to be screened are often prioritized before the screening is completed.

Specific areas to consider in family-centered screening are the specific characteristics of the child, parents, and family. Examples of child characteristics include medical risk factors and developmental skill levels across domain areas. The child's coping skills are a significant variable to assess; however, given the time constraints, these skills can be best assessed through the caregiver's report. A quick evaluation in a foreign environment with a stranger is usually stressful for the infant. Difficulty in coping with the screening might be expected. Parent characteristics include the physical and mental health of each parent, marital status, stress factors, support systems, and history. Specific family characteristics include the financial and social resources of the family, the structure of the family, and the roles of the extended family.

For the occupational therapist, the performance areas of play and activities of daily living are typical areas of focus during the screening session. Specific performance components, which comprise the previously described areas, can serve as a basis of discussion for team members when they are prioritizing the areas of focus during the screening session.

Because of the breadth and depth of focus in early intervention screening, multiple types of tools would best meet the needs of a family-centered approach. Family information might be gathered through an interview and structured observation format, while child-centered data can be gathered through a combination of norm- or criterion-referenced tools, structured observations, and interviews with family and other significant caregivers.

Examples of Screening Tools

Currently, a variety of tools are available to health and education professionals to meet the objectives of screening. Table 3-3 summarizes a sampling of screening tests used by occupational therapists and other health professionals in early intervention settings.

Tool selection criteria includes judgments on the time needed to administer, on the validity and reliability, and on the cost. In addition, the appropriateness of the tool for the intended population and the correct use of the tool is the responsibility of the examiner. Screening should neither be substituted for evaluation nor be the primary vehicle from which the child's program is planned.

The Denver Developmental Screening Test (DDST) (Frankenburg & Dodds, 1967) and its revision (DDST II) (Frankenburg, Fandal, Sciarillo, & Burgess, 1981) provide a standardized instrument to assist in the detection of developmental delay in children. Administration of the test requires a DDST worksheet and simple materials that are provided in the kit. These standardized items provide an objective method for identifying developmental delay and the opportunity to make subjective observations about the child's performance.

Table 3-3 Screening Tools used by Occupational Therapists and Other Health Professionals in Early Intervention Settings

	Milani-Comparetti Motor Development Screening Test	Chandler Movement Assessment of Infants— Screening Tests	Developmental Profile II (Interview)	Denver II	Miller Assessment for Preschoolers
Age range	B–2.5 years	1.5–12.5 mos.	3–9 1/2 years	B–6 years	2.4–5.8 years
Testing time (minutes)	4–8	5–10	20–40	10	20–30
Scoring time (minutes)	5	5–10	10–20	5	2–10
MAJOR AREAS TESTED					
Personal/social			X	X	
Communication			X	X	
Cognition			X		X
Self-help			X		
Gross motor			X	X	X
Praxis					X
Reflexes	X	X			
Fine motor				X	X
Visual-motor integration					X

Visual perception				X
Tactile				X
Vestibular				X
Tone	X			
Postural control	X	X		
Active movement	X	X		
TYPE OF TEST				
Norm-referenced		X		X
Criteria-referenced	X	X		
Informal/structured observation			Interview	X
SCORES OBTAINED				
Age level		X	X	
Percentile				X
Standard		X	X	
Quantified observation				

When a child fails items below his chronological age, the child and family are referred for further diagnostic evaluation. Subjective observations made during the testing procedures form the basis for interim recommendations that can be given to family members. When attempting to identify whether a child is developmentally delayed, validity studies have indicated that the DDST should not be the only test administered. Meisels (1989) reports that although the DDST had excellent test specificity, the sensitivity level was unacceptably low in order for the test to be used as a screening tool for at-risk children. Its use may result in the underidentification of children who would benefit from services.

Another example of a child-centered screening tool is the Milani-Comparetti Motor Development Screening Test (Milani-Comparetti & Gidoni, 1967). This test focuses on the gross motor milestones, primitive reflexes, and protective and equilibrium reactions in children from birth to 2 years of age. It can be administered in 10 minutes, which allows minimal time for observation of spontaneous movement, given that the test primarily involves physical maneuvers applied to the infant. This test was originally developed in 1967 and was revised in 1978 at the Meyer Children's Rehabilitation Institute, University of Nebraska Medical Center (Trembath, 1978). In 1987, a study of 312 children was completed at the Institute and a third revision of the screening manual was published (Stuberg, Dehne, Miedaner, & Romero, 1992; Stuberg, White, Miedaner, & Dehne, 1989).

The main strength of the Milani-Comparetti is its practicality; that is, it is administered quickly and at minimal cost, requires no special setting or equipment, and is easily learned, scored, and repeated. In addition, interobserver and test-retest reliability are moderate to high (Stuberg, White, Miedaner, & Dehne, 1989). VanderLinden (1985) conducted a retrospective study to determine the predictive validity of the Milani-Comparetti Motor Development Screening Test with a small sample of high-risk infants. Analysis of the data suggested that the accuracy of this tool in predicting motor outcome at 2 and 3 years of age is low; therefore, therapists should be cautious in their interpretation of results. The Media Resource Center at the Meyer Children's Rehabilitation Institute offers purchase or rental of training tapes and test manuals.[1]

An example of an environmental or ecological screening tool is the Home Observation for Measurement of the Environment (HOME) (Caldwell & Bradley, 1984). Items in this screening tool represent aspects of the home environment that indicate the frequency and stability of adult contact, amount of developmental and vocal stimulation, need gratification, emotional climate,

---

[1] Meyer Children's Rehabilitation Institute, Media Resource Center, 600 South 42nd Street, Omaha, Nebraska 68198-5450.

avoidance of restriction on motor and exploratory behavior, types of play materials available, and characteristics of parental concern with achievement. The manual reports positive reliability and validity, and cites various research pertaining to the construct validity of the tool. The LaDoca Publishing Company offers a training video and the manual.[2]

Summary

Family-centered early intervention often begins with the screening process. This process for identifying children who are eligible for early intervention services may occur in both medical and community settings. Occupational therapists are often involved in screening, as a team member, or an independent practitioner. Important aspects of the screening process are: (1) access to the infant's developmental and medical history; (2) use of objective evaluations in combination with subjective observations; (3) sensitivity to parent's perspectives; and (4) consideration of family, as well as child, risk factors. Screening requires that the occupational therapist be able to quickly and accurately assimilate and evaluate a child and his family, usually in a one-time interaction. Skills in identifying developmental delays, high-risk behaviors, and combinations of risk factors that may result in delays are needed. Screening may be the first opportunity for the family to interact with a pediatric occupational therapist; therefore, her active listening and sensitivity to the parents are critical in creating positive impressions. The manner in which the child is identified as appropriate for services and the parents are provided initial information about early intervention may influence future relationships between the family and the professionals who provide therapy and educational services.

References

American Occupational Therapy Association (AOTA). (1989). Uniform terminology for occupational therapy. *American Journal of Occupational Therapy, 43*(12), 808–815.

Bajnok, I. (1988, June). Specialization meets entry to practice. *Canadian Nurse, 84,* 23–24.

Batshaw, M.L., & Perrett, Y.M. (1988). *Children with handicaps.* Baltimore: Paul H. Brookes Publishing Co.

Caldwell, B., & Bradley, R. (1984). *Home observation for measurement of the environment.* Little Rock: University of Arkansas.

---

[2] LaDoca Publishing Company, 5100 E. Lincoln, Denver, Colorado 80216.

Chandler, L.S. (1990). Neuromotor assessment. In E.D. Gibbs & D.M. Teti (Eds.), *Interdisciplinary assessment of infants—A guide for early intervention professionals* (pp. 45–61). Baltimore: Paul H. Brookes Publishing Co.

Collier, T. (1991). The screening process. In W. Dunn (Ed.), *Pediatric occupational therapy—Facilitating effective service provision* (pp. 11–34). Thorofare, NJ: Slack.

Cook, D. (1991). The assessment process. In W. Dunn (Ed.), *Pediatric occupational therapy—Facilitating effective service provision* (pp. 35–72). Thorofare, NJ: Slack.

Dunn, W., & Rask, S. (1989). Nationally speaking–Entry level and specialized practice: A professional encounter. *American Journal of Occupational Therapy, 43,* 7–9.

Ellison, P.H., Browning, C.A., Larson, B., & Denny, J. (1983). Development of a scoring system for the Milani-Comparetti and Gidoni method of assessing neurologic abnormality in infancy. *Physical Therapy, 63,* 1414–1423.

Ensher, G.L., & Clark, D.A. (1986). *Newborns at risk—Medical care and psychoeducational intervention.* Rockville, MD: Aspen Publishers.

Frankenburg, W.K., & Dodd, J.B. (1967). The Denver Developmental Screening Test. *Journal of Pediatrics, 71,* 181–191.

Frankenburg, W.K., Fandal, A.W., Sciarillo, W., & Burgess, D. (1981). The Newly Abbreviated and Revised Denver Developmental Screening Test. *Journal of Pediatrics, 99,* 995–999.

Greenspan, S.I. (1981). *Psychopathology and adaption in infancy and early childhood: Clinical infant reports no. 1.* Hanover, NH: University Press of New England.

Griffith, D.R. (1988). The effects of perinatal cocaine exposure on infant neurobehavior and early maternal–infant interactions. In I.J. Chasnoff (Ed.), *Drugs, alcohol, pregnancy, and parenting.* Drodrecht, The Netherlands: Kluwer Academic Publisher.

Hanft, B.E. (1989a). Nationally speaking—Early intervention: Issues in specialization. *American Journal of Occupational Therapy, 43,* 431–434.

Hanft, B.E. (1989b). Providing family-centered occupational therapy services. *Sensory Integration Special Interest Section Newsletter, 12*(2), 1–3.

Mantovani, J.F., & Powers, J.A. (1991). Brain injury in premature infants: Patterns on cranial ultrasound, their relationship to outcome, and the role of developmental intervention in the NICU. *Infants and Young Children, 4*(2), 20–32.

Maple, G. (1987). Early intervention: Some issues in co-operative teamwork. *Australian Occupational Therapy Journal, 34*(4), 145–151.

Meier, J.H. (1976). Screening, assessment, and intervention for young children at developmental risk. In T.D. Tjossem (Ed.), *Intervention strategies for high risk infants and young children* (pp. 251–287). Baltimore: University Park Press.

Meisels, S.J. (1989). Can developmental screening tests identify children who are developmentally at risk? *Pediatrics, 83,* 578–585.

Milani-Comparetti, A., & Gidoni, E.A. (1967). Routine developmental examination in normal and retarded children. *Developmental Medicine and Child Neurology 9,* 631–638.

Palfrey, J., Singer, J., Walker, D., & Butler, J. (1987). Early identification of children's special needs: A study of five metropolitan communities. *Journal of Pediatrics, 3,* 379.

Palmelee, A.H., & Haber, A. (1973). Who is the at risk infant? *Clinical Obstetrics and Gynecology, 16,* 376–387.

Rossetti, L. (1990). *Infant-toddler assessment: An interdisciplinary approach.* Boston: College-Hill Press.

Rutter, M. (1987). Continuities and discontinuities from infancy. In J. Osofsky (Ed.), *Handbook of infant development.* 2nd ed. (pp. 1256–1296). New York: John Wiley & Sons.

Sameroff, A.J., & Fiese, B.H. (1990). Transactional regulation and early intervention. In S.J. Meisels & J.P. Shonkoff (Eds.), *Handbook of early childhood intervention.* New York: Cambridge University Press.

Sattler, J. (1988). *Assessment of children.* San Diego: Jerome M. Sattler, Publisher.

Scott, K.G., & Hogan, A.E. (1982). Methods for the identification of high-risk and handicapped infants. In C.T. Ramey & P.L. Trohanis (Eds.), *Finding and educating high-risk and handicapped infants* (pp. 69–81). Baltimore: University Park Press.

Shonkoff, J.P., & Marshall, P.C. (1990). Biological basis of developmental dysfunction. In S.J. Meisels & J.P. Shonkoff (Eds.), *Handbook of early childhood intervention.* Cambridge, MA: Cambridge University Press.

Simons, R. (1987). *After the tears.* New York: Harcourt Brace Jovanovich.

Smith, J.K. (1990). Questions of measurement in early childhood. In E.D. Gibbs & D.M. Tete (Eds.), *Interdisciplinary assessment of infants—A guide for early intervention professionals* (pp. 15–30). Baltimore: Paul H. Brookes Publishing Co.

Stangler, S.R., Huber, C.J., & Routh, D.K. (1980). *Screening growth and development of preschool children: A guide for test selection.* New York: McGraw-Hill.

Stuberg, S., Dehne, P., Miedaner, J., & Romero, P. (1992). *The Milani-Comparetti Motor Development Screening Test, Third Edition, Revised.*

Meyer Rehabilitation Institute, University of Nebraska Medical Center, Omaha.

Stuberg, W.A., White, P.J., Miedaner, J.A., & Dehne, P.R. (1989). Item reliability of the Milani-Comparetti Motor Developmental Screening Test. *Physical Therapy, 69*(5), 328–335.

Sweeney, J.K. (1986). Message from the editor. *Physical and Occupational Therapy in Pediatrics 6*(3/4), 1–2.

Thoman, E.B., & Becker, P.T. (1979). Issues in assessment and prediction for the infant born at risk. In T.M. Field, A.M. Sostek, S. Goldberg, & H.H. Shuman (Eds.), *Infants born at risk: Behavior and development* (pp. 461–483). New York: SP Medical & Scientific Books.

Tjossem, T. (1976). *Intervention strategies for high risk infants and young children.* Baltimore: University Park Press.

Trembath, J. (1978). *The Milani-Comparetti Motor Development Screening Test.* University of Nebraska Medical Center, Omaha.

VanderLinden, D. (1985). Ability of the Milani-Comparetti developmental examination to predict motor outcome. *Physical and Occupational Therapy in Pediatrics, 5,* 27–38.

4

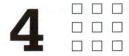

Assessment

Jane Case-Smith, EdD, OTR

An interdisciplinary approach to infant assessment is needed in order to obtain a comprehensive understanding of an infant and his family (Gibbs & Teti, 1990). Individually and then together, the discipline members of the team evaluate and interpret the child's strengths and needs so that a holistic understanding of the child and the family can be developed. In the assessment, the team gains a shared meaning of the child's issues, the family's priorities, and the interaction between the child and the caregiving environment.

Child Assessment

Early intervention assessment often begins by screening the child. If a problem is identified or suspected, screening is followed by a diagnostic developmental assessment, which provides a comparison of the child to age level skills based on a sample of average children. If the child is determined to be eligible for services, usually an interdisciplinary team obtains baseline information about the child using a developmental curriculum. This information guides development of specific child goals in the Individualized Family Service Plan (IFSP). The curriculum is used for ongoing monitoring of the child's progress and may be used with a standardized test for summative evaluation when the child transitions into another program (e.g., preschool or school). The evaluation sequence is illustrated in Figure 4-1.

The purpose of the assessment is to determine the type of test that will be administered and which disciplines are most likely to be involved. Most developmental assessments were created for a specific purpose (e.g., screening, diagnosing, and curriculum planning) and are most valid when used within that context. Table 4-1 lists the primary purposes of evaluation, the types of tests that may be used for each purpose, and examples of each type.

Multiple disciplines participate in each type of assessment. The family's role in the assessment varies according to their familiarity and comfort level

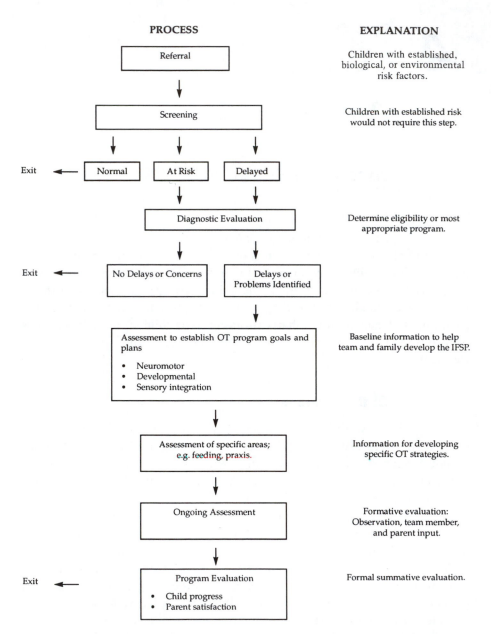

Figure 4-1 The assessment process

with the process. In general, their participation increases when the purpose of assessment is planning or evaluating the intervention program. Often, single disciplines administer screenings and an interdisciplinary team contributes to the comprehensive assessment, which serves to establish a diagnosis and plan an intervention program.

Table 4-1 Examples of Developmental Assessments

Purpose	Type of Test	Examples
Screening	Standardized	• Denver Developmental Screening Test II (DDST II)
Diagnostic tests	Standardized	• Bayley Scales of Infant Development • Neuromotor Scales: Movement Assessment of Infants, Milani-Comparetti, INFANIB
Program planning	Curricula	• Developmental Programming for Infants and Young Children (DPIYC) • Hawaii Early Learning Profile • Carolina Curriculum for Handicapped Infants
	Informal Scales	• Scales developed by individual therapists
Program evaluation	Standardized Criterion-Based	• Bayley Scales of Infant Development • Hawaii Early Learning Profile

Screening

When a child receives a developmental screening, the purpose is to identify the presence of any significant deviations from normal growth and development. Screenings are performed in community child find activities or when the caregivers, relatives, or friends identify a concern about an infant's development. Screening may also be appropriate when the infant's history includes biological or environmental risk factors (see Cook, Chapter 3). Tests for screening tend to have few items within broadly defined behavioral domains.

Formal (standardized) screening tests usually have items with standardized criteria to determine pass/fail. In general, mechanisms for scoring *how* the child performed the skill are not included. Although occupational therapists are involved in screening children, other professionals and paraprofessionals administer screenings such as the DDST II (Frankenburg, Fandal, Sciarillo, & Burgess, 1981). Screenings can be reliably administered by other individuals with minimal training in child development who study the test manual and follow the test instructions. When the results of the screening indicate a possible problem, the child is referred for further evaluation.

Diagnostic Tests

A standardized diagnostic evaluation or a criterion-based curriculum assessment may be appropriate, based on the results of the screening, the parents' desires, and the team's concerns and need for information. If eligibility for services remains a question after the screening (e.g., if a child received a borderline screening score), then further diagnostic testing may

Table 4-2 Standardized Developmental Assessments

	Bayley Scales of Infant Development (Bayley, 1969)	Gesell Developmental Schedules (Knobloch, Stevens, & Malone, 1980)	Peabody Developmental Motor Scales (Folio & Fewell, 1983)	Battelle Developmental Inventory (Newborg, Stock, Wnek, Guidubaldi, & Svinicki, 1984)
AGE RANGE	2 months–2 1/2 years	2 months–36 months	Birth–6.9 years	Birth–8 years
TESTING TIME	45 minutes	45 minutes	45–60 minutes	45 minutes–2 hours
Materials available in testing kit	x	x	x (partial)	
MAJOR AREAS TESTED				
Personal-social	x (mental)	x		x
Communication	x (mental)	x (language)		x
Cognition	x (mental)	x (adaptive)		x
Self-help		x (adaptive/personal social)	x	x
Fine motor	x (mental)	x	x	x (motor)
Gross motor	x (motor)	x	x	x (motor)
Visual motor	x (mental)	x	x	
SCORES OBTAINED				
Age level	x	x	x	x
Percentile	x		x	x
Standard	x		x	x

help in the decision regarding which program, if any, is appropriate for the child. Table 4-2 provides examples of standardized tests used by pediatric occupational therapists in early intervention for diagnostic purposes.

Bayley Scales of Infant Development

When the focus of the team is to make a diagnosis or to identify whether or not the child has a significant developmental delay, the Bayley Scales of Infant Development (Bayley, 1969) are an appropriate choice. The stated purpose of the scales is to "provide the basis for establishing a child's current status, and thus the extent of any deviation from normal" (Bayley, 1969, p. 4). The scales have norms for 2 to 30 month-old children and consist of three scales, a mental scale, a motor scale, and a behavioral record. The purpose of the mental scale is to assess maturing cognition, sensory-perceptual abilities, discriminations, memory and learning, problem solving, and receptive and expressive communication. The motor scale provides an index for physical maturation by measuring milestones of coordination and motor skill. The Infant Behavior Record (IBR) provides a means for describing naturally occurring observed behavior, as well as the child's response to his environment. The IBR helps the therapist assess the child's attitudes, interests, emotions, energy, activity, and tendencies to approach or withdraw from stimulation (Bayley, 1969).

Baseline and ceiling levels are established for each child tested. The criterion to determine the basal score for the motor scale is six successive passes. The ceiling score for the motor scale is determined by six failed items. Although the basal score for the mental scales is defined as 10 successive passes and the ceiling score as 10 successive failures, the examiner may use clinical judgment in determining whether successive items would be failed or passed and discontinue testing to prevent frustrating the infant.

Due to the strict criteria for administering and scoring items, scores on the Bayley Scales may not accurately reflect the capabilities of the child who has severe developmental delays or visual or hearing impairments. When testing children with multiple disabilities or specific sensory impairments, standardized methods for administering items often do not elicit the child's optimal performance. The child may perform an item successfully when the examiner adapts the standard method for administering the item. The nonstandardized scales described in the section on developmental curricula provide adapted methods for administering items when the child has severe disabilities or sensory impairments.

Gesell Developmental Schedules

The Gesell Developmental Schedules (Gesell, 1925; Knobloch & Pasamanick, 1974) were designed to assist in the early identification of developmental problems in infants and young children. The schedules assess infant/child development between 4 weeks and 36 months of age in the adaptive, gross motor, fine motor, language, and personal/social/behavioral domains. Most items are directly observed; however, selected items can be scored using the parents' report if the child does not comply with the test items. The schedules yield an age-equivalent level for each domain from which a developmental quotient (DQ) is then obtained by dividing the age-equivalent score by the child's chronological age.

The Gesell Developmental Schedules were originally published for the purpose of determining the neurological integrity of the young child based on performance across a number of developmental domains. The scales were revised by Knobloch and Pasamanick in 1974 and were restandardized by Knobloch, Stevens, and Malone in 1980. In the revised schedules, behavior items were achieved about 10% to 17% earlier than in the original sample (Knobloch, Stevens, & Malone, 1980). Predictive validity, using DQs of 40-week-old children from the Gesell Developmental Schedules and the IQs of 3-year-olds from the Stanford-Binet, was high (r = .87; n = 92) (Knobloch & Pasamanick, 1960). This high correlation indicates that the predictive validity of the Gesell Developmental Schedules is higher than that of other developmental assessments (Gibbs, 1990).

Battelle Developmental Inventory (BDI)

The BDI (Newborg, Stock, Wnek, Guidubaldi, & Svinicki, 1984) is a standardized assessment that evaluates the child's developmental status across five domains. These domains are personal-social, adaptive, motor, communication, and cognition. The development of the BDI was based on the concept that a child normally attains critical skills (developmental milestones) in a specific developmental sequence. Items were selected based on their overall importance to the development of the child, the critical nature of the skills, and the degree to which the behavior was amenable to educational intervention.

The test provides observation and interview methods to evaluate skills that would not ordinarily be observed in a testing session. Items are scored 0, 1, or 2, with 1 being the score for an emerging skill. The basal level for each subdomain is reached when the child scores 2 on two consecutive items and the ceiling level is reached when the child scores 0 on two consecutive items. Each domain has its own booklet and due to the length of the assessment (45 minutes to 2 hours), the process may be facilitated when each domain is assessed by a different discipline. The motor domain has 82 items and is divided into five sections as follows: muscle control, body coordination, locomotion, fine muscle, and perceptual-motor. The test items have specific instructions for children with motor, visual, and hearing impairments.

The BDI was standardized using a stratified quota sample of 800 with distribution of race and sex to reflect the United States' population. Although the test was well standardized and seems to have evidence of both reliability and validity, many of the domains have a limited number of items; therefore, the test's usefulness in treatment planning and in measuring small increments of progress is restricted.

Curricula for Intervention and Program Planning

If delays are clearly identified and the child is eligible for an intervention program, then a criterion-based assessment to determine goals and plans becomes appropriate. Most standardized diagnostic assessments (e.g., Bayley, Gesell) do not include sufficient information to formulate treatment goals and plans. Developmental curricula, such as the Hawaii Early Learning Profile (HELP) and the Early Learning Assessment Profile (E-LAP), were developed using a number of diagnostic instruments, are comprehensive within each domain, and include all or most behavioral domains. Table 4-3 provides descriptive information on developmental curricula that are frequently used in early intervention programs.

After a child has enrolled in therapy or an education program, the purpose of evaluation becomes identification of the child's strengths and needs. Comprehensive, interdisciplinary evaluation is appropriate when global delays have been identified, when delays cross domains, or when comprehensive programming is needed. An early childhood curriculum provides a survey of interrelated developmental, behavioral, and interactive competencies from which intervention goals can be derived. It forms the core of the interdisciplinary assessment. Comprehensive evaluation includes additional information from individual disciplines based on structured observations, skill analysis, and other discipline-specific instruments.

Developmental curricula contain activities that are linearly sequenced or hierarchically arranged according to the continuum of developmental milestones. Most curricula incorporate discrete behavioral tasks that are contained in normed-based measures, such as the Bayley Scales or Gesell Schedules. Some curricula measure qualitative changes in cognitive developmental processes such as cause-effect and means-end problem solving and motor developmental processes, such as reflexes, righting, and equilibrium reactions. Comprehensive curriculum include both (Bagnato & Hofkosh, 1990).

Early Learning Accomplishment Profile

The E-LAP (Glover, Preminger, & Sanford, 1978) provides a detailed task analysis for infants or children who are birth to 36 months of age. The scales are based on a number of normed tests, such as the Bayley or the Gesell. The scales survey six domains of functioning as follows: gross motor, fine motor, cognition, language, self-help, and social-emotional. An

Table 4-3 Developmental Curricula

	Early Learning Accomplishment Profile (E-LAP) (Glover, Preminger, & Sanford, 1978)	Hawaii Early Learning Profile (HELP) (Furuno et al., 1985)	Carolina Curriculum for Handicapped Infants (Johnson-Martin, Jens, & Attermeier, 1986)	Developmental Programming for Infants and Young Children (DPICY) (Schafer & Moersch, 1981)
AGE RANGE	Birth–36 months	Birth–36 months	Birth–24 months	Birth–36 months
STRENGTHS	Comprehensive assessment of cognition	Chart and checklist activity guide available	24 domains, includes guide	Includes activity guide based on recent development theories
ADAPTED TO SPECIAL NEEDS			x	x
MAJOR AREAS EVALUATED				
Social-emotional	x	x	x	x
Communication	x	x	x	x
Cognition	x	x	x	x
Self-help	x	x	x	x
Fine motor	x	x	x	x
Gross motor	x	x	x	x
Visual motor			x	
NUMBER OF ITEMS	410	685	332	299
FIELD TESTED	x	x	x	x

extensive number of items are provided and referenced from the test or tests of derivation. The greatest concentration of items are in cognition (105), gross motor (86), and fine motor (73). Basal levels are determined by eight consecutive passes and ceiling levels by three failures within five consecutive items. Emerging skills are noted as $+/-$. Although the E-LAP is a popular tool, its reliability and validity have not been investigated.

Hawaii Early Learning Profile (HELP)

The HELP (Furuno et al., 1985) surveys developmental tasks and competencies from birth to 36 months of age in six functional domains. These domains are cognition, language, gross motor, fine motor, social-emotional, and self-help. A manual lists each skill and then provides activities and instructions for professionals and parents to help facilitate the achievement of the skills by the child.

The HELP was designed to assist in planning an interdisciplinary education program for children. Each of the domains of the HELP was designed by the most expert discipline specialist in that domain; for example, an occupational therapist developed the fine motor and self-help sections. The items are clearly written and address small increments of developmental progress. The number of items and the thorough scope of the curriculum provide a foundation for comprehensive planning across disciplines. The items are not always sequenced in the hierarchy of typical development. Although the HELP has been extensively field-tested since its introduction, only one prominent research study investigated its technical adequacy and effectiveness (Bagnato & Murphy, 1989).

Carolina Curriculum for Handicapped Infants and Infants at Risk

The Carolina Curriculum for Handicapped Infants and Infants at Risk (Johnson-Martin, Jens, & Attermeier, 1986) is a Piagetian-based curriculum that assesses cognitive, affective, and sensorimotor competencies in children from birth through 24 months of age. The items are organized into 24 domains. Basic sensory systems are assessed under tactile integration and manipulation, auditory localization, and visual pursuit. The self-help area includes feeding, grooming, and dressing. The fine motor section is divided into the areas of reaching and grasping, object manipulation, and bilateral hand activity. The manual includes a chapter on motor development that gives general information about the observation and evaluation of normal and abnormal motor development and motor programming in the classroom. Adaptations of items for infants with various disabilities (e.g., visual and hearing impairments, autism, neuromotor disabilities) are also included.

The Carolina Curriculum has undergone more formal test development than the HELP and the E-LAP. The effectiveness of the curriculum in promoting changes and measuring progress was assessed in 22 programs using the change scores for a 3-month period. The field-testing indicated that interventionists found the curriculum useful for assessing infants with disabilities and developing programs for them (Johnson-Martin, Jens, & Attermeier, 1986).

Developmental Programming for Infants and Young Children (DPIYC)

Under the direction of Moersch and Schafer, an interdisciplinary team developed a curriculum that includes an adaptive scoring system for children with visual, hearing, and neuromotor impairments. The DPIYC (Schafer & Moersch, 1981) has two portions, the original curriculum for children, 3 to 6 years of age, and a more recently developed portion for children who are birth to 3 years of age. The infant assessment, entitled the Early Intervention Developmental Profile (EIDP), consists of six domains. These domains are cognition, language, perceptual/fine motor, social-emotional, gross motor, and self-care.

Although the other curricula described have more items, the EIDP provides a tool for observing and rating critical aspects of the developmental process across a wide breadth of skill domains. The scoring system allows identification of emerging skills that then become short-term goals for the child. The profile reflects current developmental theory in the motor, cognitive, and social areas. The gross motor scale and the feeding section emphasize neurodevelopmental theories of reflexive development and the integration of primitive reflexes into higher order righting reactions, protective responses, and equilibrium responses. The cognition scale focuses specifically on the acquisition of the concepts of object permanence, causal and spatial relationships, and imitation. The authors suggest that a ceiling level of six consecutive failed items be established before testing to establish a basal level of six consecutive passed items. They recommend measuring the ceiling and basal levels on the perceptual/fine motor scale prior to administering the other scales. With documented evidence of reliability and a standardized method of scoring items, the test has been selected as a measurement of efficacy in several studies of therapy for children with neurological disabilities (e.g., Bagnato & Mayes, 1986; Bagnato & Neisworth, 1985).

Program Evaluation

A final purpose of developmental assessments and curricula is program evaluation, which is critical to the intervention process. Objective measurement of goal achievement and of child progress is essential to ongoing programming, especially once baseline levels are determined, goals are established, and intervention is implemented. Evaluations of child change during and after the child's intervention program provide professionals and family members with information about the effect of therapy strategies, about the child's rate of development across behavioral domains, and about any need to change intervention methods or to reorder goal priorities.

Often the instruments selected for program evaluation are those that were used for baseline information. Strong evidence of test reliability is essential for reliable measurement of change. Therefore, tests such as the EIDP or the Carolina Curriculum, which have high reliability scores, may be more appropriate for program evaluation than the E-LAP or the HELP.

The standardized Bayley Scales have often been selected in efficacy research to measure child progress (Bagnato & Neisworth, 1985; Harris, 1981; Palmer et al., 1988). Some limitations of the Bayley Scales are its inadequate sensitivity to change due to a limited number of items and its standard scoring method of pass/fail, which does not allow a method for the scoring of emerging skills. Since the Bayley Scales are rarely the basis for formulating program goals and strategies, the skills measured may not relate to the child's goals. However, the lack of a relationship between the focus of the Bayley Scales and the focus of the interdisciplinary team may be an asset in an efficacy study, because an objective measure of the child's overall development, rather than a measure of specific goal achievement can be taken. The scales may be best suited for summative evaluation, to compare the child's developmental quotients from program entrance to program exit.

Reevaluation, using the curricula that was administered to establish goals, may provide the most helpful measure of child change in establishing new goals and in documenting the effect of the program on the child's development. Two possible disadvantages of readministering the curriculum instrument are that team members may focus on specific skills to the exclusion of others and may teach to the curriculum items. This misuse of the curriculum promotes splinter skills in the child, which do not easily generalize and do not enhance foundational skills. Another issue in measuring the effects of intervention relates to actually attributing the child change to the intervention (Simeonsson, 1988). The child's developmental changes are due to her own maturation and spontaneous changes as well as a myriad of other variables. Measures of child change increase in validity when standardized or well developed instruments are used and when the child's own developmental rate is factored into the amount of progress made. Irwin and Wong (1974) have documented methods for incorporating the child's developmental quotient (i.e., the child's rate of developmental growth) on entrance into the program into measures of the program's effectiveness.

Summary

This section describes a number of instruments that match the primary purposes of developmental assessment in early intervention. In addition to the evaluations described, measures of family concerns, resources, and priorities, evaluations of the environment (e.g., home, day-care center, or clinic), and discipline-specific tests of child behaviors and skills are essential to planning and implementing intervention. Due to the complexity of evaluation at the levels of diagnosis, intervention planning, and intervention evaluation, professionals from a number of disciplines are needed to assess and interpret the child's and family's needs and strengths. The remainder of this chapter discusses trans- and interdisciplinary assessment, the role of the occupational therapist, and the role of the family in early intervention assessment.

Early Intervention Assessment: A Collaborative Process

Infancy is the stage in human development in which skills and domains of behavior are intertwined and interdependent, necessitating a multidimensional, interdisciplinary assessment. For example, when evaluating a child with oral dyspraxia, both the speech therapist and the occupational therapist are needed to ascertain how the motor disability is affecting the child's speech (Alexander, 1990). Measurement of the infant's sensorimotor skills can provide evidence of cognitive function and neurological integrity as well as of developmental motor skills. Interpretation of subtle behaviors may lead to conclusions about multiple and related, but separate, areas of development; for example, the child who frequently arches his trunk in hyperextension may be demonstrating high extensor muscle tone related to cerebral palsy, or increased tactile defensiveness and avoidance of touch when held, or general stress due to physiological factors (e.g., respiratory distress).

When primary behaviors (e.g., rocking, stiffening, or avoidance of touch) indicate different primary problems, observation and assessment of a large sample of the child's behaviors enables an interdisciplinary team to agree on a shared understanding of the problem. Interpretation of subtle behaviors and knowledge of multiple, genetic, biological, and environmental factors results in accurate and comprehensive findings. The observations, assessments, and interpretations of an interdisciplinary team, including the family, are essential to understanding the interaction of variables and the goodness-of-fit between the child and his environment.

An Interdisciplinary Assessment Model

Early intervention assessment includes multiple forms of assessment and the gathering of information at different times by various individuals in diverse environments. These pieces become a whole when team members share the information gathered in both formal and informal meetings with the family. Then, family members and team members share their interpretations and reach consensus concerning the development of the IFSP.

Often the interdisciplinary team makes a core assessment of the developmental and the functional skills of the child to document basic knowledge. The core assessment is usually one of the curricula described in the previous section. The primary interventionist can evaluate one or two domains using parts of the curriculum or all the domains of behavior using the entire curriculum. While the curriculum provides foundational knowledge about the child's development from which the team and family develop goals, additional assessment is needed by each discipline to develop strategies for working with the child and family. In separate evaluations, each discipline involved evaluates one or two behavioral domains in-depth to determine the quality of the performance components. The primary domains evaluated are described as follows.

Cognitive Assessment

Cognitive assessment of infants reflects their abilities to acquire, store, and use information from the social and nonsocial environment. A wide range of abilities are considered within the cognitive domain including problem solving, object and person permanence, spatial relationships, causality, vocal and gestural imitation, communication, and social-emotional development (Dunst, 1984; Uzgiris, 1983). Dunst, Holbert, and Wilson (1990) describe two different strategies for assessing a child's cognitive abilities. The first method involves administering Piagetian-based cognitive scales. Dunst (1980) and Uzgiris and Hunt (1975) have developed ordinal scales based on Piaget's descriptions of the hierarchy of early cognitive development. The domains assessed in the scales are (1) object permanence, (2) means-ends abilities, (3) vocal imitation, (4) gestural imitation, (5) operational causality, (6) spatial relationships, and (7) scheme actions. Six developmental levels are defined within each domain: reflexes, primary circular reactions, secondary circular reactions, coordination of secondary circular reactions, tertiary circular reactions, and representation and foresight.

Social-Emotional Behavior Assessment

Social-emotional behaviors are another critical area for in-depth assessment beyond a core developmental assessment. The child's ability to respond to others and regulate her own behavior influences the parent—child relationship and the amount of stress in caregiving. Scales such as the Bayley Infant Behavior Record (IBR) (Bayley, 1969), the Carolina Record of Individual Behavior (CRIB) (Simeonsson, Huntington, Short, & Ware, 1982), and the Early Coping Inventory (Zeitlin, Williamson, & Szczepanski, 1988) measure child behaviors that are related to temperament and the child's ability to interact with others. Child characteristics that are known to have a strong influence on interaction patterns are activity level, attention, and behaviors that suggest excessive irritability or aggressiveness.

Carolina Record of Individual Behavior (CRIB)

The CRIB consists of two parts. The first part documents the child's level of arousal and his behavioral state. Children with disabilities often have inconsistencies in behavioral organization and lack smooth transitions from one behavioral state to another. The second part of the CRIB is divided into three sections. The first section provides for assessment of participation in interactions with others, motivation, social and object orientation, communication, endurance, and ability to be consoled. The behaviors rated in the second section are activity level, reactivity, goal directedness, response to frustration, attention span, responsiveness to caregiver, muscle tone, and responsiveness to the examiner. The behaviors in the third section are indicators of the infant's patterns of exploration, communication, and rhythmic habits. While the behaviors rated may appear unrelated and in separate domains, all the behaviors have implications for the caregiver and for the infant's ability to respond to the communication of the caregiver.

Early Coping Inventory

Other characteristics of the child help determine her ability to initiate and sustain interaction with others. The infant's ability to cope with sensory stimulation, to initiate behaviors, and to make an organized, coordinated response can be rated on the Early Coping Inventory (Zeitlin, Williamson, & Szczepanski, 1988). This scale quantifies the infant's ability to cope with the environment using organized, interactive, and effective responses. The items are divided into three categories: sensorimotor organization, reactive behavior, and self-initiated behavior.

The *sensorimotor organization* items provide a method for evaluation of the child's integration of sensorimotor processes. Coordinated movement, accommodation to touch, and visual attention are also assessed in this section.

Reactive behaviors refer to the child's responses to the demands of the physical and social environments. Sample reactive behaviors include the ability to respond to the feelings of others, to adapt to changes in the environment, and to bounce back from stressful events.

In the *self-initiated behavior* section, the child's self-generated, self-directed actions are used to meet personal needs and to interact with objects and people. The items include demonstration of persistence during activities and initiation of interactions with others. Each item is rated 1 to 5 according to the coping effectiveness of the child. The scale yields a score for the child's global coping competence and for coping effectiveness within the three categories. A chart is provided for listing the most and least adaptive coping behaviors. This list of the child's strengths and limitations in interacting with the environment provides valuable information for treatment planning (Williamson & Zeitlin, 1990).

Effect of Child's Social-Emotional Characteristics on the Family

Huntington (1988) identified three aspects of the child's behavior that have strong effects on family functioning. The first behavioral domain is temperament or individual differences in behavioral style. The temperament clusters have been identified as difficult, easy, and slow-to-warm up. The second behavioral domain is readability; that is, the extent to which an infant's behaviors are clearly defined and produce distinctive signals and cues for adults. The third domain consists of difficult behaviors that make caregiving stressful or behaviors that make the child's disability conspicuous to others, such as the mannerisms of a child with autism.

Occupational therapists may not measure these domains in a formal assessment. An early intervention team's psychologist is more likely to administer the CRIB or the IBR, while the Early Coping Inventory is often rated by the primary interventionist. Whether formal or informal assessment methods are used, it is important that the team understand and appreciate these variables to plan intervention goals and strategies. When child behaviors create stress for others and the child's coping efforts are ineffective, parent–child and professional–child interaction are inevitably affected. To improve goodness-of-fit between the child and the environment, the team helps the parent identify which behaviors are most disruptive to the home environment or seem to be a source of stress in their relationships. These behaviors can then be identified as intervention goals or the team can offer the family suggestions for compensating for the child's behaviors.

Audiology/Speech and Language Assessment

Assessment of expressive and receptive communication often begins with a hearing evaluation. If the infant's hearing is in question, an audiology evaluation will reveal the need for a hearing aid and identify which tones and pitches the child is most able to assimilate. Children with syndromes, such as Apert's, Down, and others, are particularly vulnerable to hearing loss. In addition to a hearing evaluation by an audiologist, an assessment of oral structure and oral motor skills may precede a speech and language evaluation. The integrity of oral structures and the infant's ability to coordinate and organize oral movements may be evaluated by the speech or occupational therapists (Morris & Klein, 1988). Efficient feeding and respiration relate to efficient sound production. The child's organization of rhythmic sucking, swallowing, and breathing has implications for the child's expressive language as well as for feeding.

A number of formal evaluations are available for speech and language assessment. The Bzoch League Receptive-Expressive Emergent Language Scale (REEL) (Bzoch & League, 1971) has a relatively large number of items for young children and is easy to administer. Because many of the items are based on parents' reports, the scale is frequently administered by disciplines other than the language specialist. The Bayley Mental Scale also includes a number of items that assess the child's expressive language. Receptive language is assessed through items that have verbal instructions that precede physical demonstration.

Speech and language therapists often evaluate children using a natural language sample obtained during play sessions. Ideally, samples from two different settings, such as the home and the clinic, provide a valid assessment of language skill. Picture books and imaginative toys (when age-appropriate) are typically used to create a playful environment in which speech is easily elicited. The speech therapist waits for the child to initiate communication, attends to all efforts of the child to communicate, imitates the child's gestures and vocalizations, and responds to the child's communication efforts with attention, encouragement, and praise (McDonald, Gillette, & Hutchinson, 1989). Natural language samples with the parents may differ from those with peers or objects. A variety of samples provides a clear picture as to which sources of interaction elicit the most frequent communication responses and seem to sustain that response (Warren & Kaiser, 1988).

Sensorimotor Assessment

A specific assessment of sensorimotor skills usually includes hand-eye coordination, grasping patterns, manipulation, reach, reflexes, mobility, balance, posture, and overall control of body movements. While therapists often use informal scales and naturalistic observations to assess sensorimotor skills, several normed tests are available. As previously discussed, normed scales are particularly helpful in determining eligibility for services. Following are examples of standardized motor assessment for young children.

Peabody Developmental Motor Scales (PDMS)

The PDMS (Folio & Fewell, 1983) measure fine and gross motor skills and were designed for children with motor delays, from birth through 6 years of age. The scales have standardized criteria for administering and scoring the items. A scoring system of 0, 1, and 2 allows for the measurement of emerging skills. A number of items are listed under each age category, in contrast to the Bayley Motor Scales, which has fewer items.

The test was standardized using a stratified quota sample. The manual documents the results of field-testing that provide evidence of the reliability and validity of the PDMS (Folio & Fewell, 1983). Estimates of construct and concurrent validity are high. Although not all of the items seem to be listed in the hierarchy of normal development (e.g., radial palmar grasp is listed before ulnar palmar grasp) and the test lacks sensitivity to the quality of motor skill, the test is a respected and often used instrument among occupational and physical therapists. Palisano (1986) reports that the PDMS appear to have validity with moderate to severe children with motor impairments. Its psychometric properties allow use for evaluation, reevaluation, and research of motor skills.

Movement Assessment of Infants (MAI)

The MAI (Chandler, Andrews, & Swanson, 1980) was originally developed to monitor the progress of high-risk infants. It can be used to assess infants through the first year and has normed scores available for infants who are either 4 or 8 months adjusted age. The test enables the examiner to rate the quality of muscle tone, reflex development, righting reactions, and volitional movements, using a six-point scale for each item.

The authors suggest that the MAI be used for the following purposes: (1) to identify motor dysfunction in infants up to 12 months of age, (2) to establish the basis for an early intervention program, (3) to monitor the effects of physical therapy on infants, (4) to assist in data collection and clinical research on motor development through the use of a standard system, and (5) to teach skilled observation of movement and motor development (Chandler, Andrews, & Swanson, 1980). The infant is observed in supine, prone, sitting, and standing positions; about half of the items require specific handling of the child. Time for administering the scales is minimal and the only equipment needed are toys and a tilting surface.

Sensitivity scores, indicating accuracy in identifying neurodevelopmental delay, ranged from 73.5% to 96.1%. Specificity scores, indicating accuracy in identifying normal infants, ranged from 62.7% to 78.2% (Harris, 1987).

Milani-Comparetti Developmental Examination

The purpose of the Milani-Comparetti Developmental Examination (Milani-Comparetti & Gidoni, 1967) is to screen neurological and developmental behaviors of infants and young children, from newborn to 2.5 years of age. The test provides a simple system for rating postural control, active movement, primitive reflexes, automatic reactions, parachute reactions, and tilting reactions. Five primitive reflexes, the palmar and plantar grasp reflexes, asymmetrical and symmetrical tonic neck reflexes, and Moro are included. As a screening instrument of neurodevelopmental integrity, the examination does not provide adequate information for planning intervention. The test can be administered in 10 minutes, which includes minimal time for observation of spontaneous movement. In general, the items involve physical maneuvers applied to the infant. Unlike the MAI, no training is recommended, although the manual should be studied prior to administering and scoring the test (Trembath, 1978).

Informal Observation

The sensorimotor components, such as muscle tone, reflexes, righting, equilibrium, and volitional movement, are usually evaluated informally through observation of the child's spontaneous movement in his environment and by handling the child in a variety of positions. Handling to elicit motor responses is individualized according to each infant. The qualitative aspects of sensorimotor function are discussed under the description of the occupational therapist's assessment.

Play Assessment

A play assessment rates the child's spontaneous play interactions with toys and people. Psychologists, such as McCune-Nicolich (1980); special educators, such as Fewell (1985); and occupational therapists, such as Bledsoe and Shepherd (1982) and Knox (1974) have developed play scales. The Play Assessment Scale (Fewell, 1985) determines a play age from sequenced items. The child is given opportunities to interact with various sets of toys. The play behaviors observed are scored as either spontaneous or elicited through prompting. The Preschool Play Scale (Bledsoe & Shepherd, 1982; Knox, 1974) evaluates four domains of play by age groups. These domains are space management, material management, imitation, and participation.

Play is central to the child's behavior and from play, psychological, sensorimotor, and cognitive function observations, the child can be assessed. Linder (1990) recommends that play become the basis for evaluation of all the child's developmental skills. The following section further describes a play assessment as the core of the trans- or interdisciplinary assessment.

A Trandisciplinary Arena Assessment Model

In contrast to a model of interdisciplinary assessment, in which discipline members separately administer sections of a developmental curriculum, is an arena assessment, in which all team members participate together in a core assessment of play interaction with the child. The concept of arena assessment was first developed in the National Collaborative Infant Project (Conner, Williamson, & Siepp, 1978). In an arena assessment, many professionals of differing disciplines and the parents or caregivers observe and evaluate the child together. Usually, both professionals and parents are in the same room with the child; however, a two-way mirror and an observation room may be used if the number of people frightens or distracts the child or if the parent is a source of distraction.

The purpose of the arena assessment is to achieve an integrated understanding of the child's behaviors, strengths, and needs. The context of the assessment most often involves play with the child. Developmental skills, learning styles, and interaction patterns are the focus of the observations. Parents are actively involved throughout the process (Linder, 1990).

To effectively plan an arena assessment, initial information about the child's developmental levels, acquired through the reports of the parents or others, must be gathered. This information is used to select toys and materials that will be of interest to the child. Strategies for engaging the child in play are also identified. During the arena assessment the behaviors and responses of the child are discussed. The parent is asked to comment on whether the child's behaviors are typical or atypical and to give examples of the child's responses in other environments. Opportunities for observation of parent–child interaction may be included during part of the assessment. Linder (1990) recommends that a peer be introduced into the play activities for observation of child–child interaction.

Throughout the play interactions, a facilitator who is a member of the team, imitates, encourages, and expands upon the play behaviors initiated by the child. The goal of the facilitator is to elicit the richest sample of child behaviors possible within a limited time frame. Higher level responses are continually sought by allowing the child to direct the play and by matching or imitating gestures and verbalizations. The evaluator also challenges the child with activities that tap into emerging skills as well as those that are clearly integrated behaviors. The child is more likely to respond from a sensitive, interactive contact than from a directive, didactive one (Mahoney, Finger, & Powell, 1985).

Advantages of an arena assessment, which is based on play interactions with the child in a natural environment, are functional skill observation and parent participation. Furthermore, the testing activities are flexible and may be adapted to the special needs of the child (Linder, 1990).

Although only one team member usually facilitates the performance of the child and one member facilitates the participation of the parent, all (or most) members are involved and make comments or suggestions during the session. All members participate in planning the assessment, contribute to interpreting the results, and recommend goals and intervention strategies for the child that are based on their observations and interpretations. The arena assessment can provide most of the information needed to plan intervention; however, it does not preclude specific evaluation by individual disciplines in order to have a thorough basis of program planning. Often the occupational and physical therapists benefit from an opportunity to handle the child in order to gain an understanding of her muscle tone and her movement patterns, and to appreciate how the child responds to specific handling techniques.

Arena assessments, which involve the parent and facilitate an integrated transdisciplinary approach, philosophically match the intent of the early intervention legislation. This assessment model actually crosses the lines of assessment, planning, and intervention through the use of naturalistic play and interaction opportunities to elicit and sustain the child's responses and to challenge her to the highest developmental levels. For these reasons, the arena assessment has been adopted by a great number of early intervention programs and has been recommended by leaders in the field (Foley, 1990; Garland & McGonigel, 1988; Linder, 1990; Woodruff & McGonigel, 1988).

Description of Occupational Therapy Assessment

Occupational therapists participate in all levels of evaluation from diagnosis to program planning and evaluation. Using a holistic perspective, the occupational therapist may administer a core developmental assessment for diagnostic purposes or may have a leadership role in an arena assessment. The occupational therapist brings an understanding of the interrelations of the child's function and developmental skills, of sensory perception and behavior, and of neurodevelopmental processes.

Typically, the occupational therapist analyzes the quality of performance during the scoring of items. The analysis of the quality of skill performance when shared with other team members brings an increased understanding of the problem and of the child's potential. In a diagnostic evaluation, the occupational therapist may include informal assessment of the following performance components: muscle tone, strength, coordination, motor planning, and sensory processing. Clinical judgement regarding qualitative issues, such as muscle tone and sensory processing, is essential to understanding the basis of the child's behavior. The occupational therapist often integrates information from observations of the child in a number of environments and situations in order to develop a composite picture that has meaning and represents an accurate interpretation of the child. For example, if the therapist observed that an infant boy stiffened into an extension posture when he held him, he may conclude that extensor muscle tone was high or that he had an aversion to touch. However, if the therapist then observed him relax and cuddle in his mother's arms, he would attribute the infant's stiff posture to stranger anxiety and stress. Observations in a variety of situations reveal valid information about the quality of muscle tone, posture, movement, and about the child's response to sensory input. Evaluation for program planning focuses on discipline specific areas and is multidimensional. In-depth evaluation, using a number of formal and informal methods, enables the occupational therapist to recommend appropriate child goals and to select the most effective strategies for reaching those goals.

Areas of emphasis of the occupational therapy evaluation include, but are not limited to, self-care (feeding), play, and sensorimotor skills. The primary components of assessing sensorimotor performance include sensory integration as it relates to sensory processing and perception; neuromuscular function (e.g., muscle tone, reflexes, righting responses, and equilibrium reactions); and motor components (e.g., coordination, praxis, visual-motor, and oral-motor control). Range of motion and postural alignment are biomechanical issues that relate to motor performance.

Cognition and psychosocial skills are assessed as these skills interrelate to the child's play, movement, and interaction with others and with the environment. These functional and developmental areas are the concern of various team disciplines. The role of the occupational therapist varies in different settings regarding formal and informal assessment of the child's cognitive and psychosocial skills.

Sensorimotor Performance

The occupational therapist may first administer an assessment that rates the presence or absence of motor skills. The Peabody Developmental Motor Scales (Folio & Fewell, 1983) are frequently used when a standardized test is requested by the parents or recommended by the other team members. The Peabody provides valid documentation of the child's developmental range of motor skills and can become a basis for setting goals and for communicating with the parents about the child's needs and strengths.

The curricula described in the first part of this chapter have sections for evaluating fine and gross motor skills. The skills listed in the curricula are helpful for establishing goals and for serving as a common language among the team members and parents. Identifying skills is the first step in the occupational therapist's evaluation. With a general picture of the child's strengths and limitations in the sensorimotor domain, the occupational therapist focuses on the quality of movement and posture, the child's response to tactile, vestibular, and proprioceptive input, and the child's ability to integrate sensory and motor systems into coordinated, purposeful skill. (See Appendix A for observation guidelines.)

Gross Motor Skills

Postural Control and Muscle Tone
Biomechanical and neuromuscular functions form the basis of motor skill. *Range of motion* of the extremities and trunk are issues with infants who have orthopedic or severe muscle tone problems. Range of motion is usually noted but not precisely measured unless strategies such as casting or splinting are used to increase range of motion at specific joints. In infants with spasticity, range of motion may be normal; however, maintenance of range of motion may be an appropriate goal. In infants with fused joints (e.g., arthrogryposis), range of motion may be severely limited but not a goal of therapy.

Spinal alignment is observed in all developmental positions. Alignment changes in each position; for example, an infant may fall into anterior pelvic tilt when prone and posterior pelvic tilt when sitting (Bly, 1983). Postural alignment affects the quality of motor skill by influencing the dynamic equilibrium response of the child. A child who sits with posterior pelvic tilt and a rounded trunk will inevitably use protective extension for balancing, due to lack of dynamic response and rotation of the trunk. A child who sits with a rounded trunk will also be limited in reaching patterns, particularly in the reach over her head.

Observation of postural alignment is followed by observation of *postural stability and mobility*, which is influenced by postural muscle tone. Normal postural tone is sufficiently high to support the trunk against gravity, yet at the same time allows for mobility of the extremities and dynamic adaptations of the trunk to shifts in the center of gravity. In addition, postural symmetry and midline orientation are observed in a variety of positions. The child may demonstrate high-level integration of right and left side in prone or supine versus sitting or quadruped. Consistent side preferences in different positions and asymmetries of the trunk are indications of possible neurodevelopmental problems that affect movement on one body side more than the other.

Equilibrium responses are observed in all positions. In prone, supine, sitting, quadruped, and standing, the development of postural control evolves through a similar sequence (Gilfolye, Grady, & Moore, 1990). The child first moves in axial flexion and extension. Coordination between flexion and extension depends on postural alignment and becomes a problem when trunk flexion or extension dominate the posture.

The next developmental step in the maturation of equilibrium responses is postural control in lateral righting or lateral weight shift. Observations of the child's ability to shift his weight from one side to the other requires basic integration of the two body sides and coordination of trunk flexion and extension. In a lateral weight shift (e.g., prone or sitting), the nonweight-bearing side laterally flexes and the weight-bearing side elongates. Observation of shoulder and pelvic alignment is important to the child's ability to move in the lateral (frontal) plane using smooth and well controlled movements.

After assessing that the child has achieved postural control in lateral righting, the therapist evaluates development of rotation in the transverse plane. Righting using rotation of the body axis is first observed in segmental rolling. Control of rotation requires correct postural alignment, integration of the two body sides, and coordination of the musculature that crosses the trunk in a transverse direction (Scherzer & Tscharnuter, 1992). Rotation is the hallmark of mature equilibrium and indicates that postural control has reached a sufficient level of development to support independent movement of the extremities.

Equilibrium develops in each higher level position in an overlapping and intertwined pattern (Gilfoyle, Grady, & Moore, 1990). For example, the child practices lateral weight shifts in sitting as he begins segmental rolling. The child also learns to rock in quadruped in an anterior-posterior plane as he develops control of rotation in sitting. Therefore, the occupational therapist usually reports that equilibrium skills are integrated at one postural level and are emerging in other positions that are more upright against gravity. Mature equilibrium patterns include rapid adjustments of the extremities as well as dynamic trunk movements. In mature equilibrium, both axial stability and extremity mobility support controlled body adjustment to changes in the center of gravity.

Fine Motor Skills

The first movement patterns of the upper extremities are random and reflexive. Primitive reflexes, such as the asymmetrical tonic neck reflex and grasping reflex, initially dominate arm movements. Relatively early (4 to 6 months), the primitive reflexes are integrated and voluntary control of upper extremity movement increases.

Fine motor assessment includes evaluation of reaching patterns (stability of arm in space), prehension patterns (grasp and release), and manipulation skill (bilateral and in-hand). Muscle tone and strength are key issues in the development of fine motor skills as well as postural control. Primitive reflexes that have not been integrated interfere with emerging fine motor skills. Co-contraction of muscle tone is needed to hold the arm away from the body.

Reciprocal innervation allows mobility of the arm in activity with the object. Normal muscle tone permits smooth and coordinated movements in fine motor skills (Scherzer & Tscharnuter, 1992).

Reach

The child first reaches using random arm extension in response to a visual stimulus. The stages of reaching develop from asymmetrical, imprecise, circuitous reach in a limited range of motion to accurate, well directed reach in all directions. Reach to the side precedes midline orientation. Reach at midline is initiated with humeral abduction, partial shoulder internal rotation, elbow extension, forearm pronation, and full finger extension (Exner, 1989). As scapular control and trunk stability mature, the infant uses more shoulder flexion, increased external rotation with forearm supination, and slight wrist extension. Shoulder control tends to develop prior to elbow, forearm, and wrist control.

Reach involves integration of the visual and motor systems. The child's visual focus and tracking must be sufficiently developed to maintain visual attention while reaching for the object and alternately gazing from her hand to the object (White, Castle, & Held, 1964).

In observing reaching skills, the therapist analyzes whether visual skills or shoulder and arm stability seem to be affecting the accuracy of reach. Reach is observed in prone, supine, sitting, and other developmentally appropriate positions. The object is placed at midline and to the side, at chest height, eye level, and overhead. The therapist observes whether the child visually guides his hand to the object by glancing from his hand to the object or maintains a focus on the object using proprioceptive feedback to direct his hand to the object (Bushnell, 1985; Hay, 1984). Observation of how well the hand accommodates to the size and shape of the object as it is prehended provides information about the child's proprioceptive system, motor control, and her visual discrimination of the object's features (Hall, 1990).

Grasping Skills

Grasping skills develop from primitive patterns of palmar grasp without participation of the thumb, to very precise pad prehension, to pad fingertip and thumb prehension. The Erhardt Developmental Prehension Assessment (EDPA) (Erhardt, 1982) provides a scoring system for rating the types of prehension according to their developmental sequence. The terminology for describing grasping patterns used by Erhardt offers a common language for therapists in describing prehension.

Exner (1989) and Holstein (1982) have described systems for documenting grasping patterns. Case-Smith (1989, 1991, 1992) developed an instrument that measures grasping skill of infants 2 to 7 months of age. The Posture and Fine Motor Assessment of Infants (PFMAI) provides a scoring system for documenting how the object is held in the hand, the degree of isolated thumb and finger movement, the interaction of the two hands, and the length of time the grasp is maintained (Case-Smith, 1992).

Grasping skill requires visual attention and focus on the object. A refined fingertip grasp is needed for objects that are larger or smaller than objects that fit comfortably in the palm. Prehension skill is a precursor to the ability to transfer and manipulate objects using two hands.

Another precursor to the manipulation of objects is the development of controlled release. Release occurs first in a pattern of total arm and finger extension. The first object release may be against a surface or with the hand stabilized on a surface. The child practices release by transferring an object from hand to hand and by pressing an object into a surface and opening his hand using proprioceptive input. Imprecise release through full arm and hand extension develops many months prior to the precise, well controlled release needed to stack blocks.

Bilateral Manipulation

Bilateral manipulation refers to the use of two hands together in separate and coordinated movements. To coordinate the movement of both hands together, one hand reaches and prehends without associated movements in the other hand. The hands come together at midline, then as the child learns body rotation, she freely crosses the midline. Using one hand on the opposite side of the body indicates that bilateral integration is emerging and contributes to the child's development of body scheme and manipulative skill (Gilfolye, Grady, & Moore, 1990). Bilateral manipulation may be observed by giving the child an object that requires two hands to hold, by presenting opportunities for the child to cross the midline, and by giving the child a toy easily transferred from hand to hand (e.g., a ring). Through practice in using two hands together, most children select one hand as dominant and prefer to use that hand for writing, throwing, and other fine motor skills. Laterality is generally not established until after infancy.

In-Hand Manipulation

In-hand manipulation refers to precise movements of the fingers to manipulate an object held within the hand. Exner (1989, 1992) defined three primary categories of in-hand manipulation skills and is currently developing the Test of In-hand Manipulation by Exner (TIME) (Exner, 1992). Translation is a linear movement of the object from the palm to the fingers or the fingers to the palm. Shift is a linear movement of the object between or among the fingers. Rotation is the movement of an object around its axis. Objects may be turned horizontally or end over end. In-hand manipulation requires thumb stability in opposition, isolated finger movement, and flexible stability within the palm and fingertip grasping patterns. Many of these prerequisites are not present until the child is 30 to 48 months of age. In-hand manipulation can be evaluated by asking the child to prehend several coins or small pegs one at a time, by buttoning, stringing beads, or rotating a pencil or pen.

Motor Planning

Motor planning or praxis is the ability to plan and execute purposeful, coordinated movements (Ayres, 1979). A child plans movements from an idea or in response to environmental demand. Purposeful, cognitive planning is required when a movement is unfamiliar or novel for the child. If the movement has been well practiced and is familiar, it no longer requires motor planning. Therefore, praxis is evaluated in situations that are novel for the child. Because most infants approach tasks using trial and error and physical exploration without prior mental planning, motor planning is usually not observed until 2.5 to 3 years of age. At that time, the child engages in more complex play sequences that involve planning.

Sensory Integration

A prerequisite to the infant's ability to respond to his environment is his ability to perceive sensory input. Infants who have diminished response to sensory experiences or who become overly aroused by sensory stimulation are often unable to organize an appropriate response. Because infants cannot verbally explain their sensory perceptions and preferences, the sensory evaluation is based on reading their body language and interpreting their responses to sensory stimulation.

The occupational therapist assesses which types and levels of sensory stimulation match the infant's needs and preferences. When the child is overstimulated, he is unable to demonstrate an attentive and developmentally appropriate response. The infant becomes distressed and irritable or may shut down and transition into a lower state of arousal.

A young infant may be unable to accommodate to sources of visual and auditory stimuli. Simultaneous multimodal sensory stimulation can create stress, which results in disorganized responses (Farber, 1982). To assess visual and auditory preferences, single sources of stimulation are presented to the child. A variety of stimuli at various levels of intensity are presented at midline and to the side. Combinations of auditory and visual stimuli may elicit more response in the underreactive child than a single source. Animated and nonanimated visual stimuli and a variety of bright colors, including shiny colors and black and white are used. The child may be more attentive and responsive in low light or possibly in warm-colored light; fluorescent lighting is seldom optimal for a child with visual problems (Als, 1986).

Response to auditory input provides essential information for intervention. Infants may respond to high-pitched voices more than low-toned, deep voices, often preferring musical or rhythmical sounds. Although infants may startle to a low level of auditory stimulation when drowsy or in a sleepy state, they may demonstrate pleasure to the sound when alert and awake (Als, 1986).

The child's response to touch can be evaluated by offering a variety of touch experiences to the child. A tactually defensive child may demonstrate an adverse response to light touch but enjoy deep pressure (Ayres, 1979). A child with poor discrimination of touch may be unresponsive to light touch, or touch may elicit a general, rather than specific, response. The child may also be more sensitive to touch in certain body areas than others. For example, children may be more sensitive around their mouths than on their arms or legs. A child who dislikes lying prone may be more sensitive on his anterior trunk than on other areas of his back.

In the older infant and the toddler, it is important to observe the types of tactile materials that the child seeks and prefers to use in play. A child may handle a variety of materials using only his fingertips without manipulating them in the palm of his hand. Children may also approach certain materials with great caution and may handle them quite briefly, making limited skin contact. Specific questions to the parents will verify or confirm impressions from observations of the child's interaction with materials. It is particularly important to ask how he handles food, what clothing bothers him, what objects and materials are preferred, and which textures seem irritating.

The child may demonstrate obvious enjoyment or intense fear of movement. While in a prone position, the child may enjoy slow rhythmic movement, but may be startled and begin to cry when quickly moved in an upright position. A child may respond with enjoyment when carried or held and rocked, but show fear when placed alone on an unstable surface. Young infants often have difficulty responding to rotary movements. A child who is sensitive to movement and has difficulty organizing vestibular information will tend to appear stationary and avoid movement experiences. Children who respond negatively to small movements may seek and delight in rough housing.

The therapist is alerted to difficulty in the child's ability to respond to sensory input when the parent states that the child seems most content when left alone. Sometimes a toddler will independently seek a quiet or dimly lit environment to calm an overly aroused nervous system. Often an infant overcomes excessive sensitivity to movement and touch through a combination of neurological maturation and natural caregiving experiences (e.g., rocking and massage). The parents may report this improvement and may indicate that the child's tolerance is much higher than in early infancy when environmental experiences were limited and the nervous system was developing.

Parents' reports are important in verifying the therapist's impressions. Table 4-4 presents a sensory history interview to be given to parents. Response to visual, auditory, tactile, and vestibular input varies according to the state and the mood of the child. Fear of strangers and of unfamiliar environments may affect the child's responses; for example, when in the arms of a stranger, the child may overreact to stimuli that he typically enjoys. Therefore, observations of the child do not always produce valid information about the child's reactivity to sensory input.

Table 4-4   Sensory Integration Interview Guide for Infants

Discuss the following questions and observation items with parents or teachers to examine a child's sensorimotor integration. Remember, they are intended only as a guide. If the answer to several of the age-appropriate questions is no, the child may have a sensory integration deficit, and further evaluation may be needed.

Level 1 (approximately 0 to 12 months of age)

1. Does the baby like to be held and tend to mold the body to that of the adult holding him or her? (Conversely, does the baby show arching behavior or attempt to pull or push away when held?)
2. Is the baby comfortable being moved? (Conversely, does the baby become irritable or disorganized when passively moved in space or when the body position is changed?)
3. Does the baby have favorite songs and movement games with adults and anticipate these special interactions? (Conversely, does the baby avoid any novel play situations?)
4. Does the baby explore toys orally at the appropriate age? (Conversely, does the baby avoid mouthing toys?)
5. Does the baby accept textured foods when they are introduced at the appropriate age? (Conversely, does the baby have difficulty handling textured foods, or is he or she a very picky eater?)
6. Can the baby attend to more than one stimulus at one time (e.g., look and listen at the same time)? (Conversely, does the baby "tune out" if more than one stimulus is presented at one time?)
7. At an appropriate age and motor ability level, does the baby easily move from one position to another in play? (Conversely, does the baby prefer to stay in one position and avoid transitional movements?)
8. Were the baby's sleep-wake cycles fairly well established after the first 6 weeks? (Conversely, has the baby never developed an established pattern of routines, or is the baby difficult to calm or get to sleep?)
9. Does the baby engage in a variety of progressive midline play—two hands together, transfer, and crossing the midline? (Conversely, does the baby use one hand or the other but avoid bilateral use?)

Table 4-4   *Continued*

10. Does the baby show a preference for certain sensory stimuli (e.g., music or touch)? (Conversely, do caregivers have difficulty determining the baby's preference for any sensory input?)
11. Does the baby show an appropriate response to sensory induced reflexes (e.g., rooting, protective extension, or righting responses?)

Level 2 (approximately 12 to 18 months of age)

1. Does the child enjoy exploring a variety of new textures? Will the child play with foods, textured toys, sand, etc? (Conversely, does the child avoid finger feeding or withdraw from touching new textures, even an attractive toy?)
2. Does the child's toy play progress from one level to the next in an easy flow, that is, does the child combine toys at an appropriate age? (Conversely, does the child's toy seem "stuck" at a immature level, such as mouthing, banging, or casting in a repetitive fashion?)
3. Does the child spend time exploring a toy to obtain information about all of its component parts? Does the child use touch, vision, and hearing together to assess properties of toys such as squeak toys or balls in a bowl? (Conversely, does the child show poor exploration of the component parts or details of toys? Does the child have a short attention span when given a new toy?)
4. Is the child able to follow simple directions with and without gestures? Does the child seem to be listening and looking when an adult talks to him or her? (Conversely, does the child show inconsistent responses to verbal direction and make poor eye contact when an adult talks to him or her?)
5. Does the child accept having different textures of clothing next to the skin, or is he or she more comfortable with less clothing on (e.g., no shoes or short shirts)? (Conversely, is the child very fussy about clothing? Does the child not like to be barefooted?)

Level 3 (approximately 18 months to 3 years of age)

1. Does the child seem to modulate his or her activity level appropriately to given play situations (e.g., active versus passive play, or structured play)? (Conversely, does the child have an excessive need for intense movement or proprioception, such as jumping, rocking, and swinging, or does the child avoid movement altogether?)
2. Does the child explore new play equipment with anticipation and show good motor planning and balance skills? (Conversely, does the child avoid novel play situations or show difficulty getting on and off age-appropriate play equipment? Is the child clumsy, or does he or she want to remain on the ground at all times?)
3. Does the child demonstrate an ability to remain focused on a task despite moderate levels of environmental visual and auditory activity? (Conversely, does the child seem to be auditorily or visually distractible when playing with other children?)
4. Can the child participate well in group or circle activities? Does the child seem to understand the sequence of and changes in activities? (Conversely, does the child seem lost when in group or circle activities?)
5. Is the child comfortable trying new things or with changes in plans? (Conversely, does the child become upset if routines or plans are changed?)

Source: From Jirgal D, Bouma K: *Sensory Integration Special Interest Section Newsletter,* 1989, p. 5, reproduced with permission of the publisher.

Family and Environmental Variables

Family variables are the concern of all team members and the family, itself, has a critical role in the evaluation process. By requiring that each early intervention system develop a process for writing IFSPs, the early intervention legislation (PL 99-457; PL 102-119) ensures a family-centered approach. The purpose of the IFSP is for families and professionals to work together as a team to identify and mobilize formal and informal resources to help families reach their chosen goals. Part H of PL 99-457 and its accompanying regulations require that the IFSP, with the concurrence of the family, include a statement of the family resources, concerns, and priorities. These are to be determined by the family (Kaufmann & McGonigel, 1991).

Family Resources, Concerns, and Priorities

Assessment of a family's resources, concerns, and priorities may begin by asking open-ended questions about the aspects of the family life that help their child grow and develop. When parents have difficulty identifying specific strengths and needs, checklists or surveys may be used. The Family Needs Survey, Revised (Bailey & Simeonsson, 1990) and the Family Needs Scale (Dunst, Cooper, Weeldreyer, Snyder, & Chase, 1988 in Dunst, Trivette, & Deal, 1988) are examples of such instruments. The written checklist may stimulate the parents' identification of the issues and may increase their understanding of what services the early intervention program can offer. When used with the checklists, open-ended questions can reveal details about the needs of a family. Turnbull and Turnbull (1986) suggest that early intervention professionals ask if the family desires information about (1) teaching the child at home, (2) advocacy and working with professionals, (3) planning for the future, (4) helping the family relax and enjoy recreational activities, and (5) finding and using more support.

In assessing family concerns, the occupational therapist can describe the kinds of services offered by the early intervention program. She may suggest areas in which additional information or help may be needed. Potential areas of concern that are identified by Bailey (1988) can guide the interview with the parents. These areas are listed as follows:

Categories	*Examples*
Need for information	Information about the child's disability
Need for support	Opportunities to meet and to talk with other parents
Explaining to others	Explaining the child's problem to her siblings or grandparents
Community services	Help in locating respite care or day-care

Categories	Examples
Financial needs	Help in paying for therapy
Family functioning	Help in supporting one another

The concerns that the parents would like to work on become part of the IFSP. When concerns fall outside the functions of the agency (e.g., provide financial assistance for special equipment), the staff should provide assistance in helping the parents locate and access the needed service from other community agencies.

Most of the scales available to assess family concerns and resources focus on family needs. Yet, as discussed in chapter 1, the strengths and resources of the family unit should become the building blocks of the intervention program. Parents are often reluctant to verbalize a list of their family's strengths. For example, a mother may naturally handle her infant in gentle ways that facilitate the infant's ability to organize incoming sensory information and to attend to surrounding activity. Another example is the mother who feeds her child at a good pace and who appropriately positions her child. These skills should be acknowledged as being a strong base for further enhancing the child's abilities.

When the family feels awkward about sharing their strengths or does not recognize them, the team can help by identifying the resources they perceive as valuable assets that can serve as a foundation for the intervention program. For example, family time together and open communication among family members might be identified as important family resources. Family strengths are measured informally through observation and interview (Kaufmann & McGonigel, 1991). Table 4-5 provides a list of open-ended questions that can elicit the family's resources, concerns, and priorities.

Table 4-5 Open-Ended Questions To Ask When Assessing the Family's Concerns, Resources, and Priorities

---

- What information would you like from the agency?
- Can you explain the kinds of support systems that are important to your family?
- How have friends or extended family provided support?
- How might the program be of support to your family?
- Do you have any financial concerns related to the expenses incurred in your child's care?
- Is arranging child care an issue?
- Can you identify any community services that we can help you access (e.g., a dentist who treats children with special needs)?
- What strengths do you see in your family?
- What do you want for your family in the future?
- How can our program help you achieve your dreams for your family?
- What are your priorities for your family?

Cultural Background

Throughout the assessment and intervention process, sensitivity to cultural differences is essential. Cultural values influence how family members respond to a child with a disability and how they respond to external sources of support (Wayman, Lynch, & Hanson, 1990). In many cultures, the family is extended to include numerous relatives and nonrelatives. Family membership may be somewhat fluid. Distant relatives or friends may be considered family members as situations and relationships change. The extended family may be the most important support network for the parents and should be included in the assessment process. Cultural background also influences the relationship and the communication established between the family and the team. Evaluations should be adapted to match the family's native language and cultural differences should be considered in interpreting the results.

Although the assessment process heightens the team's awareness that the family's cultural beliefs differ from their own, the cultural beliefs and values of a family are usually learned after an extended period is spent working with the family. Any assumptions about the family's response to services or about their willingness and desire to participate in the program should be avoided. In best practice, sensitivity to and competence in the family's culture are priorities of the early intervention team (Anderson & Fenichel, 1989).

Home Environment

Many of the variables described in the previous sections are learned by interviewing the parents, whose responses are encouraged by active listening, reflecting on what is said, and indicating support and understanding. A home visit can provide information about the home environment, about the interactions among family members, and about the resources and sources of stimulation available. The team member who makes the home visit brings a picture of that environment to the other team members. All team members need to understand the home setting and the learning environment of the child, whether services are home- or clinic-based.

The HOME (Caldwell & Bradley, 1978) is a systematic method for measuring key aspects of the environment known to relate to caregiving and child development. The HOME measures the content, quality, and responsiveness of the home environment for children birth to 36 months of age. Using clusters of variables, the HOME is a method to assess the parents' emotional and verbal responsivity, avoidance of restriction and punishment, organization of the physical environment, provision of adequate play materials, and opportunities for variety in daily stimulation. An environment with several siblings, pets, and age-appropriate toys may be more stimulating than an environment with a plentiful supply of toys that appears sterile and does not include siblings or readily available playmates. Particular concern is raised if the home environment appears unsafe and intervention is needed to protect the child from injury.

Occupational therapists have particular interest in visiting the home environment as part of the evaluation process. They evaluate the fit of the home environment to the needs of the child. Sensory needs are an important consideration. If the child is hyporesponsive and delayed, a stimulating environment is beneficial. Interactions that involve developmentally appropriate visual and auditory stimulation can promote responses in the infant. Opportunities for one-on-one interaction with toys and others is important in fostering developmental skills. An environment without toys and siblings that does not offer opportunities for developmentally stimulating interactions may become a concern of the therapist. Recommended strategies for play with the child would need to consider and compensate for lack of resources within the home.

If the child is easily overstimulated or is sensory defensive, a highly busy, noisy environment can be stressful to the child. As a result, the child may be continually distressed and may be unable to respond to the caregivers or the environment. The therapist identifies particular areas of sensory defensiveness and stress; she then recommends adapting those aspects of the home environment to promote the infant's comfort level and ability to calm, to attend, and to successfully interact with others. Aspects of the home that may be stressful to a sensory defensive infant are noise levels, lighting, the amount of time people touch and hold the child, and the daily activity level within the home.

A Typical Day

Occupational therapists are also interested in the daily routines of the infant and the parents. By asking the parents to describe a typical day, the therapist gains knowledge that assists in planning intervention. Specifically, a description of the parents' daily routine reveals the amount of caregiving required by the child. It also provides the therapist with information about which caregiving activities seem to be frustrating or stressful for the parents. Activities that seem to take an unusual amount of time (e.g., dressing) or activities that must be repeated at frequent intervals (e.g., feeding every 2 hours) can be sources of stress for the parents. These activities may become priority goals for therapy.

Information about the family's routine also allows the occupational therapist to design activities that will fit into the family's routine (Rainforth & Salisbury, 1988). Exercises or activities to foster developmental skills are recommended according to the family's interest and are to be implemented

Table 4-6 Assessing the Typical Day

• "I would like to learn more about your typical routine. It is most helpful if you describe what you do day to day in detail."

• "Tell me about a typical day. You might pick a weekday, if that is more routine." When parents report that weekend days and weekdays are completely different, both should be described.

• "When do you wake up?"

• "What do you typically do first?"

• "When are family times, when are quiet times?"

Additional information may be sought if not spontaneously offered by the parent.

• "Who participates in bathing the child?" "Dressing?" "Feeding?" "Other caregiving?"

• "When are difficult times with the child?"

• "When do recreational activities fit into the day?"

• "How much time is needed to complete specific tasks (e.g., feeding)?"

---

at times that are convenient and easily fit into the family's schedule. Table 4-6 lists questions that may be asked when assessing the family's typical day.

Family Structure and Support Systems

Other characteristics that have strong implications for family function, parenting style, and priorities in caregiving relate to the structure, background, and experience of the family. The family's support system also has important implications for the therapist's recommendations (see Case-Smith, Chapter 2). Information about these family variables is gathered by a social worker, a service coordinator, or a primary instructor. Relevant information about family characteristics learned through informal conversation should be shared with the team. The number of nearby family and extended family members relates highly to the amount of support available to the parents. Family composition influences the amount and quality of caregiving and stimulation the child receives. Single parent families may need more support and may be more stressed by the responsibility of a child with a disability; however, assumptions about the child's environment cannot be made from knowledge of one or two variables. Although a single parent may appear to be in a stressful situation he may have the continual support of parents or may have a devoted and supportive friend. Some single parents have developed coping mechanisms and nontraditional support systems that enable them to meet their own needs while offering caregiving, attention, and developmental stimulation to their infants.

Parent–Child Interaction

Social interaction between parents and their child becomes the foundation for the child's future relationships with siblings and peers (Comfort, 1988). Such interactions affect the development of cognitive ability (Bee et al., 1982; Ramey, Farran, & Campbell, 1979) and psychosocial skills (Macoby & Martin, 1983; Tronick & Gianino, 1986). The early social interaction between the parent and the child encourages the child's responses and heightens her interest in the environment. The goodness-of-fit between the child and the caregiver can lead to the building of optimal relationships and to positive opportunities for the child's overall development (Simeonsson, Bailey, Huntington, & Comfort, 1986). The mother's warmth and affection, contingent responses, sensitivity to the child's interests, and encouragement of achievement have been found to relate to positive child outcomes in studies of children without disabilities (Clarke-Stewart, 1973; Yarrow, Rubenstein, Pedersen, & Jankowski, 1972). The quality of infant development appears to increase when parents respond to the infant frequently and provide the infant with developmentally appropriate experiences (Hanzlik, Chapter 9; Stern, 1977).

Although formal assessments are available for measuring parent–child interaction, occupational therapists often informally assess the quality of parent–child interaction based on experience, observation skills, and clinical judgment. The content of these assessments may provide the basis for the therapist's informal evaluation of parent–child interaction.

Examples of Parent–Infant Interaction Scales

Examples of the formal interaction scales frequently used by therapists and other disciplines in early intervention programs are described in Table 4-7. As one of the original parent–infant interaction scales, the Parent Behavior Progression (Bromwich, 1981) recognized the importance of the parents' interactions with the child. The scale assesses maternal behaviors and attitudes related to parent–infant interaction. The parents' behaviors are described according to the six levels of the scale. The levels are (1) enjoyment of the infant, (2) sensitivity/responsiveness, (3) mutuality in interaction, (4) developmental appropriateness, (5) initiation of new activities based on those presented previously, and (6) independently generating new developmentally appropriate activities.

Two scales that have undergone more instrument development and provide a more sensitive scoring system than the Bromwich Scale are the Nursing Child Assessment Teaching Scales [Nursing Child Assessment Satellite Training (NCAST), 1978a] and the Nursing Child Assessment Feeding Scales (NCAST, 1978b). These scales have 73 and 76 yes/no items, respectively. In the teaching scale, the parent is observed teaching the child how to use a

Table 4-7 Parent–Child Interaction Scales

Scale	Intended Populations	Content	Scoring System	Administrative System	Reliability
Nursing Child Assessment Teaching Scale (1978a) and Feeding Scale (NCAST, 1978b)	Mothers at medical risk during pregnancy, delivery, or postnatally; prematurity; failure to thrive; neglect and abuse. Infants ages 6–36 months.	Rates parents' behaviors in teaching or in feeding related to sensitivity to cues, response to distress, social-emotional, and cognitive growth fostering. Rates child behaviors in feeding and in teaching, related to clarity of cues and responsiveness to parents.	Binary scale for occurrence/nonoccurrence of 149 total behaviors.	Natural feeding situation for dyad and structured session with two tasks for mother to teach, one at age level and one higher. Can be administered at home or in clinic.	During training, 65% agreement with one of four practice tapes; 85% agreement in three of five field home visits. Certificate awarded when these levels are achieved. Correlations of .70–.83 for two observers for feeding scale and .79–.83 for teaching scale.
Maternal Behavior Rating Scale (Mahoney, 1985)	Infants with mental retardation. Infants ages 12–36 months.	Rates interactive behaviors, including cognitive and social stimulation of the mother. Rates child's reaction to maternal stimulation.	Eighteen behaviors rated on a 1–5 scale; each point on the scale is behaviorally anchored.	Twenty minutes, code ten minutes only. Free play with standard set of toys. Videotaped home observations.	Correlations of .76–.81 between two observers across all behaviors of exact agreement. Correlations within one point of .93–1.00.
Parent Behavior Progression (Bromwich, 1981, 1983)	Disabled and developmentally delayed; premature and low birth weight. Infants from birth to 36 months.	Rates parents' behaviors believed to facilitate attachment. Behaviors important for facilitating cognitive growth.	Binary checklist for reported or observed behavior under each level.	Naturalistic observation during 2–3 home visits of 1–15 hours each.	Interrater agreement ranged from 33% to 100% across all behaviors. Correlations between consecutive ratings made at 4-month intervals ranged from .31 to .78.
Parent/Caregiver Involvement Scale (Farran, Kasari, & Comfort, 1986)	Normative; families with children who have disabilities; poverty; adolescent mothers. Infants ages 3–36 months.	Rates parents in interaction with child related to cognitive and emotional growth (vocalizations, proximity, mutual play). Rates five general items rate overall interactive pattern.	Eleven behaviors rated along each of the dimensions: Amount, Quality, Developmental Appropriateness. Behaviors rated on a 1–5 scale; odd-numbered points behaviorally anchored.	Mothers are instructed to play with infant as they would at home. Twenty minutes of continuous interaction are observed.	Intraclass reliability correlations range from .77 to .87 in home observations and from .53 to .93 in laboratory observations.

new toy; in the feeding scale, the mother is observed while feeding the infant. The scales measure both the mother's behavior and the infant's ability to respond to the mother. The mother's behavior score summarizes maternal sensitivity, alleviation of infant distress, and activity to foster infant development. The infant behavior score summarizes the clarity of infant cues and responsiveness to caregivers (Barnard & Bee, 1984). Training to use the scales is strongly recommended. The training uses videotapes and requires that trainees achieve .85 reliability with a partner on five observations. The NCAST scales, as well as the Bromwich scale, are appropriate for infants, birth to 36 months of age.

A more recently developed scale, which assists early intervention professionals in assessing the quality of parent–child interaction, is the Parent/Caregiver Involvement Scale (Farran, Kasari, Comfort, & Jay, 1986). This scale provides a method for describing the quality and appropriateness of the parents' interactions with the child. The scale was specifically developed to be used with delayed or at-risk children who are served by an early intervention team. The parents' behaviors are rated according to the amount, quality, and appropriateness of involvement. Some examples of the 11 behaviors are physical and verbal involvement, responsiveness, initiation of activity, control, playfulness, goal-directed assistance, and positive and negative verbalizations. The mother or father is instructed to play with the child, and a set of toys is usually provided. The scale is rated after a 20-minute observation of free play. The test developers recommend that therapists practice rating tapes with a partner and achieve .85 reliability prior to administering the scales.

Informal Assessment of Parent–Child Interaction

When a formal scale is not used, several considerations should be given to how parent–child interaction is informally assessed. A naturalistic setting, such as the home, is important to ensure that the parent and child feel comfortable. The examiner structures the observation by asking the parent to play with the child as she normally would. The therapist might say, "I would like to observe how your infant plays with toys. You can help him if you like." Toys should be available, only some of which are developmentally appropriate. The most natural play interactions may occur with toys available in the home or with toys familiar to both parent and child. Ten to twenty minutes seems to be an ideal observation time (Comfort, 1988). After 10 minutes of observation, the parent should reach a comfort level with the therapist's presence and may become less aware that she is being observed. More than 20 minutes becomes an unreasonable length of time for the parent and child to engage in play. Observations of parent and child play for several minutes before or after therapy can provide a wealth of information, especially when observations occur in a number of different contexts.

Summary

The caregiving environment is assessed by observing the parent–child interactions and the child interacting within the home environment. Assessment of parent–child interaction is most appropriate when the relationship is at-risk, either due to parent variables (e.g., an adolescent, single mother) or child variables (e.g., a hyperresponsive, irritable child). The purpose of informal observations of the parent and child together is to understand the parenting style so that recommendations and suggested activities can be tailored to that style. Understanding how the parent and infant interact also assists the therapist to identify activities that both will enjoy and that will enhance their relationship.

Integrating Assessment Information

Therapists use their own mental images of the home, family activities, and parent–child interaction to design therapy for the child. Images of the child and family in a number of contexts heighten the therapist's awareness of what issues are important for both the infant and the family. They form the background for the direction and priorities of therapy and guide the activities and recommendations of the therapist. Although not always recorded as part of the formal evaluation, conversations with the parents about home life and experiences with their child do form the background and basis of the therapist's intervention. Since the therapist's actions and suggestions evolve from the complexity of this dynamic relationship between infant and family, additional information is continually needed. Parental feedback, in addition to child response, guides the direction and the content of therapy.

Early intervention assessment includes all the variables described in this chapter (i.e., aspects of the child's developmental function and information about the family's priorities); however, analysis of the variables that affect or reflect the child's development is not the equivalent of a comprehensive evaluation. Synthesis or integration of the variables is necessary. A synthesized assessment includes understanding the home environment and the family's daily routine, as well as assessment of the parent–child interaction and of the child and his environment.

The Parents' Role in Evaluation

The parent, as a team member, has a variety of roles in the assessment, to include being involved in the planning of the assessment process. Figure 4-2 provides a form that may be used to elicit the family's preferences in the planning process. The family may want standardized testing to be included. When possible, they should be given the option of an arena

1. Questions or concerns others have (e.g., babysitter, clinic, preschool) about my child:

2. Other places you can observe my child:

    Place: _____   Place: _____

    Contact person: _____   Contact person: _____

    What to observe: _____   What to observe: _____

3. I want others to see what my child does when:

4. I prefer the assessment take place:

    _____ at home   _____ at another location   _____ at the center

5. A time when my child is alert and when working parents can be present is:

    _____ morning   _____ afternoon   _____ early evening

6. People who I would like to be there other than parents and early intervention staff:

7. My child's favorite toys or activities to help her/him become focused, motivated, and comfortable:

8. During the assessment, I prefer to:

    ___ a. Sit beside my child
    ___ b. Help with activities to explore her/his abilities
    ___ c. Offer comfort and support to my child
    ___ d. Exchange ideas with the facilitator
    ___ e. Carry out activities to explore my child's abilities
    ___ f. Permit facilitator to handle and carry out activities
    ___ g. Other:

Figure 4-2 Preassessment planning: The setting (Project) [Reprinted from Kjerland L, Kovach J: Family-staff collaboration. In Gibbs ED, Tete DM: *Interdisciplinary assessment of infants*. Baltimore: Paul H. Brookes Publishing Co., 1990, p 292, reproduced with permission of the publisher.]

assessment and of individual discipline assessments. The parent may appreciate an opportunity for the entire team to observe the child together or may feel threatened in a group situation and know from experience that the child becomes overly stimulated or atypically inhibited in the presence of a group of adults. If the parents have a priority concern (e.g., that the child is not yet talking), it should be addressed first in the assessment process. While it is often appropriate to investigate all developmental domains and behaviors, the team needs to respond to the primary concerns of the parent.

The parents participate in all aspects of the assessment, although their roles differ according to the focus of the assessment. In addition to providing information about their family and their resources, concerns, and priorities, the parents provide information about the child that is not available through assessment, observation, or past records. Understanding of the child's temperament, personality, and social-emotional needs is best learned through the parents' experiences. They describe the child's likes, dislikes, fears, and pleasures to help the other team member successfully approach and interact with the child. When parents articulate their intimate knowledge of the child, the team members can integrate their understanding of the child from the perspective of a discipline into a whole.

The parents are also essential to the interpretation of the assessment data. Many teams meet without the parents to discuss the assessment results, particularly when medical or social concerns necessitate a preliminary discussion by the disciplines involved. While preliminary team discussions are appropriate at times, the team needs to recognize that planning of the program must include the parents. The team may individually establish concerns and priorities; however, these need to be presented to the parents in order to collaborate on goals and activities. The parents should offer a final interpretation of what is important and identify the priorities of their child's program. The effectiveness of the intervention program relies on team and parent collaboration throughout the evaluation and planning process.

References

Alexander, R. (1990). Language assessment. In E.D. Gibbs & D.M. Teti (Eds.), *Interdisciplinary assessment of infants: A guide for early intervention professionals* (pp. 77–89). Baltimore: Paul H. Brookes Publishing Co.

Als, H. (1986). A synactive model of neonatal behavioral organization. Framework for the assessment of neurobehavioral development in the premature infant and for support of infants and parents in the neonatal intensive care environment. *Physical and Occupational Therapy in Pediatrics,* 6(3/4), 3–54.

Anderson, P.P., & Fenichel, E.S. (1989). *Serving culturally diverse families of infants and toddlers with disabilities.* Washington, DC: National Center for Clinical Infant Programs.

Ayres, A.J. (1979). *Sensory integration and the child.* Los Angeles: Western Psychological Services.

Bagnato, S.J., & Hofkosh, D. (1990). Curriculum-based developmental assessment for infants with special needs: Synchronizing the pediatric early intervention team. In E.D. Gibbs & D.M. Teti (Eds.), *Interdisciplinary assessment of infants: A guide for early intervention professionals* (pp. 161–176). Baltimore: Paul H. Brookes Publishing Co.

Bagnato, S.J., & Mayes, S. (1986). Patterns of developmental and behavioral progress for young brain-injured children during interdisciplinary intervention. *Developmental Neuropsychology, 2,* 213–240.

Bagnato, S.J., & Murphy, J.P. (1989). Validity of curriculum-based scales with young neurodevelopmentally disabled children: Implications for team assessment. *Early Education and Development, 1*(1), 50–63.

Bagnato, S.J., & Neisworth, J.T. (1985). Efficacy of interdisciplinary assessment and treatment for infants and preschoolers with congenital and acquired brain injury. *Analysis and Intervention in Developmental Disabilities, 5,* 81–102.

Bailey, D.J. (1988). Assessing family stress and needs. In D.J. Bailey & R.J. Simeonsson (Eds.), *Family assessment in early intervention* (pp. 95–118). Columbus, OH: Charles E. Merrill.

Bailey, D.J., & Simeonsson, R. (1990). *The Family Needs Survey.* Chapel Hill: Frank Porter Graham Child Development Center, University of North Carolina.

Barnard, K.E., & Bee, H.L. (1984). The assessment of parent–infant interaction by observation of feeding and teaching. In T.B. Brazelton & B. Lester (Eds.), *New approaches to developmental screening in infants.* New York: Elsevier North Holland.

Bayley, N. (1969). *Bayley Scales of Infant Development.* New York: The Psychological Corporation.

Bee, H.L., Barnard, K.E., Eyres, S.J., Gray, C.A., Hammond, M.A., Spietz, A.L., Snyder, C., & Clark, B. (1982). Prediction of IQ and language skill from perinatal status, child performance, family characteristics, and mother–infant interaction. *Child Development, 53,* 1134–1156.

Bledsoe, N., & Shepherd, J. (1982). A study of reliability and validity of a preschool play scale. *American Journal of Occupational Therapy, 36,* 783–788.

Bly, L. (1983). *The components of normal movement during the first year of life and abnormal motor development.* Oak Park, IL: Neurodevelopmental Treatment Association, Inc.

Bromwich, R. (1981). *Working with parents and infants: An interactional approach.* Baltimore: University Park Press.

Bromwich, R. (1983). *Manual for the Parent Behavior Progression and Supplement.* (Available from Michael Moore, California State University, Northridge, CA 91330.)

Bushnell, E.W. (1985). The decline of visually guided reaching during infancy. *Infant Behavior and Development, 8,* 139–155.

Bzoch, K., & League, R. (1971). *Assessing language skills in infancy: A handbook for the multi-dimensional analysis of emergent language.* Baltimore: University Park Press.

Caldwell, B., & Bradley, R. (1978). *Home observation for measurement of the environment.* Little Rock: University of Arkansas.

Case-Smith, J. (1989). Reliability and validity of the Posture and Fine Motor Assessment of Infants. *Occupational Therapy Journal of Research, 9,* 259–272.

Case-Smith, J. (1991). *The posture and motor assessment of infants.* Rockville, MD: American Occupational Therapy Foundation.

Case-Smith, J. (1992). A validity study of the Posture and Fine Motor Assessment of Infants. *American Journal of Occupational Therapy, 46*(7), 597–606.

Chandler, L., Andrews, M., & Swanson, M. (1980). *The movement assessment of infants: A manual.* Rolling Bay, WA: Infant Movement Research.

Clarke-Stewart, K.A. (1973). Interaction among mothers and their young children: Characteristics and consequences. *Monographs of the Society for Research in Child Development, 38,* 153.

Comfort, M. (1988). Assessing parent–child interaction. In D.J. Bailey & R.J. Simeonsson (Eds.), *Family assessment in early intervention* (pp. 65–94). Columbus, OH: Charles E. Merrill.

Connor, F., Williamson, G., & Siepp, J.M., Eds. (1978). *Program guide for infants and toddlers with neuromotor and other developmental disabilities.* New York: Teachers College Press.

Dunst, C.J. (1980). *A clinical and educational manual for use with the Uzgiris and Hunt Scales of Infant Psychological Development.* Austin, TX: PRO-ED.

Dunst, C.J. (1984). Toward a social-ecological perspective of sensorimotor development among the mentally retarded. In P. Brooks, R. Sperber, & C. McCauley (Eds.), *Learning and cognition in the mentally retarded* (pp. 359–387). Hillsdale, NJ: Lawrence Erlbaum Associates.

Dunst, C.J., Holbert, K.A., & Wilson, L.L. (1990). Strategies for assessing infant sensorimotor interactive competencies. In E.D. Gibbs & D. M. Teti (Eds.), *Interdisciplinary assessment of infants: A guide for early intervention professionals* (pp. 91–112). Baltimore: Paul H. Brookes Publishing Co.

Dunst, C.J., Trivette, C., & Deal, A. (1988). *Enabling and empowering families: Principles and guidelines for practice.* Cambridge, MA: Brookline Books.

Erhardt, R.P. (1982). *The Erhardt Developmental Prehension Assessment (EDPA).* Tucson, AZ: Therapy Skill Builders.

Exner, C. (1989). Development of hand functions. In P. Pratt & A. Allen (Eds.), *Occupational Therapy for Children.* 2nd ed. St. Louis, MO: Mosby Company.

Exner, C. (1992). In-hand manipulation. In J.Case-Smith & C. Pehoski (Eds.), *Development of hand skills in children.* Rockville, MD: American Occupational Therapy Association.

Farber, S. (1982). *Neurorehabilitation: A multi-sensory approach.* Philadelphia: W.B. Saunders.

Farran, D.C., Kasari, C., Comfort, M., & Jay, S. (1986). *Parent/caregiver involvement scale.* Unpublished rating scale. (Available from Continuing Education, University of North Carolina, Greensboro, NC 27412.)

Fewell, R.R. (1985). *Play Assessment Scale.* 5th ed. Unpublished document. Seattle: University of Washington.

Foley, G.M. (1990). Portrait of the arena evaluation: Assessment in the transdisciplinary approach. In E.D. Gibbs & D.M. Teti (Eds.), *Interdisciplinary assessment of infants: A guide for early intervention professionals* (pp. 271–297). Baltimore: Paul H. Brookes Publishing Co.

Folio, M.R., & Fewell, R.R. (1983). *Peabody developmental motor scales and activity cards: A manual.* Allen, TX: DLM Teaching Resources.

Frankenburg, W.K., Fandal, A.W., Sciarillo, W., & Burgess, D. (1981). The Newly Abbreviated and Revised Denver Developmental Screening Test. *Journal of Pediatrics, 99,* 995–999.

Furuno, S., O'Reilly, K.A., Hosaka, C.M., Inatsuka, T.T., Allman, T.L., & Zeisloft, B. (1985). Hawaii Early Learning Profile. Palo Alto, CA: VORT Corporation.

Garland, C.W., & McGonigel, M.J. (1988). The individualized family service plan and the early intervention team: Team and family issues and recommended practices. *Infants and Young Children, 1*(1) 10–21.

Gesell, A. (1925). *The mental growth of the preschool child.* New York: Macmillan Publishing Co.

Gibbs, E.D. (1990). Assessment of infant mental ability: Conventional tests and issues of prediction. In E.D. Gibbs & D. M. Teti (Eds.), *Interdisciplinary assessment of infants: A guide for early intervention professionals* (pp. 77–89). Baltimore: Paul H. Brookes Publishing Co.

Gibbs, E.D., & Teti, D.M., Eds. (1990). *Interdisciplinary assessment of infants: A guide for early intervention professionals.* Baltimore: Paul H. Brookes Publishing Co.

Gilfoyle, E.M., Grady, A.P., & Moore, J.C. (1990). *Children adapt: A theory of sensorimotor development.* 2nd ed. Thorofare, NJ: Slack.

Glover, M.E., Preminger, J.L., & Sanford, A.R. (1978). *Early Learning Accomplishment Profile.* Winston-Salem, NC: Kaplan School Supply.

Hall, S. (1990). Observation of sensorimotor development. In T. Linder (Ed.), *Transdisciplinary play-based assessment: A functional approach to working with young children* (pp. 201–248). Baltimore: Paul H. Brookes Publishing Co.

Harris, S. (1981). Effects of neurodevelopmental therapy on motor performance of infants with Down's syndrome. *Developmental Medicine and Child Neurology, 23,* 477–481.

Harris, S. (1987). Early detection of cerebral palsy: Sensitivity and specificity of two motor assessment tools. *Journal of Perinatology, 7*(1), 11–15.

Hay, L. (1984). The development of movement control. *The Psychology of Human Movement.* New York: Academic Press.

Holstein, R.R. (1982). The development of prehension in normal infants. *American Journal of Occupational Therapy, 36,* 170–176.

Huntington, G.S. (1988). Assessing child characteristics that influence family functioning. In D.B. Bailey & R.J. Simeonsson (Eds.), *Family assessment in early intervention* (pp. 45–64). Columbus, OH: Charles E. Merrill.

Irwin, J.V., & Wong, S.P. (1974). Compensation for maturity in long-range intervention studies. *Acta Symbolica, 5*(4), 33–45.

Jirgal, D., & Bouma, K. (1989). A sensory integration observation guide. *Sensory Integration Special Interest Newsletter.* Rockville, MD: American Occupational Therapy Association.

Johnson-Martin, N., Jens, K., & Attermeier, S. (1986). *The Carolina Curriculum for Handicapped Infants and Infants at Risk.* Baltimore: Paul H. Brookes Publishing Co.

Kaufmann, R.K., & McGonigel, M.J. (1991). Identifying family concerns, priorities, and resources. In M.J. McGonigel, R.K. Kaufmann, & B.H. Johnson, (Eds.), *Guidelines and recommended practices for the Individualized Family Service Plan.* 2nd ed. Bethesda, MD: Association for the Care of Children's Health.

Knobloch, H., & Pasamanick, B. (1960). An evaluation of the consistency and predictive value of the fourth-week Gesell Developmental Schedule. In G. Shagass & B. Pasamanick (Eds.), *Child Development and Child Psychiatry, 13,* 10–31.

Knobloch, H., & Pasamanick, B. (1974). *Gesell and Amatruda's developmental diagnosis.* 3rd ed. New York: Harper & Row.

Knobloch, H., Stevens, F., & Malone, A. (1980). *Manual of developmental diagnosis.* Houston, TX: Developmental Evaluation Materials, Inc.

Knox, S. (1974). A play scale. In M. Reilly (Ed.), *Play as exploratory learning: Studies in curiosity behavior* (pp. 247–266). Beverly Hills: Sage Publications.

Linder, T.W. (1990). *Transdisciplinary play-based assessment: A functional approach to working with young children.* Baltimore: Paul H. Brookes Publishing Co.

McCune-Nicolich, L. (1980). *A manual for analyzing free play.* New Brunswick: Douglas College, Rutgers University.

McDonald, J., Gillette, Y., & Hutchinson, T. (1989). *ECO Scales Manual.* San Antonio, TX: Special Press, Inc.

Macoby, E.E., & Martin, J.A. (1983). Socialization in the context of the family: Parent–child interaction. In P.H. Mussen (Ed.), *Handbook of child psychology* (Vol. 4, pp. 1–101). New York: John Wiley & Sons.

Mahoney, G. (1985). *Maternal Behavior Rating Scale Manual.* (Available from UCONN Health Center, Pediatric Department, Farmington, CT 06032.)

Mahoney, G., Finger, I., & Powell, A. (1985). The relationship between maternal behavioral style to the development of organically impaired mentally retarded infants. *American Journal of Mental Deficiency, 90,* 266–302.

Milani-Comparetti, A., & Gidoni, E. (1967). Routine developmental examination in normal and retarded children. *Developmental Medicine and Child Neurology, 9,* 631–638.

Morris, S.E., & Klein, M. (1988). *Prefeeding skills.* Tucson, AZ: Therapy Skill Builders.

Newborg, J., Stock, J.R., Wnek, L., Guidubaldi, J., & Svinicki, J. (1984). *Battelle Developmental Inventory.* Allen, TX: DLM Teaching Resources.

Nursing Child Assessment Satellite Training (NCAST). (1978a). *Nursing Child Assessment Teaching Scale.* Seattle, WA: University of Washington.

Nursing Child Assessment Satellite Training (NCAST). (1978b). *Nursing Child Assessment Feeding Scale.* Seattle, WA: University of Washington.

Palmer, F.B., Shapiro, B.K., Wachtel, R.C., Allen, M.C., Heller, J.E., Harryman, S.E., Moslier, B.S., Meinert, C.L., & Capute, A.J. (1988). The effects of physical therapy on cerebral palsy. *New England Journal of Medicine, 318,* 803–808.

Palisano, R.J. (1986). Concurrent and predictive validities of the Bayley Motor Scale and the Peabody Developmental Motor Scales. *Physical Therapy, 66*(11), 1714–1719.

Rainforth, B., & Salisbury, C.L. (1988). Functional home programs: A model for therapists. *Topics in Early Childhood Special Education, 7*(4), 33–45.

Ramey, C.T., Farran, D.C., & Campbell, F.A. (1979). Predicting IQ from other-infant interactions. *Child Development, 50,* 804–814.

Schafer, D.S., & Moersch, M.S. (1981). *Developmental programming for infants and young children.* Ann Arbor: University of Michigan Press.

Scherzer, A.L., & Tscharnuter, I. (1992). *Early diagnosis and therapy in cerebral palsy: A primer on infant developmental problems.* New York: Marcel Dekker, Inc.

Simeonsson, R.J. (1988). Evaluating the effects of family focused intervention. In D.B. Bailey & R.J. Simeonsson (Eds.), *Family assessment in early intervention* (pp. 251–268). Columbus, OH: Charles E. Merrill.

Simeonsson, R.J., Bailey, D.B., Huntington, G.S., & Comfort, M. (1986). Testing the concept of goodness of fit in early intervention. *Infant Mental Health Journal, 7,* 81–94.

Simeonsson, R.J., Huntington, G.S., Short, R.J., & Ware, W.B. (1982). The Carolina record of individual behavior: Characteristics of handicapped infants and children. *Topics in Early Childhood Special Education, 2*(2), 43–55.

Stern, D. (1977). *The first relationship: Infant and mother.* Cambridge, MA: Harvard University Press.

Trembath, J. (1978). *The Milani-Comparetti Motor Development Screening Test.* Omaha: Meyer Children's Rehabilitation Institute, University of Nebraska Medical Center.

Tronick, E.Z., & Gianino, A. (1986). Interactive mismatch and repair: Challenges to the coping infant. *Zero to Three, 6*(3), 1–6.

Turnbull, A.P., & Turnbull, H.R. (1991). *Families, professionals, and exceptionalities: A special partnership.* 2nd ed. Columbus, OH: Charles E. Merrill.

Uzgiris, I. (1983). Organization and sensorimotor intelligence. In M. Lewis (Ed.), *Origins of intelligence.* 2nd ed. (pp. 135–189). New York: Plenum Press.

Uzgiris, I., & Hunt, J.Mc V. (1975). *Assessment in infancy.* Urbana: University of Illinois Press.

Warren, S., & Kaiser, A. (1988). Research in early language intervention. *Early intervention for infants and children with handicaps.* Baltimore: Paul H. Brookes Publishing Co.

Wayman, K.I., Lynch, E.W., & Hanson, M.J. (1990). Home-based early childhood services: Cultural sensitivity in a family systems approach. *Topics in Early Childhood Special Education, 4,* 56–75.

White, B., Castle, P., & Held, R. (1964). Observations on the development of visually directed reaching. *Child Development, 35,* 349–364.

Williamson, G.G., & Zeitlin, S. (1990). Assessment of coping and temperament: Contributions to adaptive functioning. In E.D. Gibbs & D.M. Teti (Eds.), *Interdisciplinary assessment of infants: A guide for early intervention professionals* (pp. 215–226). Baltimore: Paul H. Brookes Publishing Co.

Woodruff, G., & McGonigel, M.J. (1988). Early intervention team approaches: The transdisciplinary model. In J.B. Jordan, J.J. Gallagher, P.L. Hutinger, & M.B. Karnes (Eds.), *Early childhood special education: Birth to three.* Reston, VA: Council for Exceptional Children, Division for Early Childhood.

Yarrow, L., Rubenstein, J., Pedersen, F., & Jankowski, J. (1972). Dimensions of early stimulation and their differential effect in infant development. *Merrill-Palmer Quarter, 18,* 205–218.

Zeitlin, S., Williamson, G.G., & Szczepanski, M. (1988). *Early Coping Inventory.* Bensenville, IL: Scholastic Testing Service.

5

Models of Service Delivery and Team Interaction

Jane Case-Smith, EdD, OTR
Barbara Burris Wavrek, MHS, OTR

Services to infants, young children, and their families are provided through both hospital programs and community-based programs. These programs have significant differences and considerable variety in their structures, organizations, funding sources, and purposes. However, although there are significant, intrinsic differences between models of service delivery in hospitals and in community-based programs, both are concerned with the provision of high-quality services responsive to the needs of children and their families. Hospital programs and community programs may be considered complementary in the provision of a continuum of early intervention services, with each offering a unique and important contribution.

Community programs include public and private agencies, outpatient clinics, schools, and private practices. The programs that receive state and federal funding must comply with the state and federal regulations and policies for early intervention legislation. Hospital services are most often provided in pediatric hospitals, in general hospitals, or in rehabilitation facilities that have inpatient units for children. Privately funded agencies and medical facilities follow internally developed policies and meet standards established by private accrediting agencies, such as the Joint Commission for the Accreditation of Healthcare Organizations (JCAHO) or the Commission for the Accreditation of Rehabilitation Facilities (CARF). In response to current legislation and accepted best practice, both community-based early intervention programs and pediatric medical facilities provide family-centered services.

Hospitals are structured to meet the immediate or long-term health care needs of children and their families. Community-based programs are structured to meet the social, educational, and developmental needs of children and their families, with medical considerations being a secondary issue. When a child's medical needs take precedence, hospitalization for short or prolonged periods of time becomes necessary. During hospitalization, the child's and family's social and developmental needs are also considered important; however, the emphasis on service provision shifts to meeting these needs within the context of the child's total medical care. A family with a child who has a newly diagnosed medical condition may be exposed to the concept of and need for early intervention for the first time in the hospital setting. A child with a chronic medical problem may, over a period of time, receive both hospital- and community-based early intervention services, depending on changes in his health status. Enabling smooth, effective transitions of the child and family between hospital programs and community-based programs becomes a challenge for both the family and the professionals involved.

The focus of this chapter is to explore the characteristics of hospital programs and community-based programs, to describe team functions and models of service delivery in these settings, to describe the role of occupational therapy in these settings, and to depict a model of collaboration between hospital programs and community programs for infants, young children, and their families.

Hospital-Based Programs

A hospital is ". . . an institution providing medical, surgical, or psychiatric testing and treatment for people who are ill, injured, pregnant . . . on an inpatient, outpatient or emergency care basis: often involved with public health programs, research, medical education. . . ." (*Webster's New World Dictionary of American English*, 1989). Hospitals, major components of the health care delivery system, may be private, nonprofit facilities or may be for-profit facilities, which are part of a larger organization or multihospital system (Levy, 1988). Private, nonprofit hospitals may also choose to affiliate with similar institutions for exchange of information, program development, and achievement of common goals. Multihospital systems enable coordination of services, consolidation of services, and maintenance of financial viability (Levy, 1988).

Children may be served in either general hospitals, where individuals of all ages and with various diagnoses are served, or in facilities dedicated solely to the evaluation and treatment of children. Hospitalization may be required for acute problems or for periodic care of chronic problems. The type of facility and length of hospital stay influences the services the child receives and the type of occupational therapy services that are provided. During an acute hospital stay, for example, occupational therapy emphasis may be placed on assessment, program planning, and recommendations rather than ongoing treatment. Some children who are hospitalized for prolonged periods of time receive daily occupational therapy intervention.

The type of facility also affects services available to children and their families. Children hospitalized in pediatric facilities have access to a broad range of professionals in various specialties who have had experience in treating complex medical problems. Occupational therapy services tend to be highly specialized in a pediatric facility and well developed in specialty areas (e.g., neonatal care, upper extremity anomalies, and burns). In addition, the hospital stay tends to be longer in a pediatric facility, perhaps enabling more in-depth intervention than would be possible in a general hospital.

Another factor affecting services to children is the geographic region served by the hospital. Pediatric hospitals tend to serve broad geographic regions and are usually equipped to diagnose and treat conditions that require the expertise of pediatric specialists or that are life-threatening. Unfortunately, a facility of this type may be located quite a distance from the child's home, complicating the issue of hospitalization for families and creating additional stress due to frequent visitations. The child who is hospitalized a significant distance from home is not only separated from his familiar environment, belongings, and friends, but may also be separated from one or both parents and other family members. The parents may feel torn between staying with the hospitalized child and caring for other children at home. Hospital personnel, such as chaplains or social workers, may be called upon to provide support for parents who are too far from home to receive support from family members and friends.

Community-Based Programs

Community-based early intervention programs represent a wide continuum of services that offer a variety of resources to young children and their families. Early intervention programs may focus on the parent (e.g., mental health agencies) or on the child (e.g., day-care centers, rehabilitation centers). Some agencies have programs for both the child and family (e.g., early education programs, public health departments). The missions of these agencies differ, based on their primary funding source, the administrative body, and the communities that they serve. The types and numbers of programs that are available vary according to the community's resources. Programs tend to reflect the size and composition of the community. In general, programs are more available and accessible in urban areas versus rural areas.

Often the state agencies who funnel state and federal dollars to local programs determine the structure, the organization, and the size of community programs. Each state has a lead agency for administering Part H of PL

99-457, the early intervention legislation (e.g., Department of Health, Department of Education, or Department of Human Services). As a result, early intervention programs may be housed in education settings, public health departments, mental retardation/developmental disabilities agencies, or others. Such wide disparities in administrative bodies and organizations result in programs with very different staffing structures and organizations. For example, early intervention programs in the public health departments may have nurses as service coordinators and those housed in education settings may have special education instructors as service coordinators. The role of the occupational therapist changes according to these differing missions and organizational structures. Although education programs focus more on classroom instruction, private clinics and rehabilitation centers that serve young children tend to emphasize therapy services. This difference in emphasis is influenced by the types of children who attend the programs and the funding sources that are received, as therapies are reimbursed by medical insurance and Medicaid, and special education is not. Privately funded programs that depend on third party reimbursement tend to offer more direct therapy services than publicly funded programs.

Children must be medically stable in order to attend community programs. When primary health issues are not the family's major concern, the child and family can focus on functional and developmental issues. Once the infant is discharged from the neonatal intensive care unit (NICU), the infant's growth and development usually accelerate and the parents gradually become more comfortable in play interaction and less intimidated about handling. The priorities of community programs also shift from those of the hospital setting. Healthy children, who have more energy to play and more interest in interaction than children with serious medical problems, need active and dynamic treatment approaches (e.g., that emphasize sensorimotor skills) rather than passive treatment modalities (e.g., positioning, splinting). The focus of therapy is on the infant's ability to function and interact and to support the family in the promotion of optimal infant development within the family context. As a result, community programs develop services to support families, to meet their education needs, and to assist in community integration. For example, certain community programs establish services such as parenting classes and support groups for parents who have special needs (e.g., developmental disabilities).

In addition to having different missions, community agencies are usually smaller than hospitals and tend to serve fewer numbers of children and families. The family is involved with a community early intervention team for a relatively long time period (e.g., 2 to 3 years) compared to the length of time they are involved with the hospital team (e.g., several months) (Gilkerson, 1990). When families participate in community programs for extended periods of time, they generally form relationships and bonds with the professionals serving their child. Relationships and friendships between professionals and parents are facilitated in a relaxed and informal atmosphere, which is more likely to occur in a small community program than in an institutional setting. Although the parents are typically appreciative of the medical professionals who helped their child through the medical crisis, they are often more capable of forming relationships with professionals when the acute medical crisis has passed. For these reasons, community teams that provide long-term care may have more opportunities to form collaborative relationships with families than hospital-based teams.

Intervention is made available for all of the subsystems of the family in community settings; therefore, the family is served as a whole. This broader focus of intervention may include programs for siblings as well as ongoing programs for parents. In addition, a broader scope of resources are used to meet the needs of the infant and family. Programs may offer social supports through parent-to-parent networks or through respite care, using persons who are trained in caring for children with special needs. Play groups may include parents and siblings, as well as children with special needs. In order to help the family identify and access comprehensive resources, community programs link together through interagency collaborative efforts. Interagency collaboration is the hallmark of comprehensive services for families. Collaboration between agencies includes sharing of referrals and information, and planning together with the family. Occupational therapists and all the team members are responsible for helping families make these linkages. Later in this chapter a model for collaboration between medical- and community-based programs is presented.

Early Intervention Teams

In both medical and educational settings, professionals work together as a team to meet the needs of their clients. A *team* is an organized body of individuals that share goals and interests. Usually a team has a leader, although often in early intervention programs, the leadership of the team changes according to the identified needs of the client (e.g., the occupational therapist may be the team leader for a child with sensory integration dysfunction). The team leader is also determined by the composition of members (e.g., does the team include a physician or an administrator?) and the nature of the task (e.g., planning intervention with a family or revising the preschool curriculum). Furthermore, the structure of the team is highly dependent on the nature of the organization. In medical-based teams, the leader is most often a physician. The physician may be the team leader in name only, while true leadership is shared among several team members. This biomedical model is a linear team organization, with the physician directing the child's intervention and the other disciplines responding to this direction (McClellan, 1991). In community programs, the service coordinator or teacher may be the team leader. Educational programs tend to use a biosocial model, which is best depicted by a circle reflecting that all disciplines contribute to the planning and decision making. The parent becomes a team member in addition to being the recipient of care. While some authors have suggested that parents can lead the team, this rarely occurs in practice unless the parent is knowledgeable and comfortable with the system.

Importance of Communication

Because communication and collaboration are essential to the provision of early intervention services, it is important for the team to have formal lines of communication. Methods for sharing information include team meetings, collaborative intervention sessions, written evaluations, and progress notes. The need for collaboration and a working system of communication within the early intervention team is influenced by the following variables:

1. The early intervention team is likely to be the family's first experience in the arenas of health care, social services, and special education. This team prepares the family's entry into the system of services for children with developmental disabilities.
2. The parents are unfamiliar with the technical language used by professionals, as well as the rules of the system.
3. Since the parents lack knowledge as to how the team functions, they have difficulty in becoming team members. Learning the team's rules and the system's organization requires time and experience.

Shared Meaning

The most important outcome of the communication system created by the early intervention team is that professionals and family members develop shared meanings about the child and her needs and strengths. For example, when the child is given a definitive diagnosis, such as cerebral palsy, the meaning of the diagnosis varies among team and family members. To the occupational therapist, the diagnosis of cerebral palsy implies specific therapeutic approaches and techniques, and a focus for intervention. To other professionals, cerebral palsy means that certain educational and medical problems can be anticipated. To the parents, the diagnosis of cerebral palsy often has a social meaning and the disability becomes defined in its social context.

Parents are concerned with the effects that the illness will have on interpersonal relationships; for example, how it will affect family members and how it will affect their child's peer relationships. Parents are also concerned about the child's developmental function, her success in school, and her ability to fit into the community. These overriding concerns may be more important than the developmental steps that are often the focus of the therapists.

Communication between the parents and the therapists helps clarify how the therapist's goals match the parents' concerns and facilitate the best outcomes for the child. Even when professionals and parents have the same goals for the child; the meaning of those goals and the approach for reaching them may differ.

Common Language

Mcanings differ because parents and professionals speak different languages. During team meetings with the parent, professionals typically communicate at two different levels, one technical and one nontechnical. The use of specific medical terminology, while helpful to the physician, can be baffling to the parent. Translation of technical terms for the parents should be complete and should be offered without intimidating the parents. Although continual translation of terms can be both a challenge and a source of stress to the occupational therapist, at the same time, it helps the parents understand the intervention and builds their trust in the team.

Parents are most likely to reinforce intervention suggestions when team members explain them in sufficient depth, reinforce each other's suggestions, welcome parents' feedback, and incorporate the parents' ideas into a suggested activity. Such collaboration requires time and willingness to negotiate in order to develop a shared meaning of what is best for the child.

Characteristics of Collaborative Teams

Teams that have a high level of communication and who have the support of the organization to develop collaborative programs for children and families are likely to have the following characteristics:

1. The team membership is stable over time and the members develop relationships that include appreciation of each other's skills.
2. The team members share a common philosophy and express common values.
3. The team as a whole is supported by the organization's administration. This includes being granted the time to meet as a team as well as having the opportunity to train together. Ideally, the team has the privilege of meeting for reasons other than client care.

4. The administration does not place team members in a position of competition. Collaboration is fostered and reinforced.
5. Members perceive each other as similar in status and power (Bailey, 1984).

Team Development

Teams change and evolve over time. When teams remain intact by maintaining the same members, they generally become more cohesive and begin to work together as a whole. Healthy and cohesive teams have the opportunity to spend time together and have frequent and open communication (Spencer, 1986). The opportunities for communication may be few in high-pressure, fast-paced settings. Poor communication or lack of interaction almost always affects team cohesion and interactions within the family. While agreement and harmony among team members is not necessary in working with families, frequent, open communication *is* essential to best practice. Teams that offer integrated and coherent services to families have probably evolved through a developmental process. In the developmental process, the team devotes time and energy to learning about each other, to communicating their values and goals, and to building consensus with families regarding goals, plans, and service delivery (Blechert, Christansen, & Kari, 1987). Development of a cohesive team requires a commitment from individual members to the team as a whole. When members acknowledge that the whole is greater than the sum of the parts, they become motivated to move toward open communication and shared roles.

One aspect of the team that is essential to its development is stability of the team's membership (Bailey, 1984; Golin & Duncanis, 1981). Team composition often changes because a number of consultants move in and out of the team structure. Frequently, the occupational therapist is contracted as a consultant. The administration may not contract for the therapist's time to attend team meetings, particularly those related to team process. Without the opportunity to become part of the team building process, members do not achieve cohesive team function. In hospital programs and large community programs, the therapist may serve on a number of teams comprised of a mix of disciplines within the agency. While multiple teams may be necessary in large agencies that serve hundreds of families, administrators should appreciate the value of enabling core teams to work together.

Another potential reason for team membership instability is staff turnover. Research indicates that turnover of early intervention personnel, particularly therapists, is high (Yoder, Coleman, & Gallagher, 1991). Every time a new member is introduced into the team, a new cycle of team development is initiated. When team members are reshuffled for administrative reasons, the team begins a rebuilding process.

The growth of an early intervention team must be nurtured and nourished. Team collaboration is fostered with administrative support for team process time, opportunities for team training, and reasonable caseloads. Teams that have stable memberships have opportunities to build relationships that can include the family. Team stability should be valued as an important factor in the interdisciplinary collaboration that supports and empowers families. The following sections discuss team interaction in hospital and community settings.

Team Interaction Models

Teams are generally organized into multidisciplinary, interdisciplinary, and transdisciplinary models. These models have been widely described in the literature (Fewell, 1983; Golin & Duncanis, 1981; Lyon & Lyon, 1980; McCollum & Hughes, 1988; McCormick & Goldman, 1979). In reality, teams move from model to model and often function as a hybrid of the models defined in Table 5-1. A team may function using a transdisciplinary model when the child has mild delays in only one domain and using an interdisciplinary model when the child's delays cross several behavioral domains. Table 5-1 describes the differences among these models.

Multidisciplinary Medical Teams

A child and family enter a medical system, such as a hospital, in order to identify a disability or dysfunction or to follow-up the diagnosis. The purpose of hospitalization is to define strategies for restoring health and function. Care is provided by various health care professionals under the direction of a physician who specifies the services (i.e., occupational therapy) to be involved (Stephens, 1989). Communication among the disciplines involved in child care tends to be informal and may best be described as a multidisciplinary model of interaction (Fewell, 1983).

The medical team within the hospital tends to organize care around the individual as a patient, rather than using a systems approach that includes the family and the community in child care. The emphasis is on hospital personnel within the institution providing all the needed services (Gilkerson, Gorski, & Panitz, 1990).

The primary physician is usually perceived as the leader of the medical team and the manager of services for the child, determining the evaluation and intervention services needed and outcomes desired prior to the child's

Table 5-1 Project Trans/Team—Three Models for Team Interaction in Early Intervention

Component	Multidisciplinary	Interdisciplinary	Transdisciplinary
Philosophy of team interaction	• Team members recognize the importance of contributions from several disciplines.	• Team members are willing and able to share responsibility for services among disciplines.	• Team members commit to teaching, learning, & working across disciplinary boundaries to plan & provide integrated services.
Family role	• Generally, families meet with team members separately by discipline.	• Families meet with the team or team representative and have varying roles on the team.	• Families are full team members with primary decision-making authority—the team captain if so desired.
Lines of communication	• Lines of communication are typically informal. Members may not think of themselves as part of a team.	• The team meets regularly for case conferences, consultations, etc.	• The team meets regularly to share information and to teach and learn across disciplines, as well as for case conferences, consultation, team building, etc.

Staff development	• Staff development generally is independent and within individual disciplines.	• Staff development is frequently shared and held across disciplines.	• Shared staff development across disciplines is critical to team development and role release.
Assessment process	• Team members conduct separate assessments by disciplines.	• Team members conduct separate assessments by discipline, but share results.	• Staff and family participate in an arena assessment, observing and recording across disciplines.
Service plan development	• Team members develop separate plans for intervention within their own disciplines.	• Goals are developed by disciplines, but are shared with the rest of the team to form one service plan.	• Staff and family develop plan all together, based on family needs, resources, priorities, and values.
Service plan implementation	• Team members implement their plan separately by discipline.	• Team members implement parts of the plan for which their disciplines are responsible.	• Team members share responsibility & are accountable for how the plan is implemented by one person.

Source: Child Development Resources, Project Trans/Team Outreach: *The transdisciplinary model of service delivery.* 1990, reprinted with permission.

discharge. The physician's decisions are, however, influenced by the input of the various professionals involved (Gilkerson, Gorski, & Panitz, 1990). The physician first determines who participates on the child's team and then the general purpose of their participation, based on the observed needs of the child and family. For example, a 6-month-old infant is hospitalized for poor weight gain, refusal to eat, and obvious distress experienced at and following mealtimes. The nurse caring for the child encounters the same difficulties in feeding the child. The child's primary physician orders the necessary medical tests to evaluate for gastroesophageal reflux, consults occupational therapy for an oral-motor and feeding evaluation, consults a clinical dietician to determine an appropriate diet and monitor weight gain, and consults the clinical social worker for evaluation of family and parent–child dynamics. The occupational therapist determines that the infant's oral-motor and feeding skills are age-appropriate and notes the infant's behavioral responses to feeding. The dietitian discovers that the family has provided an appropriate and adequate diet for the child. In addition, the social worker notes that although the child's difficulties are causing both parents to experience anxiety, the parents are concerned about the child and interact with the child in a highly positive and appropriate manner.

The medical diagnostic tests indicate that the child is experiencing significant reflux, which is causing serious discomfort and interfering with the feeding experience. As a result, the physician (1) synthesizes the information from the different professionals and tests, (2) provides the necessary intervention in the form of medication to alleviate the child's reflux, (3) requests that the occupational therapist teach the parents ways to position the child after feeding to minimize reflux, (4) schedules follow-up appointments in his office, and (5) discharges the child and family from the hospital. The intervention provided is specific to the child's medical problem and involves providing the parents with direction and recommendations to alleviate the medical condition. This directive approach results in efficient resolution of the identified problem.

Under the medical model, the team consists of a physician, a nurse, and persons from other health care disciplines, depending on the child's and family's needs. Consequently, the team members and their specialties vary as the child's needs are identified and as those needs change. For example, an infant with a single, teenage parent may be admitted to the hospital for failure-to-thrive and may initially be given a medical diagnostic test to evaluate whether a physiological cause exists. If a physiological cause for the failure to gain weight is eliminated, psychosocial variables in the family are then explored as possible factors. Lack of positive parent–child interaction or a highly stressful family situation can necessitate the involvement of the clinical social worker. Simultaneously, delays in the child's development, low muscle tone, depressed interactive skills, poor exploratory or play skills, and questionable feeding problems can lead to a referral to the occupational therapist. By contrast, a child hospitalized for a lower extremity fracture may have the physician, nurse, and physical therapist as members of his medical team.

A multidisciplinary hospital-based team is influenced by the changing team composition, the level of commitment of the physician to use a team approach, the availability of staff to participate in team activities, and the initiative of the professionals involved (Bailey, 1984; Golin & Duncanis, 1981). The changing composition of the team affects the relationships of the team members and overall team cohesion. Individual disciplines may function separately, communicating with each other informally or through documentation in the hospital chart. The level of the physician's commitment to a team approach determines which disciplines are consulted during the child's hospitalization, as well as how and to whom information about the child is communicated.

The availability of team members and the initiative of those members also affects how the team functions. Fluctuations in caseload, staff absences, and shortages affect the availability of health care personnel to provide services or to participate in care conferences, family conferences, or other patient-related meetings. These problems particularly affect team function when lines of communication are informal and depend on the initiative of the individual. When time pressures and staff shortages limit participation in team-related activities, the ability of the health professionals to develop and to function as a team is severely hampered. In multidisciplinary teams, individual initiative in seeking out team members—to discuss issues of common importance, to ask questions, and to participate in planning—is critically important to team functioning. Despite the various influences that can limit the teamwork of health professionals in the hospital, those who are committed to providing quality services do develop positive relationships with colleagues, patients, and families.

A cohesive hospital team is most likely to develop when the program is highly defined, the need for specific disciplines is clearly delineated, and the members of the team remain constant. Acute, inpatient rehabilitation programs are one example where teams tend to be highly developed and cohesive. Inpatient rehabilitation programs, which follow CARF guidelines, have clearly defined admission and discharge criteria, well delineated program components, a program evaluation mechanism, and an identified need for the involvement of various disciplines. Usually, the physician in the rehabilitation program is knowledgeable about the roles of the different disciplines and is committed to a team approach. An interdisciplinary model of interaction is followed (Fewell, 1983; McCormick & Goldman, 1979). Team members work together toward mutually agreed-upon functional outcomes for their clients. Family conferences, team meetings, and team projects foster interaction and communication among team members. All members of the team participate in program planning, parent and patient instruction, and discharge planning. In addition, each patient has a case manager or patient program manager who facilitates coordination of services and communication among team members. One model, which rotates this responsibility among team members, also helps establish equality within the team and contributes to team development. Under this interdisciplinary model, the occupational therapist, the physical therapist, the speech pathologist, and other team members may each have the opportunity to become a program manager for a given child during the child's hospital stay.

In a hospital, parent participation on the child's medical team does not usually occur, although the parent may develop close relationships with the individual health care professionals who are involved with the child. The relationship between the physician, other health care professionals, and the parents tends to be asymmetrical, with the health care professionals, especially the physician, assuming responsibility for the direction of the child's care (Gilkerson, Gorski, & Panitz, 1990). Several factors contribute to this asymmetry. The physician, by nature of his specialized knowledge and training, is perceived by the parents as the expert who has access to the necessary resources to diagnose and treat the child's illness or disability. The parent may be willing to defer to the physician or other health care personnel because of their expertise and professional prestige (Gilkerson, Gorski, & Panitz, 1990).

Other factors that may affect parent participation are the stress induced by the child's illness/disability and hospitalization, external demands on the parent, and the logistics of convening meetings with the parents and the professionals involved. Families of children newly diagnosed with an illness or disability may find it difficult to understand or to accept their child's condition. In addition, families are often not prepared for hospitalization and for the uncertainty of the child's outcome (Affleck & Tennen, 1991). They may also be struggling to care for children at home while attending to the needs of the hospitalized child, and may be unavailable to participate in team discussions or planning. As a result, parents often rely on individual relationships with the various health care professionals to make decisions and plans, and use informal lines of communication to meet their need for information.

In summary, it is apparent that the medical team's structure, cohesion, and development may be affected by various factors in the hospital. These factors include the type of hospital unit and program, the acuity of the patient's health problem, and the commitment of the physician and other health professionals to a team approach. Team dynamics and interaction (i.e., multidisciplinary or interdisciplinary models) are also determined by these factors.

Interdisciplinary Community-Based Teams

The interdisciplinary model is used in many community programs, particularly in agencies that have primarily occupational, physical, and speech therapists (e.g., out-patient clinics or rehabilitation centers). In this model, the occupational therapist and other team members perform separate evaluations and then develop goals based on the assessment results. These goals are discussed among the team members and with the parents and a coordinated program is developed. When appropriate, the child and family receive direct occupational therapy services. Simultaneously, the occupational therapist provides consultation to the other professionals who work with the child. The advantage of the interdisciplinary approach is that the child and family receive coordinated direct care and instruction from a number of individuals with expertise in different areas (Fewell, 1983; McGonigel & Garland, 1988). This approach works particularly well when common goals have been agreed upon and the professionals collaborate on the strategies to be used. Formal lines of communication (e.g., through regular team meetings) provide opportunities to discuss the family's changes in priorities or circumstances, so that the team members give ongoing consideration to the family's wishes (Peterson, 1987). This approach seems to be particularly helpful when the child and family have a number of diverse needs (e.g., when the mother has a history of drug abuse, when the child has multiple disabilities) or when the family desires such an approach. Effective implementation of this model includes changing the team members that have direct contact with the child and family as their needs change. For example, a child with Down syndrome may first be seen by the occupational therapist to encourage the child's early motor and play skills. When the child begins speech therapy at 12 months of age for more emphasis on communication skills, occupational therapy may be discontinued. Occupational therapy may begin again at 24 months of age to encourage preschool play skills and self-care skills. During these first 24 months, the child may have received ongoing physical therapy for activities to improve posture and gross motor skills.

Interdisciplinary models in which the occupational therapist provides consultation and direct services to the child and family are most likely to meet their evolving needs. A young child who was exposed to cocaine in utero may benefit from sensory integration procedures in the first several months of life. As the infant demonstrates increased adaptation to the environment and is able to initiate and maintain interactions, direct occupational therapy may discontinue and the therapist instead provides consultation regarding oral-motor and feeding issues. The therapist assists the team in identifying which model is most appropriate for each infant and family. The family's preferences for direct or indirect therapy services are respected. Family-centered services are flexible regarding the role of team members throughout the course of intervention. A flexible model works best when the team members have opportunities for both informal and formal communication. Meetings with the family result in group decisions about plans and revisions to plans. Informal communication allows members to share experiences, successes, and disappointments when they are not at formal meetings, which promotes continuity and consistency in the intervention program.

Transdisciplinary Community-Based Teams

The transdisciplinary approach is based on the assumption that coherence is promoted when the family primarily interacts with one professional (Lyon & Lyon, 1980; McGonigel & Garland, 1988). The approach allows the family to develop a relationship with one individual, as well as increase their comfort with and decrease their confusion about the early intervention program (Woodruff & McGonigel, 1988). The transdisciplinary approach is appropriate for the infant who is medically fragile and does not tolerate multiple sources of stimulation. It is also a selected choice when problems in parent–child interaction have been identified. In this model, all team members assess the child, usually together in an arena assessment (United Cerebral Palsy National Collaborative Infant Project, 1976). Then, the team, which includes the family, assembles to plan the intervention services. One primary service provider is designated to implement the plan with the family. At this point, the roles of the other team members are to monitor progress either through the observation of primary service providers or through a hands-on reassessment (Maple, 1987; Woodruff & McGonigel, 1988).

In the transdisciplinary approach, all team members commit to teaching, learning, and working across disciplinary boundaries (Peterson, 1987). They share the information and the skills that meet the child's needs from the perspective of their discipline skills. After the team develops the plan, one or two persons become responsible for carrying out the recommendations and activities. The primary interventionist and the parents learn to recognize when the expertise of the occupational therapist or of another discipline is needed. Therefore, this model requires that team members are well versed in the skills and resources of the other disciplines on the team (McGonigel & Garland, 1988; Woodruff & McGonigel, 1988).

The transdisciplinary approach involves a process called role release (Foley, 1990; Lyon & Lyon, 1980; Woodruff & McGonigel, 1988). In this process, the occupational therapist's role is taught to the primary interventionist. Sufficient explanation and details are needed so that the strategies can be effectively implemented. The occupational therapist acknowledges the skills of the primary interventionist by providing strategies that can be realistically applied. She recognizes when techniques should be modified in order to be applied correctly. At times, prior to application in the home, recommendations for handling the infant are modeled and then practiced with the therapist. Successful role release occurs after the occupational therapist has had the opportunity to teach the methods on several different occasions with children who present different needs and adaptations. Role release also involves skills in consultation, which are discussed later in this chapter.

Although, the occupational therapist sometimes serves as a consultant to the instructor based on the family's and team's discretion, she may assume the role of primary interventionist, which results in her taking on the roles of the other disciplines. Activities designed by speech and physical therapists become part of the occupational therapist's intervention. This role exchange or expansion requires the therapist to learn to skillfully implement language and physical therapy techniques and to make the transition from a focus on occupational therapy to a global, holistic approach in order to meet the needs of the child and family. When assuming primary responsibility for the intervention, the occupational therapist needs a heightened awareness of when advice and consultation from other disciplines is needed. As the team matures and members become more comfortable implementing a transdisciplinary approach, roles become more blended and the skills of the professionals cross discipline lines (Woodruff & McGonigel, 1988). The transdisciplinary approach was never intended to promote the development of a team in which each discipline member has the same skills or in which one discipline can be exchanged for another. Nor does the approach imply that the primary interventionist provides all of the resources needed by the child and family. Rather, the sharing of knowledge and skills related to the child's and family's individual needs is continual and frequent. Regular opportunities for sharing among the team members are needed so that joint problem solving and consultation characterize each family's intervention program.

The intention of the transdisciplinary process is for individual members to add to their own expertise by incorporating the information and skills offered by the other members of the team into their discipline repertoires (United Cerebral Palsy National Collaborative Infant Project, 1976). The transdisciplinary process does not mean that the hands-on skills of the therapists can be implemented by any other team member. For children with cerebral palsy who benefit from hands-on sessions and from demonstrations for the parents, the occupational or physical therapist may be the lead interventionist. The team recognizes when hands-on skills are important and when occupational therapy services are needed as an adjunct to the primary intervention role versus when the occupational therapist should become the primary interventionist. Often children with cognitive delays have the special educator as their primary interventionist. However, the occupational therapist consults on issues such as self-feeding delays or delays in prewriting and manipulation skills. The transdisciplinary approach is frequently used when the child and family receive services in the home. The use of numerous professionals is not cost effective for the early intervention program, due to travel expenses, and the amount of time required of the professionals.

The therapist uses a process of clinical reasoning to continually formulate and adapt treatment strategies that are responsive to the child and family (Fleming, 1991; Shaaf & Mulrooney, 1989). In the clinical reasoning process, the therapist synthesizes experiences with the child into a fluid and dynamic treatment process. Clinical reasoning, as defined by Schoen (1987) and Mattingly (1991), is based on ongoing, direct experiences with families and infants. The transdisciplinary approach, which relies only on consultation by specialists, poses difficulties in the implementation of the clinical reasoning process when therapy recommendations are based on pieces of the whole rather than on a comprehensive picture. It is often difficult to individualize recommendations when the problem is verbalized by another professional rather than experienced by the therapist. Therefore, the transdisciplinary approach should be implemented carefully with complete recognition of when an alternative model of intervention is appropriate (Woodruff & McGonigel, 1988). Whether the occupational therapist has multiple opportunities to observe the child, or whether she bases recommendations on a single evaluation, she must be highly skilled in analyzing the child's developmental function and synthesizing the family and home situation given a limited amount of information.

Models of Service Delivery

Center-Based Services

Center-based services in hospital or community-based programs follow numerous rules that are instituted by the administration or are agreed upon by the team members. These rules include where evaluations and therapy occur, when they occur, and all of the processes required for the family to enter the system. Rules may be written—for example, assessments and planning are scheduled on Wednesdays—or may be unwritten—the social worker is always the last to arrive to the meeting. The family is unfamiliar with these unwritten rules and norms and, therefore, is naturally uncomfortable with the clinical environment. The parents learn the rules over time when they regularly attend the program, yet they always have an incomplete picture of the program's rules and policies because they are outsiders to the system. When the rules change frequently, adjusting to the program is more difficult. Both the parents and the child seem to feel most comfortable when they come to the center regularly and the rules remain unchanged with time. The familiarity of surroundings, the specific interests of each of the professionals, the variety of activities, and the logistics of time and place are all factors in the parents' adjustment to the program.

The advantages of center-based programs for families are often the social opportunities. The family members meet other parents and observe other children who are in similar situations. Such opportunities provide a perspective of other children's problems and increase the family's understanding of developmental disabilities. Friendships and interactions with other parents can provide emotional support and helpful information. Parents have explained the advantages of informally discussing their children with the other families that they meet in the clinic or in preschool. Naturally occurring, informal conversations can mean more to parents and be of greater support than formalized parent groups (Dunst, Trivette, & Deal, 1988). In home-based services, the parent may not have these informal opportunities. Feelings of isolation may increase when the parents do not have opportunities to meet other parents who have children with disabilities. Parents often note how much they learn from other parents; therefore, the community program offers a natural environment in which parent-to-parent interaction can occur.

What does this model of service delivery mean to the occupational therapist who works in a center-based early intervention program? Usually this model provides daily opportunities for learning from other occupational therapists and other professionals. Therefore, it may be an ideal environment for the novice therapist. Because this model typically gives therapists more control over their schedule and their time than home-based services, the therapist may have more time to spend in direct care and therapy services. Greater opportunities for informal communication are present on a day-to-day basis with the staff located directly in the center rather than working in isolated home settings.

Center-based programs also present more opportunity for the young child to develop social skills and to form peer relationships. Interaction with other children becomes particularly important for children who are 3 to 5 years of age. For this reason, children who receive home-based services during infancy are often encouraged to attend preschool when they are 3 years old.

Center-based teams that have frequent opportunities for both formal and informal communication have the flexibility to use the model of service delivery that is most appropriate to the family's needs. These teams are most likely to witness successful outcomes. Kjerland and Kovach (1987) demonstrated the effectiveness of services that are tailor made to suit the specific strengths, needs, and resources of each child and family. Project Dakota proposed a service menu format to stimulate creativity and flexibility in deciding the who, what, how, and where of interventions in the home, the community, and the clinic (see Case-Smith, Chapter 2). The location, frequency, and nature of early intervention services may need to be as diverse as the children and families (Kjerland & Kovach, 1987).

Community Home-Based Services

The normal environment of an infant is usually the home. Home-based services are advocated in the literature (Halpern, 1984; Hinojosa, Anderson, & Strauch, 1988). The majority of early intervention programs offer home services in addition to center-based services as options for intervention (Bailey & Simeonsson, 1988). After hospital care, services in the home are often instituted for children who are medically unstable or who need to avoid the possibility of infection posed by exposure to other children. Children who are technology-dependent also receive therapy at home. Such home-based services are common in rural areas where travel to distant medical centers is expensive and difficult for families.

The occupational therapist can have the lead responsibility for implementing home-based services or he can share this responsibility with a number of other professionals. The occupational therapist may act as a consultant to a home-based instructor; therefore, he makes few visits to the home and provides input to the instructor based on periodic team assessments.

In working with families, home-based services offer several advantages to the occupational therapist. Once inside the home, the therapist has a clear picture of the child's environment. During the course of intervention, the therapist has multiple opportunities to gather information on the child's interactions with the family in their natural environment. This information enables him to adjust and adapt therapy strategies so that they are congruent with the family's everyday life. When parents are taught methods to facilitate developmental skills, materials from the everyday environment can be used. The therapist suggests that household materials be used in play activities with the child. By visiting the family in their home, the therapist becomes aware of the materials that can be used to promote child development and can subsequently recommend use of specific toys. The therapist can also help the family establish special play areas for the child and adapt seating and positioning devices (e.g., add footrests and lateral supports to the child's high chair).

When the parent takes a primary role in directing and implementing intervention, more opportunities for the child to be involved in therapeutic activities occur. However, a number of disadvantages should be considered before asking the parents to become responsible for implementing the child's therapy. First, parents often do not have the needed skills to implement therapy activities. They may not have interest in or the necessary education to learn therapeutic techniques. Second, many parents prefer not to be their children's teachers because involvement in therapy may detract from more important roles that they have as parents (Winton & Turnbull, 1981). Kogan, Tyler, and Turner (1974) demonstrated that when parents implement therapy, negative interactions between the parent and child may result. Serving as the child's teacher can place the parents' attentions on developmental skills and progress; therefore, their enjoyment of other aspects of the child's personality is decreased. Hinojosa (1990) found that mothers of children with cerebral palsy did not have the time, energy, or confidence to implement a therapist-directed home treatment program.

Home-based services may offer the most ideal way to match therapy goals to the family's daily living activities. Once the therapist learns the methods used and resources available, he can tailor recommendations to match what is already occurring in the home (e.g., feeding and bathing) (Case-Smith, 1993). If the evening meal times are chaotic, feeding interventions are recommended for times other than the family's evening meal together. The therapist can recommend physical arrangements that best promote the child's play and movement in the home and that allow the parent and child to focus on the interaction and the activity (Shaaf & Mulrooney, 1989). Simulation of bathing and hygiene activities in the clinic is unrealistic, and as a result, suggestions made in the clinic may not be relevant to the home setting or may be difficult, if not impossible, to implement. It is noted that regular home visits promote successful problem solving, especially concerning issues of daily living (Case-Smith, 1993; Rainforth & Salisbury, 1988).

One goal of therapy is to promote the goodness-of-fit between the child and the environment; therefore, assessing the attributes of the home environment and observing the interactions of the child within that environment are essential to improving the fit. For example, a sterile, noncluttered environment may not fit the needs of a child with developmental delays who needs regular exposure to toys and play activities. In contrast, the child who is highly distracted and easily stressed may not be able to attend to play in a cluttered, highly stimulating environment. The therapist may appraise home-based services as an opportunity to improve the fit between the child and her environment and between the child and her family.

The home can also offer an optimal context for evaluating parent–child interaction. Interactions between the parent and child that appear stressed and negative in the clinic may appear more relaxed, warm, and positive in the home. Intervention related to enhancing interaction occurs naturally through discussions of the child's responses to her environment and to family members.

It has been suggested that interaction within the home facilitates a positive therapist–parent relationship. The home is a much more intimate environment than the clinic or the hospital; thus the home may provide a more relaxing atmosphere for therapy (Bailey & Simeonsson, 1988). The family members feel as if they are sharing an important part of themselves. They also may acknowledge that the therapist has driven to their home at his time expense.

The normal activity level of the home tends to set the pace of therapy. In homes with many family members and high activity levels, this environment may actually be a disadvantage to the therapy sessions. For example, when other small children are present during therapy, the parent may be distracted and unable to attend to the activities (Bailey & Simeonsson, 1988).

Occupational Therapy Roles in Medical- and Community-Based Early Intervention Programs

Occupational therapists are called upon to fill many roles. These roles have been explained in various sources (AOTA, 1989, 1991). Practice in early intervention requires advanced skills and expertise beyond the knowledge base of the entry-level practitioner (Hanft, 1988). The roles of the therapist as both a specialist and consultant in early intervention are discussed as follows.

Specialty Practice in Hospitals

In a pediatric hospital, the occupational therapists are expected to be pediatric specialists with a thorough understanding of and expertise in areas pertinent to the evaluation of and intervention with the child. The therapists typically treat infants and young children as inpatients and outpatients, and may assist community agencies with problem solving or diagnostic issues. For example, a 20-month-old child with cerebral palsy; spastic quadriplegia; episodes of coughing and choking during feeding; and a history of feeding problems and respiratory infections is receiving services in an early intervention program in the community. The occupational therapist of the early intervention program has concerns about the child's coughing and choking episodes during feeding and the child's frequent respiratory infections. Following his recommendation, the child and family are referred to the area pediatric hospital for a videofluoroscopic swallowing study to evaluate the child's swallow and to rule out aspiration. As a member of the team who addresses feeding and swallowing disorders, the occupational therapist may assess the child's oral-motor and feeding skills prior to the videofluoroscopic study, position and feed the child during the study and, with the radiologist and speech therapist, analyze the child's swallowing with different food consistencies. Based on the outcome of the study, the hospital-based team may make recommendations to the child's referring physician, parents, and community program as to the consistencies of foods that the child is capable of eating without aspirating, as well as other strategies for making feeding a safe and pleasant experience. This example of gaining access to specialized services through the hospital is one illustration of collaboration between hospital-based and community-based programs for infants and young children.

The specialized skills of the hospital occupational therapist may be provided through ambulatory programs, such as hospital clinics. For example, a 3-year-old child with myelomeningocele is referred to a hospital-based seating clinic for evaluation by the multidisciplinary team. The team in the clinic includes a physician specializing in physical medicine and rehabilitation, an occupational therapist, a physical therapist, and a clinical social worker, as well as the clinic nurse. The clinic team, after obtaining information from the community program and the family, evaluates the child and discusses options for seating and mobility and obtains the prescription for the seating device. They also identify vendors for purchase of the chair and assist the family with financial matters related to the purchase. In specialized clinics, the therapists' expertise, in conjunction with input from the community therapists and the family, results in the best outcome for the child and family.

Consultation in Community-Based Programs

The examples of the clinic visit and the swallowing evaluation suggest ways in which the occupational therapist functions as both a specialist and a consultant. In community-based programs, the occupational therapist may hold expertise in a number of specialty areas but primarily functions as a generalist in a system of comprehensive intervention. Her role within the program is often that of a consultant. The following section describes the skills needed to function as a consultant and how therapy goals can be met through a consultancy model.

As the pattern of service delivery changes in community programs, the role of the therapist on the team alters. When the occupational therapist is the primary interventionist and provides most of the direct services, she usually functions as the team leader for that child and family. Additional responsibilities of team leadership include organizing team meetings regarding the child's programs and initiating discussion with other team members about changes in the family's situation and the child's status. The therapist may function as service coordinator for the family, helping them access additional resources and facilitating communication among service providers. She may be instrumental in assisting the family to obtain equipment, such as wheelchairs, adapted devices, orthotics, and prosthetics.

The occupational therapist often provides the impetus for developing new strategies and new approaches for the child's program. The occupational therapist may assist the team to understand the child better by reframing the problems using a framework of neurodevelopment or sensory integration. Based on an in-depth understanding of neurophysiology related to function, the occupational therapist suggests strategies using neurophysiological principles that match the child's underlying problems. She also guides the primary interventionist in evaluating the effectiveness of new strategies.

Providing consultation to a home-based or center-based instructor requires well developed communication skills. To effectively offer consultation, the occupational therapist should participate in the initial assessment of the child and team planning. As a consultant, the therapist analyzes the child's developmental strengths and needs and the child's interactions with the environment in the contacts that she has with the child and family. Analysis of the critical issues and an understanding of the family's priorities are also important. Consultation is also based on past experience with similar children and an inventory of ideas that have been effective in other situations. From the initial evaluation, the therapist holds a picture of the child and formulates a list of recommendations that are given to the primary interventionist as needed, or when requested. Consultation after the initial planning involves sensitive listening to the home-based instructor as she describes the child's responses and behaviors. In addition, probing the situation with questions elicits information that is helpful to solving the problem.

When the occupational therapist is not the primary interventionist and an occupational therapy problem is identified, the therapist may consult with the primary interventionist during a home visit in which both are present with the family. The two professionals and parents collaborate in joint problem solving by discussing past behaviors of the child, observing the child's responses to new methods, and discussing the parents' priorities and concerns. As a result of this collaboration, new strategies can be tried, responses of the child can be evaluated, and adaptations can be made with the child. When the occupational therapist serves primarily as the consultant, opportunities to observe and interact with the child are essential in evaluating the effectiveness of recommendations and in monitoring any changes in the child. The occupational therapist builds on direct experiences with the child and family to maintain a clear and current picture from which recommendations and suggestions can be made.

A number of models are identified in the literature on consultation (Babcock & Pryzwansky, 1983; West & Idol, 1987). The model that is most likely to result in a lasting relationship is the collaborative model. The model seems most appropriate for team members who work together in a variety of situations and who collaborate and communicate frequently. In collaborative consultation, the therapist and instructor work together to identify the problem and solutions, to formulate a plan, and to evaluate the recommendations. Both are responsible for portions of the plan (Dunn, 1985). This process involves extensive follow-up and evaluation. It involves the commitment of both the consultant and the consultee to the child and family, and to solving the problem. Researchers of the efficacy of consultation stress the importance of the consultant's collaboration skills to successful consultation (Idol, Paolucci-Whitcomb, & Nevin, 1986). Most professionals prefer collaborative consultants and tend to initiate consultation contacts when the consultant uses collaboration. The following section provides a description of a model for collaborative consultation.

Steps in Collaborative Consultation

Step 1: Identify the Problem

In order to identify the problem, the consultant requests information through open-ended statements that elicit detailed, descriptive information. Examples are as follows: "Tell me what you observe when mother feeds him" or "Describe how he sits in the high chair." The consultant listens to the inflection and emotional tones of the consultee. *Listening* to the consultee's emotional tone helps identify the primary concern. At times, the occupational therapist needs specific clarification of the description. A clarifying statement is helpful when the description is ambiguous or unclear.

Paraphrasing is another method for clarifying that the consultant heard what the consultee meant to say. The consultant paraphrases by rewording the consultee's response. When paraphrasing or clarifying, language and terms that are specific to occupational therapy are avoided. Introduction of discipline-specific terminology tends to create more confusion than clarification.

Once the primary issue is identified, the consultant may probe the situation by asking specific questions that assist in comprehensive understanding of the issue. An *open question* elicits greater amounts of information; a closed question is usually answered by yes, no, or a single-word response. One-answer questions may be used when specific information is desired (e.g., "Is his head resting forward or backward during feeding?"). By probing into the problem, the occupational therapist puts the issue into a theoretical framework from which intervention strategies are generated. Examples of probes are as follows: "Does he sound raspy before or after his feeding?" or "Does he lose food from his mouth when the mother feeds him in his infant seat as well as when she holds him?" The resulting information helps the therapist identify the causes and the parameters of the problems.

Step 2: Generate Possible Solutions

In the second stage, the occupational therapist generates a list of alternative ideas that may become solutions to the problem. The consultee and consultant work together in this *brainstorming phase.* The consultant may initiate this phase by asking what the instructor has done to solve the problem. Then, the consultee and consultant can produce a range of possible solutions. Suggestions made during the brainstorming phase are possibilities rather than recommendations. The consultant may use probing methods, ask open-ended questions, or attempt to clarify the problem; however, the ideas generated during this stage are not evaluated in order to prevent inhibiting additional brainstorming.

Paraphrasing and expressing understanding are important methods of communication used to increase the consultee's comfort and confidence in generating solutions. Encouragement and support can also increase the instructor's willingness to pose alternatives to the problem.

Step 3: Evaluate the Solutions

Both the consultant and consultee participate in evaluating the list of possible solutions. The occupational therapist evaluates the solutions based on his expertise and experience with other children. The instructor evaluates the solutions based on experience with the child and family and insights into the home environment. Additional information on solutions that have already been tried may be provided at this stage. The consultant analyzes the solutions in an attempt to predict probable outcomes. The list of recommendations is refined and revised so that the agreed-upon solutions are appropriate and are optimal strategies for solving the problem.

Step 4: Devise a Plan for Implementation and Evaluation

A list of recommendations is not a satisfactory outcome for a consultation. The occupational therapist and instructor should *develop a plan* for how the strategies will be implemented, how often and for what time period the strategy or technique will be used, and how its effectiveness will be evaluated. Not all strategies are time bound. For example, a positioning method recommended by the consultant may be appropriate for a long period of time. The effectiveness of a recommended position is evaluated during a range of activities. Consideration is given to the child's comfort or discomfort, to the child's respiratory patterns, and to the child's level of endurance in the new position. The consultant should describe expected outcomes and specific observations that would give evidence of the position's effectiveness.

Step 5: Monitor and Evaluate the Recommendations

Successful consultation involves more than one interaction between the occupational therapist and the primary interventionist. In the collaborative model of consultation, both persons have responsibility for implementing the solution. Either person may initiate further discussion of the program after implementation has begun.

Again, helpful descriptive information is elicited by open-ended statements (i.e., "Tell me how he responds when you place the toy midline as he is lying prone.") A more general statement may elicit new concerns or related problems (i.e., "Tell me how it is going."). Such a statement may be the best way to elicit the spontaneous overall impressions of the instructor. Then, the consultant can ask more specific and directed questions regarding the agreed-upon plan. It is important that in evaluating the effectiveness of the solution, the occupational therapist does not appear to be evaluating the skills of the instructor. If the instructor implemented the solution incorrectly or incompletely, the consultant adapts to this situation by offering alternative solutions that are easier to implement. Further instruction and detail may be needed or alternative solutions generated.

Communication that is supportive and encouraging to the instructor and the parents and evaluation of the child's responses and the effectiveness of the recommended strategies are appropriate during this phase. The occupational therapist should express explicit interest in the outcome and in the additional problem that resulted. The instructor's evaluation gives the therapist feedback as to the effectiveness of the solutions; this feedback is helpful for future consultations. Collaborative consultation is characterized by a trusting relationship in which each partner appreciates and respects the skills and ideas of the other.

Hospital and Community Program Collaboration: A Model

Hospital and community-based services for infants and their families may be considered complementary components of a comprehensive service delivery system. The types of intervention, team structure and organization, focus of care, and level of family involvement usually differ, yet many infants with chronic illness or disability are served at different times in both of these settings. Collaboration and cooperation between hospitals and community programs is essential for comprehensive provision of services and smooth transitions for the infant and family.

An early intervention project at a children's hospital in a midwest city provides an example of a partnership between a tertiary care facility and a community-based agency. In this project, the children's hospital and the county early childhood education (ECE) program have collaborated to provide early intervention services for hospitalized children from birth to 3 years of age. The purposes of the program are to (1) provide early intervention to promote developmental skills in hospitalized infants, (2) facilitate an interdisciplinary team process involving the family as part of the team, (3) create a linkage with community early intervention programs to which children and their families are referred upon discharge, and (4) allow a smooth transition for children and their families from the hospital to home and to services in the community. The partnership has resulted in the ECE providing funding for an early intervention teacher/coordinator at the children's hospital. The teacher/coordinator provides the educational component for infants and their families in conjunction with the hospital's health care professionals. The child's and family's health care team becomes the physician, nurse, occupational therapist, physical therapist, teacher, and other disciplines, such as social work dieticians, or speech-language pathologists. Because the program is offered within a medical model, some accommodations must be made to the system in which the services are offered. Consequently, the teacher/coordinator requests a referral from the physician for the child's participation in the early intervention program prior to contacting the family to ensure that the child is considered medically able to participate.

Children in the hospital may be identified as candidates for early intervention from a number of sources. The teacher/coordinator attends weekly case disposition meetings for the newborn intensive care unit and bimonthly meetings for the newborn developmental unit in order to identify infants who may benefit from the early intervention program. Other disciplines in the hospital, including occupational therapy and physical therapy, also identify infants in the medical and surgical units who may benefit from early intervention.

Once a child and family have been identified and the physician has agreed upon the child's participation, the teacher/coordinator approaches the family, describes the program to them, and offers them the opportunity to participate. When the parents agree to participate and eligibility has been determined, the child and family are enrolled in the ECE program. To determine eligibility for the program under the developmental criteria, a developmental assessment must be completed. If the infant recently received a developmental assessment and the results indicate eligibility (delay in any developmental domain), further evaluation is not needed. If an assessment has not been completed, the teacher/coordinator and the therapists collaborate on the developmental evaluation to assure comprehensive services without duplication of effort. Diagnoses of enrolled children vary but may include bronchopulmonary dysplasia, short-gut syndrome, traumatic brain injury, failure-to-thrive, and other neurological disorders.

Individualized Family Service Plan (IFSP)

Within 2 weeks of enrollment, a meeting is held to develop and discuss the IFSP. Attending team members usually include the family, teacher, nurse, occupational therapist, and physical therapist, although other disciplines may attend as well. Once again, the medical nature of the environment must be considered; for example, if a child's condition becomes unstable before the IFSP meeting, the meeting is postponed until he is once again medically stable.

The family's goals for the child may relate to his medical condition. Parents may prioritize a goal such as oral feeding in lieu of using a gastrostomy tube. Goals that have a medical focus must include the physician's perspective and approval. The IFSP is updated every 3 months or sooner if discharge is imminent or the child's progress warrants changes in the program.

Ongoing intervention is quite intense (compared to the standards of community programs) and includes therapies three to five times per week for approximately 30 to 45 minutes and educational services approximately two to five times per week for 45 minutes. Because many of the children have complex needs, joint sessions between therapists or between a therapist and the teacher often occur. Parents may participate if present; however, many parents are only able to visit in the evening.

As typifies the medical setting, most communication among team members is informal in nature, with parents developing relationships individually with team members. However, in addition to the IFSP meetings, care conferences involving families and other team members are held as needed. Discharge planning for early intervention services often begins at the IFSP meeting and continues through care conferences or other meetings as discharge approaches.

Transition

One benefit of this program is coordination of discharge planning. Prior to discharge, the team identifies the child's developmental needs and the options for meeting those needs in the child's home community. Since the children's hospital is a regional center, many children will return to homes in rural areas or in towns where service delivery options may be limited. In addition, the child's ongoing medical needs may require special equipment, home nursing, or other special services. The hospital's continuity of care department works with the family and the team to identify the necessary resources. Once options have been identified, the family chooses the services they feel will best meet their needs. The early intervention teacher/coordinator makes the appropriate contact in the child's home community for developmental intervention, and, if possible, obtains an enrollment packet from the early intervention agency that will serve the child. Therefore, enrollment materials may be completed by the family and pertinent health care professionals prior to discharge, enabling an efficient entry into community-based services. At the same time, the family is asked to sign a release of information so that therapy reports and other hospital information can be sent to the community agency. If possible, a representative of the community program visits the hospital to meet the child and family in preparation for the transition. At this time, the family may be informed about the community parent support groups and other services (e.g., financial assistance) when relevant to the family's needs.

Following discharge, most families are contacted by the community program within 2 weeks to initiate intervention. The teacher/coordinator from the hospital communicates with the family by phone 2 weeks postdischarge to confirm whether contact has been made with the community program. In some cases, the family may indicate that the services are different than expected and that they would like to change to a different program. At this point, the members of the hospital team may assist the family in locating other resources.

What occurs if a child is readmitted? Once a child has been enrolled in the county early intervention program, the enrollment remains in effect for 1 year. Children who are readmitted within the year may once again receive services through the hospital-based early intervention program; however, since most subsequent hospitalizations are of short duration, the child's IFSP does not change. The child's community program provides the hospital with information concerning the child's goals in order to assist the staff in program planning while in the hospital. Often, the child's hospitalization can serve as an opportunity to use the available specialized services as identified by the community program or the parents. For example, provision of splints or special adaptive equipment that is not readily available in the child's home community may be requested. At discharge, reports of services provided are once again sent to the community program with the parents' permission.

The partnership between the hospital and ECE represents an effort to develop interagency collaborative relationships to meet the needs of infants and families. The program exemplifies a formalized linkage between medical- and community-based services. This partnership provides opportunities for communication, family involvement, and collaboration between hospital and community resources that enable smooth transition and continuity for families and their children.

References

Affleck, G., & Tennen, H. (1991). The effect of newborn intensive care on parents' psychological well-being. *Children's Health Care, 20*, 6–14.

American Occupational Therapy Association (AOTA). (1989). *Guidelines for occupational therapy services in the school systems.* Rockville, MD: Author.

American Occupational Therapy Association (AOTA). (1991). *Guidelines for occupational therapy services in early intervention and preschool services.* Rockville, MD: Author.

Babcock, N.L., & Pryzwansky, W.B. (1983). Models of consultation: Preferences of educational professionals at five steps of service. *Journal of School Psychology, 21*, 359–366.

Bailey, D.B. (1984). A triaxial model of the interdisciplinary team and group process. *Exceptional Children, 51*(1), 17–25.

Bailey, D.B., & Simeonsson, R.J. (1988). Home-based early intervention. In S. Odem & M. Karnes (Eds.), *Early intervention for infants and children with handicaps.* Baltimore: Paul H. Brookes Publishing Co.

Blechert, T.F., Christiansen, M.F., & Kari, N. (1987). Intraprofessional team building. *American Journal of Occupational Therapy, 41*(9), 576–582.

Case-Smith, J. (1993). Self care in children with developmental disabilities. In C. Christiansen (Ed.), *Ways of living.* Rockville, MD: American Occupational Therapy Association, Inc.

Dunn, W. (1985). Therapists as consultants to educators. *Sensory Integration Special Interest Section Newsletter, 6*(1), 1–4.

Dunst, C.J., Trivette, C., & Deal, A. (1988). *Enabling and empowering families: Principles and guidelines for practice.* Cambridge, MA: Brookline Books.

Fewell, R.R. (1983). The team approach to infant education. In S.G. Garwood & R.R. Fewell (Eds.), *Educating handicapped infants: Issues in development and intervention* (pp. 299–322). Rockville, MD: Aspen.

Fleming, M. (1991). The therapist with the three track mind. *American Journal of Occupational Therapy, 45*, 1007–1015.

Foley, G.M. (1990). Portrait of the arena evaluation: Assessment in the transdisciplinary approach. In E.D. Gibbs & D.M. Teti (Eds.), *Interdisciplinary assessment of infants.* Baltimore: Paul H. Brookes Publishing Co.

Gilkerson, L. (1990). Understanding institutional functioning style: A resource for hospital and early intervention collaboration. *Infants and Young Children, 2*(3), 22–30.

Gilkerson, L., Gorski, P., & Panitz, P. (1990). Hospital-based intervention for preterm infants and their families. In S. Meisels & J. Shonkoff (Eds.), *Handbook of early childhood intervention* (pp. 445–468). Cambridge: Cambridge University Press.

Golin, A.K., & Duncanis, A.J. (1981). *The interdisciplinary team.* Rockville, MD: Aspen.

Halpern, R. (1984). Home-based early intervention: Emerging purposes, intervention approaches and evaluation strategies. *Infant Mental Health, 5,* 206–220.

Hanft, B. (1988). The changing environment of early intervention services: Implications for practice. *American Journal of Occupational Therapy, 42,* 724–731.

Hinojosa, J. (1990). How mothers of preschool children with cerebral palsy perceive occupational and physical therapists and their influence on family life. *Occupational Therapy Journal of Research, 10*(3), 144–162.

Hinojosa, J., Anderson, J., & Strauch, C. (1988). Pediatric occupational therapy in their home. *American Journal of Occupational Therapy, 42,* 17–22.

Idol, L., Paolucci-Whitcomb, P., & Nevin, A. (1986). *Collaborative consultation.* Rockville, MD: Aspen.

Kjerland, L., & Kovach, J. (1987). *Structures for program responsiveness to parents.* Eagan, MN: Project Dakota, Inc.

Kogan, K.L., Tyler, N., & Turner, P. (1974). The process of interpersonal adaptation between mothers and their cerebral palsied children. *Developmental Medicine and Child Neurology, 16,* 518–527.

Levy, L. (1988). The health care delivery system today. In H.L. Hopkins & H.D. Smith (Eds.), *Williard and Spackman's occupational therapy.* 7th ed. (pp. 153–164). Philadelphia: J.B. Lippincott.

Lyon S., & Lyon, G. (1980). Team functioning and staff development: A role release approach to providing integrated educational services for severely handicapped students. *Journal of the Association for the Severely Handicapped, 5,* 250–263.

Maple, G. (1987). Early intervention: Some issues in cooperative team work. *Australian Occupational Therapy Journal, 34*(4), 145–151.

Mattingly, C.F. (1991). What is clinical reasoning? *American Journal of Occupational Therapy, 45,* 979–987.

McClellan, M. (1991). The discourse of interdisciplinary health care assessment: Toward a biosocial model. Dissertation at the Ohio State University, Columbus.

McCollum, J.A., & Hughes, M. (1988). Staffing patterns and team models in infancy programs. In J.B. Jordan, J.J. Gallagher, P.L. Hutinger, & M.B. Karnes (Eds.), *Early childhood special education: Birth to three.* Reston, VA: The Council for Exceptional Children, Division for Early Childhood.

McCormick, L., & Goldman, R. (1979). The transdisciplinary model: Implications for service delivery and personnel preparation for the severely and profoundly handicapped. *AAESPH Review, 4,* 152–161.

McGonigel, M.J., & Garland, C.W. (1988). The individualized family service plan and the early intervention team: Team and family issues and recommended practices. *Infants and Young Children, 1*(1), 10–21.

Peterson, N. (1987). *Early intervention for handicapped and at-risk children: An introduction to early childhood special education.* Denver, CO: Love.

Rainforth, B., & Salisbury, C.L. (1988). Functional home programs: A model for therapists. *Topics in Early Childhood Special Education, 7*(4), 33–45.

Schoen, D. (1987). *Educating the reflective practitioner. How professionals think in action.* New York: Basic Books.

Shaaf, R., & Mulrooney, L. (1989). Occupational therapy in early intervention: A family centered approach. *American Journal of Occupational Therapy, 43*(11), 745–754.

Spencer, P. (1986). Team dynamics relative to exemplary early services. In *Project Bridge: Decision-making for early services: A team approach.* Elk Grove Village, IL: American Academy of Pediatrics.

Stephens, L.C. (1989). Occupational therapy in the school system. In P.N. Pratt & A.S. Allen (Eds.), *Occupational therapy for children.* 2nd ed. (pp. 593–611). St. Louis: C.V. Mosby Co.

United Cerebral Palsy National Collaborative Infant Project. (1976). *Staff development handbook: A resource for the transdisciplinary process.* New York: United Cerebral Palsy Associations of America.

Webster's New World Dictionary of American English. (1989). Springfield, MA: Merriam-Webster Inc.

West, J.F., & Idol, L. (1987). School consultation (part 1): An interdisciplinary perspective on theory, models, and research. *Journal of Learning Disabilities, 20*(7), 388–409.

Winton, P. & Turnbull, A. (1981). Parent involvement as viewed by parents of preschool handicapped children. *Topics in Early Childhood Special Education, 1,* 11–19.

Woodruff, G., & McGonigel, M.J. (1988). Early intervention team approaches: The transdisciplinary model. In J.B. Jordan, J.J. Gallagher, P.L. Hutinger, & M.B. Karnes (Eds.), *Early childhood special education: Birth to three.* Reston, VA: The Council for Exceptional Children, Division for Early Childhood.

Yoder, D.E., Coleman, P.P., & Gallagher, J.J. (1990). Personnel needs—Allied health personnel meeting the demands of Part H, PL 99-457. A report. Chapel Hill: Frank Porter Graham Child Development Center, University of North Carolina.

Approaches and Strategies in Early Intervention

6

□ □ □
□ □ □
□ □ □

Early Emotional Development and Sensory Processing

Elise Holloway, MPH, OTR

Early conceptualizations of infant and child development emphasized cognitive and motor competence, which were thought to automatically unfold. However, in the 1940s and 1950s, the psychoanalytic concepts of intrapsychic processes and of early experience as mediators of development changed this emphasis. This influence of psychoanalytic thought resulted in an increasing interest in early emotional development and in closer examination of the caregiver's role in the child's early development (Minde & Minde, 1986; Tyson, 1984).

Psychoanalytic theory has provided the basis for empirical research that examines the infant's experience of interpersonal relatedness. While theorists and researchers differ in their views of the parent–infant relationship, they all agree that the infant's first relationship with the caregiver is the basis for the child's later social, emotional, and personality development (Teti & Nakagawa, 1990).

In general, there is little reference within the occupational therapy literature to early emotional development other than brief mention of Freud and Erickson. However, there are several other theorists, clinicians, and researchers from other disciplines whose work has relevance for occupational therapy in early intervention. This body of work dovetails nicely with the work of

The author gratefully acknowledges Robin Doran, PhD, Randall Ramirez, LCSW, and Lois Wainstock, MA for contributing their ideas to the formulation of this chapter.

For ease of reading, the words *mother* and *she* will be used to denote a parent or a consistent caregiver and the word *he* will be used to denote the infant.

A. Jean Ayres and with the focus of occupational therapy on sensory processing as a foundation for purposeful activity. The purpose of this chapter is

1. to provide a brief overview of the sensory integrative theory
2. to acquaint the reader with other psychoanalytic theories and with the empirical data that has grown out of interest in the earliest relationships from historical and developmental perspectives
3. to pose questions to the reader that will stimulate critical thinking about the ways in which difficulties in sensory processing may impact the development of the infant's sense of self

It is not the purpose of this chapter to provide a study of sensory integrative theory. For an understanding of sensory integrative theory, in-depth reading of Ayres' original work and of the neurobiological literature is recommended. Also, there are several aspects of the parent–infant relationship that are not addressed in this chapter. In the parent–infant relationship, parents bring with them their own histories, fantasies, and expectations of the infant and of the parenting experience. Their perception of the infant and attribution of meaning to the infant's behaviors are as important as the infant's actual behaviors (Brazelton & Cramer, 1990; Fraiberg, 1980). Certainly, a stressful social situation such as poverty or substance abuse also affects the parents' abilities to be emotionally available to the child. While important to the infant's developing sense of self, these areas are beyond the scope of this chapter.

Overview of Sensory Integrative Theory

Sensory integrative theory describes how individuals develop the capacity to perceive, learn, and organize sensations from the body and from the environment to accomplish self-directed, meaningful activities. An important component of this theory is Ayres' explanation of how the infant develops the capacity to organize sensory input. She suggested that initially, the newborn infant experiences sensations but is not able to attach meaning to them. Through the child's innate drive to master his body and his world and through his ongoing interactive experiences, he begins to attach significance to the sensations that he is receiving. As the infant continues to experience various amounts, types, and combinations of sensory information in his environment, he responds by producing an adaptive response, a goal-directed purposeful response to the environment. Each time the infant responds adaptively, his nervous system stores the perception or knowledge of this experience. It is then in place to guide future organization of differing sensory experiences and environmental demands. Each time the infant is able to successfully meet the challenges of his environment, there is an increase in his brain's ability to organize sensation for production of increasingly complex adaptive responses. This process is termed sensory integration (Ayres, 1972, 1979; Clark, Mailloux, & Parham, 1989).

Ayres proposed that adequate sensory integration is not only the basis for learning but also for emotional development. She pointed out that emotion is a function of the nervous system, and that processing and integrating sensation to produce adaptive responses supports emotional growth. When the child experiences challenges to which he can respond effectively, he has fun, which may be interpreted as an affective state of joy. The child with difficulties in sensory modulation may have negative affective associations since his emotional and physical experience of the world may be one of distress rather than of fun (Ayres, 1979; Clark, Mailloux, & Parham, 1989).

Ayres emphasized the importance of the tactile and vestibular systems as unifying systems in that their efficient operation promotes the development of the individual's relationship to gravity and to his environment, and his overall organization of behavior (Ayres, 1979). Two commonly mentioned sensory modulation disorders with emotional consequences, gravitational insecurity and tactile defensiveness, are thought to be based in inefficient functioning of these two systems.

Gravitational security is vital to emotional security. The infant needs to develop the "trust that he is firmly connected to the earth and that he will always have a safe place to stand" so that he can, in a sense, move out into the world (Ayres, 1979). To this end, the child is endowed with an inner drive to explore and master gravity and he pursues this via his motor skills acquisition. Those children who have gravitational insecurity, which is defined as an intense anxiety and distress in response to movement or to a change in head position, experience a primal threat when asked to move (Clark, Mailloux, & Parham, 1989). The child prefers to stay in physical contact with a secure base and to avoid play that involves movement.

Another example of hyperresponsivity to sensory input that can have social-emotional implications is tactile defensiveness, which is defined as an aversive reaction to touch. Those naturally occurring emotionally based sensorimotor play experiences in a young child's life, such as hugging, tickling, and wrestling, may be imbued with the negative rather than the positive affective meaning that would be expected (Ayres, 1979; Clark, Mailloux, & Parham, 1989).

With the tactile and vestibular systems efficiently working together, the infant learns that he is separate and distinct from his mother and every other person and thing. The child can begin to take emotional command of his life only to the extent that his body sensations allow him to move freely, effectively, and without negative affective associations as he interacts with his world (Ayres, 1979).

The Importance of Parent–Child Relations to Early Emotional Development

Good Enough Holding

Physician and psychoanalyst D.W. Winnicott strongly influenced the study of the infant's early emotional development by suggesting that the infant cannot be studied in a vacuum. A number of researchers report that their work has been guided by Winnicott's suggestions that "a baby cannot exist alone, but is essentially part of a relationship" (Winnicott, 1964) and that the mother's *good enough holding* of the infant in both a physical and psychological sense helps to establish the foundation for the infant's sense of self (Winnicott, 1971).

Winnicott repeatedly stressed that the care the infant receives from his mother allows him to have a sense of personal existence and build a sense of *continuity of being* (Winnicott, 1986). To illustrate this, he used the metaphor of the mother holding the infant. Initially, the infant is held at his mother's breast, given total support and nourishment. As the infant matures, he is then held in his mother's lap. He is able to begin to sit more independently but still needs some support. He begins to look out at the world and to look at his mother from a different perspective. Holding continues in a larger sense as the child then moves to sit and play on the floor in the presence of the mother. His mother remains both physically and emotionally available to him.

Winnicott felt that good enough holding protects the child from physical and psychological danger. The mother takes into account her infant's skin sensitivity, auditory sensitivity, visual sensitivity to falling, and response to the action of gravity (Winnicott, 1986). For Winnicott, holding includes the child's and mother's daily routine of care with its frequent adaptations for the infant's growth and development in both the physical and psychological realms. Through holding the infant, the mother supports the infant's natural abilities to develop. As the mother allows more physical space between herself and the infant to match his maturing motor and cognitive needs, she provides the infant with more emotional space. This balance of physical and psychological separation provides a space for play, creating a figurative as well as a literal space for the child's emerging sense of self.

Winnicott described the infant's sensory experience during daily activities as an important part of allowing the infant to move away from his mother emotionally in order to create a space for himself. The occupational therapist might ask: Would the tactually defensive infant perceive his mother's holding as protective in both a real and emotional sense? How does the infant interpret his mother's response to his tactually defensive behaviors? Would an infant be able to move out of his mother's lap emotionally if he is unsure of his body due to deficiencies in processing vestibular and somatosensory input? What would it mean to the child if emotionally he is ready to move out of his mother's lap but because of motor planning difficulties he is unable to do so? What would the child's psychological sense of self be if physically he does not really know where he is in that play space without his mother's grounding?

These questions may be answered differently by each mother–infant pair; there is no one correct way of interpreting them. These types of questions must be asked alongside other, more frequently asked, treatment-oriented questions, such as How much tactile input is too much for this child? Does graded proprioceptive input help him to tolerate touch and better modulate his behaviors? How does he transition from one position to another?

One possible scenario for the tactually defensive infant may be that he does not perceive his mother's touch or holding as pleasurable or protective, rather he perceives it as threatening. He may pull back, arch, or fuss. He does not receive the secure good enough holding that he needs emotionally to begin to learn about himself and his world. Reciprocally, his mother may also pull back, possibly feeling rejected by the infant and not able to move beyond this feeling to determine how she can hold him so that he is comfortable, thus, providing the emotional holding that he needs. These types of interactions can bring about an unfulfilling cycle of distress and missed opportunities for building the infant's sense of self and furthering the parent–infant relationship in a positive manner.

Separation and Individuation

Margaret Mahler, a pediatrician and psychoanalyst, furthered the understanding of early emotional development by contributing the theoretical notion of the "psychological birth of the infant" (Mahler, Pine, & Bergman, 1975). She synthesized theory with a methodology for observation of infants and their mothers, interpreting observable interactions as correlates of interpersonal relations, thereby describing the separation-individuation process. This process is one in which the infant establishes a sense of separateness from and a sense of relation to his real world. This separateness is in relation to his own body experiences and in relation to his mother.

Mahler states that, like any intrapsychic process, this continues throughout the life cycle. However, the main aspects of this process take place during the first 3 years of life (see Table 6-1). Separation is thought of as the child's emergence from a symbiotic fusion with the mother. Individuation is the child's assumption of his own individual characteristics. These two processes are intertwined.

Initially, Mahler reported her belief that after birth, the baby's first experiences are of his internal sensations and that he generally does not respond

Table 6-1   Stages of the Separation-Individuation Process

Age	Stage	
2 to 4 months	Normal symbiosis:	Infant experiences dual-unity with mother
4 to 8 months	Differentiation:	Infant's somatosensory-based development of body image and awareness of self as separate from mother begins
8 to 18 months	Practicing:	Infant begins to engage in independent exploration but returns to mother for emotional refueling
18 to 24 months	Rapprochement:	With growing sense of separateness, infant struggles between autonomy and dependence
24 to 36 months	Individuality:	Infant establishes internal representation of self as separate and shows beginning emotional object constancy

Source: Data from Mahler MS, Pine F, Bergman A: *The psychological birth of the human infant.* New York: Basic Books, 1975, pp. 1–119.

to external stimuli. With the growing empirical research, she acknowledged that the infant does indeed respond to external stimuli (Stern, 1985). However, theoretically, the infant does not completely distinguish between stimuli coming from outside and from within. Through the experience of the mother's caregiving acts, the baby emerges from this inturning to enter a state of what she called *normal symbiosis*, generally around 1 to 2 months of age.

It is during this normal symbiotic period that the infant, largely through his mother, becomes interested in the outside world. However, the infant only experiences himself as part of his mother, a dual-unity , because a well-delineated sense of self has not yet emerged (Mahler, 1986). Mahler points out that she does not intend symbiosis in the biological sense but in the sense that the infant has not yet become an *I* as differentiated from the *not-I* of the rest of his world, primarily his mother. She strongly suggested that the perceptual experience of body contact, or what she termed the experience of the sensoriperceptive organ, is the main contributor to the infant's ability to begin to separate self from the object world (Mahler, Pine, & Bergman, 1975). The infant's inner sensations contribute to forming the *feeling of self*. It is these two intrapsychic processes that contribute to the infant's increased perceptual and affective investment in the sensory input coming from the outside world, but which the infant does not yet recognize as coming from outside. The infant requires a balance of stimuli coming from outside and from within. This psychophysiologic balance depends on the matching of behavior patterns of mother and infant. Winnicott's concept of good enough holding behavior promotes this equilibrium. In essence, Mahler, Pine, &

Bergman (1975) suggest that the mother is the mediator of the infant's earliest sensory and affective experiences.

The symbiotic phase leads into the *separation-individuation* process. This process is divided into subphases, the first of which is termed *differentiation/development of body image* and occurs generally between 4 to 8 months of age. The infant remains more awake and alert; his attention is more and more directed outward. With increasing motor skill, the infant tentatively explores his mother's face, hair, and body. He also moves out of the mother's lap and then checks back with the mother. These actions are what Ayres might term early adaptive responses. Combined with the infant's memories of his daily routines and interaction experiences, this leads to the somatopsychic differentiation of self from mother.

Overlapping differentiation is the *practicing* subphase that usually occurs with the onset of the earliest locomotion (i.e., crawling). The mother now becomes the home base to which the infant returns after exploring his world. The baby returns for emotional refueling through physical contact with the mother. As independent cognitive functions and walking skills mature, the infant takes one of the largest steps in individuation. He begins to explore at some distance from his mother, enjoying his own greatness of skill and his widening world. He shows a growing interest in practicing his skills and in exploring further. This experience of independent exploration is exhilarating for the child but ultimately leads to the child's awareness of his separateness and relative helplessness in the world. As this awareness grows, stimulated by his maturationally acquired ability to move away from his mother physically and by his cognitive growth, the child shows an increased need to share his new skills and experiences with his mother, as well as to share in love. This period, occurring around 18 months of age, is termed *rapprochement*.

At this time, there is a revival in the child's concern about his mother's whereabouts, decreasing frustration tolerance, and an increased need for her emotional availability to support him. No longer just home base, mother is someone with whom the child wants to share the world. His emphasis changes from locomotion-exploration to social interaction with mother. At the same time, however, the toddler continues to struggle with the need for independence. The child shows both a kind of shadowing-of-mother behavior and a darting-away-from-mother behavior that indicates his ambivalence between his need for her love in a physical and psychological sense and his need for autonomy and separateness.

Between 18 and 24 months of age, Mahler reports an important emotional turning point for the toddler . He begins to gradually experience obstacles in his way of anticipated "conquest of the world" (Mahler, 1986). Along with increasing motor skills, cognition, and perception, there is an increasing differentiation between himself and his mother. He begins to learn that he is a separate individual who is no longer able to command relief or assistance merely by feeling the need for them or giving voice to his needs. The child employs all kinds of mechanisms to resist separation from his mother but can no longer go back to that dual-unity. Verbal communication becomes more necessary. The toddler gradually realizes that his parents are separate individuals with their own interests. This is termed the *rapprochement crisis.* By 21 to 24 months of age, many toddlers resolve this rapprochement crisis and once again can function at a relative distance from the mother.

The practicing and rapprochement subphases may proceed very differently for the toddler who is gravitationally insecure. He may not be able to begin to move away from his mother, his secure base, if indeed he needs her to help keep him grounded in the primal way described by Ayres.

The last subphase is *consolidation of individuality/beginning of emotional object constancy.* It is made possible by the toddler's increasing language development, which seems to give the child a greater sense of control over his environment; the internalization of parental rules and demands; and the ability to express wishes, fantasies, and mastery through symbolic play. During this phase, which lasts until 30 to 36 months of age, the child can gradually accept separation from the mother once again due to beginning emotional object constancy. This is more than solely Piaget's concept of object permanence; it implies internal representation of the mother in an affective sense. Now, at times, this image can substitute for the emotional availability of the infant's actual mother; thus, he can maintain his emotional equilibrium for longer separations. This fourth subphase is characterized by the unfolding of the complex cognitive functions of verbal communication, use of time, fantasy play, and reality testing. Mental representations of the self, as distinctly separate from internal representations of the mother and other objects, pave the way for the formation of self-identity (Mahler, 1986).

The development of a body percept may support the development of those internal representations of self as separate in that one's own physical boundaries are more defined. The child who has irregularities in processing bodily sensations may not have a well developed body percept or body map (Ayres, 1979). With an inadequate body percept, the child may continue to have more of a physical rather than a solely emotional connection to the mother, possibly interrupting or slowing the separation-individuation process.

A Break with Tradition

John Bowlby's studies of early social-emotional relationships began a new tradition of psychoanalytic thinking (Bowlby, 1969, 1988a). His theory of attachment explained infant behaviors such as the infant's distress upon separation from his mother, the infant's tendency to follow the mother and to use her as a home base for exploratory excursions, and the infant's tendency to return to the mother's presence upon arrival of an unfamiliar adult. He deemphasized the psychoanalytic notion that early infant–mother attachments resulted from an association made between the mother and the provision of food.

Harlow's studies of infant monkeys contributed to Bowlby's shift away from tradition. In Harlow's study (1961), infant monkeys were separated from their mothers at birth and reared with surrogate mothers; one mother was made of wire with a feeding tube and the other was covered with terrycloth but without a food source attached. When distressed, the monkeys went to the cloth-covered surrogate for consolation even though it played no role in feeding. Harlow's findings argued against the role of feeding in the development of early attachments and emphasized the importance of physical contact.

With the increasing empirical evidence as support, Bowlby proposed that the child's tie to the caregiver develops as a result of the activation of a preadapted, biologically based, goal-corrected, motivational system. His conceptual breakthrough concerning the biological function of attachment was important because it showed that the infant's tie to the primary caregiver could not be explained solely in terms of cognitive and socioemotional development.

In Bowlby's attachment theory, the newborn infant is said to be predisposed to engage in behaviors that will ensure proximity to the caregiver. Behaviors such as crying, clinging, smiling, visual tracking, and vocalizing elicited in caregiving were given importance. Caregivers are also said to be biologically predisposed to respond to such signals and provide appropriate care. During the first months of the infant's life, these species-specific behaviors become more complex and coordinated. The infant begins to direct these signals toward specific persons. It is in the context of these early interactions that an attachment bond to the caregiver develops (Malatesta, Culver, Tesman, & Shepard, 1989).

The occupational therapist may ask how these signaling and responding behaviors may be affected if the infant has difficulties in sensory modulation. Is it possible that caregiving activities may not be well timed if the overall interaction's timing is off due to hypersensitivity or hyposensitivity to the environment's sensory messages?

Bowlby hypothesized that there is a regulatory system, or an attachment system, that exists within a person. Its goals are to regulate behaviors that maintain proximity and contact with a selected protective person or attachment figure in order to provide a feeling of security. Based on observation of infants' separation responses, Bowlby determined that this regulatory system becomes well organized around 9 months of age. The system prevents an infant from straying too far from a caregiver in an unfamiliar world and initiates the infant's search when the protective caregiver is absent. It is this proximity-security regulating system that Bowlby refers to as attachment.

This system was seen to make evolutionary sense due to its basic survival value by helping to protect the helpless infant from potential dangers.

Bowlby suggested that even though attachment exists between two individuals, the system is organized within the attached person and organized preferentially around a specific partner. This internal attachment system monitors and processes information taken in via the sensory systems, regarding danger signals and accessibility of attachment figure, on a physical and psychological level. While Bowlby felt that the system was activated by perceived danger versus safety, others have suggested that it may be continually active, always regulating activation/deactivation (Bretherton, 1987). When no danger signals are present and the attachment figure is accessible, the child feels secure and is able to explore. The system continuously monitors the caregiver and sets limits on how far from the secure base the child will move. When the environment is alarming to the child due to unfamiliarity or to another perceived threat, the regulatory system resets and the child may engage in proximity-seeking behavior or may need physical contact.

The hypersensitive child perceives that his environment is threatening; conversely, the hyposensitive child does not register enough consistent information about the environment. In either case, is it possible that irregularities in sensory processing may affect the distance that he will move away from his secure base? If the therapist sees clinginess on the part of the child with sensory integrative dysfunction, it may indeed be appropriate attachment behavior. How emotionally threatening might it be to move the child away from his mother during occupational therapy intervention in the clinic setting?

Returning to psychoanalytic tradition, Bowlby suggested that in the course of interacting with the physical and social world, the infant constructs internal representations, or working models, of the mother in addition to internal models of the self and the world. This occurs late in the first year of life, concomitant with maturing cognitive capacities. These representations are imbued with affective meaning and are shaped by the quality of care that the infant has received in terms of the mother's emotional and physical availability. These working models are used by the infant to plan, understand, and guide behavior relative to the caregiver (Bowlby, 1969; Bretherton, 1987; Malatesta, Culver, Tesman, & Shepard, 1989; Teti & Nakagawa, 1990).

Infants who have had sensitive, consistent caregiving are thought to develop a working model of the caregiver as warm and responsive, and a working model of themselves as worthy of love and support. Infants who had caregivers who were inconsistently available or rejecting are thought to develop an internal representation of the caregiver as unresponsive and of themselves as unworthy of love. These working models can be shaped by ongoing environmental circumstances and are believed to have a strong organizational influence on future behavior, including resolving future psychosocial adaptations. Those infants who develop trust in relationships with their responsive caregivers would be expected to adapt to future challenges more successfully than those infants who did not develop this trust (Teti & Nakagawa, 1990).

Bowlby's conceptualization of the working model as helping the infant to plan, understand, and guide his behaviors may be a cognitive-emotional correlate of the adaptive response described by Ayres. Is it possible that some toddlers with sensory processing difficulties develop working models that are distorted by inefficient modulation of sensation? Would the child's working model of his parent or of himself be distorted if his parent is not perceived as consistently available or as threatening at times due to sensory defensiveness?

The Infant's Contribution: Individual Capacities

Bowlby's work is generally considered to be theoretical in nature although his clinical observations of infants contributed to it. He noted that the earlier contributions of theoreticians, such as Freud, Erickson, Winnicott, and Mahler, provided the skeleton for understanding the infant's earliest emotional development (Bowlby, 1988b). The empirical research that has taken place subsequent to the development of these theories contributes the clothing for that skeleton. This next section will provide a selected overview of the research, which begins to elucidate this theory.

Clinicians and researchers in the field of infant development have continued to refine and reorganize certain aspects of the early theories and apply them to practice, stressing different components of the infant–parent relationship. One such area has been in the examination of early infant capabilities.

Several researchers have focused on the role that emotion plays in organizing behaviors (Barrett & Campos, 1987; Fox, 1989; Izard, 1982; Malatesta, Culver, Tesman, & Shepard, 1989). They all agree that emotion serves an adaptive function but they differ in their definition of emotion, in their view of the association between the infant's internal feeling experience and overt behavior, and also in the degree to which they believe biologically controlled systems versus cognitive systems influence emotional development.

Differential Emotions Theory

Drawing on the early work of Darwin, Izard observed infants across several cultures and noted consistent, discrete facial expressions (Malatesta, Culver, Tesman, & Shepard, 1989; Izard, 1982; Izard & Malatesta,

1987). Specific facial expressions for fear, anger, joy, and surprise have been described. These innate facial, vocal, and body expressions seen in young infants are believed to reflect internal feeling states. Izard (1982) suggests that they play a crucial role in the early infant–mother signaling system that was described by Bowlby and others. In this view, called the *differential emotions theory*, emotions are believed to be neurophysiologically grounded behaviors, suggesting that early affective behavior is innate and somewhat stereotyped. The distinct neurophysiological processes subserving each of the fundamental emotions are activated by biologically and psychologically meaningful stimuli. Izard (1982) also suggested that this innate wiring and preadaptation for signaling may be modified via socialization experiences. On the other hand, the cognitive-constructivist approach proposes that cognition, rather than biology, acts as a central mechanism in the infant's growth and differentiation of emotion. From this perspective, the facial expressions described by Izard are not true emotions. Cognitive maturation and beginning differentiation of self from others, occurring around three months of age, is required (Malatesta, Culver, Tesman, & Shepard, 1989).

Action Tendencies

Barrett and Campos (1987) offer a relational view of emotion, placing less of an emphasis on the unifying role of a central feeling state and more importance on what the child is doing to adapt his goals to the environment and to modify the environment to fit his goals. Because different actions have different affective meanings, or *action tendencies*, they feel that the research emphasis should be on what the child does rather than on what he feels. This relational emphasis should shift the study of emotion away from the individual to the study of the person-environment transaction (Barrett & Campos, 1987; Campos, Campos, & Barrett, 1989). A young infant's action tendency in regulating his emotional arousal may be vocalization, self-distraction, manipulating a body part, playing with an object, or leaving the scene (Kopp, 1989). Barrett and Campos (1987) feel that emotions are not mere feelings but rather a process that establishes, maintains, or disrupts meaningful interactions between the person and his environment. Action tendencies help organize the child's emotional experience. In addition, they may have a relationship to Ayres' adaptive response in that both emphasize the importance of the child's purposeful response to the environment. Is it possible that when an adaptive response is elicited during occupational therapy intervention, it may help the child to organize his emotional states?

Cross-Modal Studies

With a different view of infant capabilities, another group of investigators have been examining the young infant's ability to utilize and to discriminate between various sensory inputs (Rose & Ruff, 1987). Early infant oral exploratory behavior may provide the basis for later perceptual discrimination as shown in a variety of cross-modal studies. In cross-modal studies, the infant receives sensory information about an object through one sensory system to make inferences about other sensory aspects of the object. By changing their sucking rates, infants have been shown to discriminate between smooth and nubby spheres that they have mouthed. Auditory perception and temporal grouping studies show that 1.5- to 3-month-old infants can discriminate between patterns of auditory tones while preferential visual scanning of infants younger than 2 months of age has been reported. Infants appear to be predesigned to be able to perform a cross-modal transfer of sensory information that permits them to recognize a correspondence between tactile and visual information. In one study, 3-week-old children were given two tactually different pacifiers to suck on while blindfolded. They had contact with the pacifier using only their mouths. When the blindfolds were removed, the infants reliably looked more at the last pacifier on which they sucked.

It appears that early in life, infants have an innate general capacity to take information received in one sensory modality and translate it into another sensory modality. This is most likely not a simple transfer, but requires encoding of information in the nervous system at a different level than is recognized in any of the sensory modalities. This suggests that young infants experience a world of perceptual unity (Stern, 1985). At the present time, only inferences have been made from observation of overt infant responses in these areas. Establishing the presence of infant cross-modal and amodal perception now provides the basis for investigating the underlying mechanisms of these processes that contribute so significantly to infant–mother interaction (Rose & Ruff, 1987).

Psychophysiologic Aspects of Emotion

Some investigators have been examining the psychophysiologic aspect of emotion. In a study of 10-month-old infants who were separated from their mothers and approached by a stranger, EEGs differentiated hemispheric asymmetries during facial expressions of anger and sadness (Fox & Davidson, 1988). Other investigations regarding heart rate variability or vagal tone, as related to emotional reactivity, suggest that there are individual differences in infants' responses to novel and mildly stressful events and that these are associated with varying degrees of parasympathetic and possibly brain stem influence (Fox, 1989). Fox (1989) reports that in the infant's early months of life, differences in vagal tone may be associated with heightened responsivity to sensory stimulation. With maturation, he suggests that there may be increased cortical inhibition and an increase in sustained attention. These findings suggest that infants may be better able to regulate their arousal and emotional level by controlling their attention to modulate their physiological reactivity.

Reciprocal Interactions of Mother and Child

Microanalysis of parent–infant interactions, such as those by Fox (1989) and Fox & Davidson (1988), have led to more global and contextual approaches (Brazelton & Cramer, 1990). Supported by the growing knowledge of infant and toddler perceptual and affective abilities, this line of investigation relates to the notion of the dyadic relationship as the setting for the infant's development of attention and affective tone. The mother–infant social system is believed to be maintained by dynamic processes and continuous cycling of feedback; in fact, each partner has been observed to make finely tuned adjustments to each other's behaviors (Brazelton & Cramer, 1990; Brazelton, Koslowski, & Main, 1974; Brazelton, Tronick, Adamson, Als, & Wise, 1975). Infants have been noted to actively process social signals. They respond in specific and appropriate ways to their mothers' communicative signals.

Initially, it was thought that these reciprocal interactions were brought about by entrainment of both the mother's and the infant's rhythms in that each partner would slow down or speed up his internal clock to fit the other's pattern (Lester, Hoffman, & Brazelton, 1985). However, it has been shown that early mother–infant face-to-face interactions have a conversation-like pattern with a bidirectional influence. These interactions are not periodic and do not appear to cycle on and off at regular, precise intervals, but are regulated by the mother and the infant themselves over the course of the interaction (Cohn & Tronick, 1988).

The way in which the infant and mother go about using their interactive capacities to achieve their communicative goals has been termed the mutual regulation model (Brazelton, 1982; Gianino & Tronick, 1988). Often, the goal of the mother–infant dyad's interchange is the affective process of interaction in and of itself. It is this mutually rewarding interactional synchrony achieved by infant and mother that fosters the infant's development of an internal working model of the mother as available and responsive (Isabella, Belsky, & von Eye, 1989). At times in this process of reciprocity and mutual joint regulation, there may be mismatches. However, Gianino and Tronick (1988) feel that these mismatches allow the infant the opportunity to broaden and develop his interactive and self-regulatory skills, and that this facilitates the infant's coping capabilities when the mother is briefly not available.

Temperament

Temperament, as conceptualized by Thomas and Chess (1977), is described as the stylistic component of a child's behavior. It helps determine how actions are performed rather than why or what is performed. Temperament is believed to have a biological basis and is evidenced in behavioral tendencies rather than discrete actions. It is thought that these biological tendencies are continuous over time, but that they may be shaped or modified by the child's experience. Understanding a child's temperamental tendencies in various situations contributes to understanding his constitutional responsivity to the environment and his self-regulation of emotion (Williamson & Zeitlin, 1990). While there are differences in definition of temperament between researchers, there is consensus that important variables of temperament are activity, reactivity, emotionality, and sociability (Goldsmith et al., 1987). In studies of parent–infant interaction, infant–parent attachment, and of the child's use of the parent to cope when encountering novel situations, the child's temperament has been seen to influence the interchange (Bates, 1987; Crockenberg, 1981; Kagan, Reznick, & Snidman, 1987).

In addition to bringing their affective state with them to an interchange, infants and toddlers will seek out emotional information from a significant other (i.e., a parent). This social referencing starts around the middle of the child's first year. When he encounters an ambiguous or threatening situation that is beyond his own abilities to assess, the child will check back with his parent for help in assessing the situation and in regulating his behavior. In studies with the visual cliff, for example, infants checked their mothers' facial expressions to determine if it was safe to cross the cliff. If they saw a happy facial expression, they approached; when they saw fear on their mother's face, they avoided the cliff (Campos & Stenberg, 1981; Klinnert, Campos, Sorce, Emde, & Svejda, 1982).

Summary

This cursory overview demonstrates that a wide range of research into the child's early affective experience has been undertaken. This affective experience primarily takes place within the give-and-take of the parent–infant relationship.

Bridging the Gap: Developing an Affective Core

As a result of these research findings, it is now generally accepted that infants and their caregivers are biologically organized to engage in relationships that are regulated by affective interchanges. Infants and parents are known to have built-in capacities for initiating, maintaining, and terminating social interactions (Brazelton, Tronick, Adamson, Als, & Wise, 1975; Emde, 1980; Izard, 1982; Stern, 1985; Termine & Izard, 1988). The work of Emde and Stern has begun to bridge the gap between empirical research and psychoanalytic theory by linking this knowledge of infant capabilities with the theoretical concept of the development of a sense of self.

Emde (1980) and Stern (1985) propose that throughout the day's activities, the infant's experience is monitored by the parent who interprets and assigns an affective meaning to it and then reacts. The baby begins to differentiate the parent's actions, how his mother acts as this relates to his state of arousal or his bodily experience, and then he incorporates this into his working models (Call, 1984). In essence, the mother responds to what she thinks and feels about what she hears and sees the baby doing. The baby perceives her actions in the context of his own needs and bodily experience and then incorporates this into his own subjective bodily experience. This patterned emotional signaling system is dependent on both partners' emotional availability, which is essential for the infant's ongoing development (Emde, 1980, 1988, 1989; Stern, 1985).

In the latter half of the infant's first year, the infant and his mother begin to engage in what Stern calls *affect attunement* (Stern, 1984, 1985; Stern, Barnett, & Spieka, 1983). This is a mutual matching of internal feeling states, not just matching or imitating overt behaviors. The shift of both the mother's and the infant's focus is to the inside, to the quality of the feeling that is shared. Affect attunement is a balancing of emotional tone between the parent and the baby. This balance promotes interest and pleasure in the current situation. If there is no balance the infant may disengage, showing distress, avoidance, and a turning off of affective interchange.

This process that the mother and infant repeatedly go through together reinforces the infant's gradual knowledge of his own affectivity and sense of self. Emde terms this the *development of the infant's affective core.* By linking his past and current experiences, the infant's affective core provides him with a sense of coherence and connection with others (Emde, 1988). If the parent's emotional availability is not optimal, it does not play the facilitating role in the infant's affective experience, limiting his emerging sense of self and his ongoing emotional development (Emde, 1988, 1989; Sameroff, 1989; Stern, 1985, 1984; Stern, Barnett, & Spieka, 1983).

Once again, the occupational therapist may be concerned with the impact of inefficient sensory modulation on the infant's overall internal feeling state. If he is not emotionally available because he is engaged in coping with inconsistent or overwhelming sensory input, he may not be able to put out the energy to participate in the attunement process. If his internal affective state fluctuates from situation to situation due to changes in the amount or variety of sensory stimulation but this is not apparent to his mother, how does she negotiate these differences in the infant?

A Synthesis of Theory and Clinical Practice

Greenspan and colleagues synthesized psychoanalytic theories and Piagetian theory with the infant/toddler clinical research to construct the developmental-structuralist approach (Greenspan, 1981, 1988; Greenspan & Greenspan, 1985, 1989; Greenspan & Lieberman, 1980; Greenspan & Lourie, 1981). This perspective describes infant emotional behavior in developmental levels which are broad, overlapping categories (see Table 6-2). It is based on the assumptions made from empirical research and theory: for example, from birth, the infant is capable of adaptive responses to the environment; behavior becomes progressively more organized during the first 2 years of life; infants show individual differences that are related to the development

Table 6-2 Emotional Milestones of Infancy and Toddlerhood

Age	Task
0 to 3 months	Homeostasis: To achieve internal regulation and establish interest in the world
2 to 7 months	Attachment: To become involved in the animate world
3 to 10 months	Somatopsychologic differentiation: To engage in purposeful communication with others; to begin to differentiate self from others
9 to 24 months	Behavioral organization, initiative, and internalization: To establish a complex sense of self through organization and internalization of multisensory experiences
18 to 48 months	Representational capacity: To create ideas and engage in emotional thinking by integrating experience over the sensory, emotional, and motor realms

Source: Data from Greenspan SI: Fostering emotional and social development in infants with disabilities. *Zero to Three*, 1988, 9(1), 8–18.

of coping skills and are precursors of basic ego functions (Greenspan & Lieberman, 1980).

The first level is one of *regulation*. One of the infant's first tasks is to be able to adapt to his external environment while maintaining his internal homeostasis. Over the first 3 months of the infant's life, he matures in his ability to regulate his states of arousal and develops rhythms of sleep and wakefulness. He begins to discriminate external events from his internal experiences. He then integrates these experiences with his actions to produce beginning adaptive responses, such as bringing his hand to his mouth for self-consoling. Once he is able to maintain smooth neurobehavioral regulation while interacting with his world, the infant is then able to become more involved in interpersonal relations.

The next stage, ranging from 2 to 7 months, is the beginning *capacity for human attachment.* This beginning relatedness to others is based on the infant's ability to experience and express affect and to use multiple sensory modalities in a reciprocal manner during his interactions. Establishing a primary attachment with a caregiver occurs parallel to the infant's growing interest in his inanimate world. Due to these events, the infant begins to participate more frequently in more complex communication patterns.

Somatopsychologic differentiation, from 3 to 10 months, follows the attachment stage. At this time, infant differentiation processes are occurring at both the somatic and psychological levels but these are not yet fully demarcated areas of the infant's experience and continue to have some areas of overlap. The infant begins to differentiate himself from the rest of his world in the affective, behavioral, and sensorimotor realms of experience. He knows one somatic-physiologic state, (i.e., hunger) from another. He begins to discriminate his caregiver's moods and communications, and he can discriminate one person from another. It is during this stage that the infant begins to know that he is a separate person.

Behavioral organization, initiative, and *internalization* characterize the period of 9 to 24 months as the toddler develops a complex sense of self. The child's internal sensations and images become organized into mental representations. He is able to string together several related behaviors rather than the simple causal linking of two events. Greenspan (1981, 1988) defines this as the child's ability to organize and evoke his internal multisensory experiences of animate objects, such as his mother. He internalizes his experiences in organized interrelated units within his emotional system. Because of these emotionally based internal representations, he is able to take initiative in exploring his world. This capacity depends on the continuing maturation of the infant's central nervous system and the availability of appropriate experiences.

The ability to integrate experience across the sensory, motor, and affective realms; to practice ideas through pretend play and language use; and to consistently differentiate the I from the not-I and to express emotions via language constitute the stage of *representational capacity, differentiation,* and *consolidation.* This process of using emotional ideas to guide behavior continues and matures between 18 months and 4 years.

In addition to these developmental levels, Greenspan (1988) has identified four interactional processes that occur between infants and parents. He suggests that these are essential for promoting healthy emotional and social development. These are processes that occupational therapists can facilitate during their intervention programs.

The first process is *attention and engagement.* This involves face-to-face contact, a sense of connectedness, and shared attention between the infant and another person within the context of warm feelings. It is very important that the infant be able to process sensory information so as to find the world interesting and pleasurable. The therapist may ask, how can I adapt my treatment activity to help the child engage in an affective sense? Am I encouraging a full range of emotional expression? How do I structure the environment to provide pleasure and interest? How can I connect with this infant in a meaningful way rather than just handle him?

A second process is establishing *intentionality* and *two-way communication.* This involves reciprocity or the give-and-take of information in both verbal and nonverbal ways. Emotional messages are communicated via movement and movement patterns, facial expression and gesture, vocal tone and rhythm, and combinations of all of these. Interventions may be aimed at facilitating processing of visual, spatial, and auditory information so that the child may interpret the affective cues of others.

Sharing of meaning is the third core process described by Greenspan (1981, 1988). The ability of the child to begin to use words, gestures, and pretend play to communicate his intentions is essential if he is to be able to create ideas and engage in emotional thinking on his own. Using symbols in an interchange with another person is considered crucial to developing personality characteristics such as creativity, imagination, and self-awareness. The therapist working with a child who has a sensory processing-based dyspraxia, for example, may want to encourage the child to incorporate his own emotional themes into the therapeutic activity to help promote this process much in the way that traditional intervention structures the environment but allows the child to set the course of activities.

The fourth process is *categorizing meanings.* Greenspan (1981, 1988) suggests that the child's ability to categorize emotional and impersonal experience is the foundation for basic personality functions. The most elemental category is the I and not-I. Others are what is real and pretend, what happens now versus in the future, and here and there. This ability to categorize meaning promotes a sense of reality, the ability to accept responsibility for one's own actions, and a stable mood. If inefficient sensory processing delays the child's first categorization of I versus not-I, then it might also impact the other areas of categorizing meanings. Would this then affect the child's emerging sense of reality and time as well as his regulation of mood?

A Sense of Self within the Context of Occupational Therapy

The previous sections of this chapter are intended to give the reader a small sample of the range of theoretical and clinical work related to early emotional development and to begin to look at the possible relationships between this body of knowledge and sensory integrative theory. The empirical research relating to the infant's capabilities generally supports the theorists' constructs. While it is important to examine theories and clinical research separately, it is most useful when it is integrated into a whole. Greenspan's work (1988) in this area can be very helpful to the occupational therapist in clinical practice. Another, visual representation integrating these perspectives can be seen in Figure 6-1.

Overall, these psychoanalytic theorists and the following clinical research support the importance of daily routines and interactions as the bases for providing appropriate sensory experiences that allow the infant's early emotional development to unfold. This nicely complements the therapist's knowledge of sensory integrative theory as proposed by Ayres.

General principles may be drawn from these perspectives for application when providing occupational therapy services to a young child with sensory processing dysfunction.

1. The parent or caregiver is the mediator of the infant's sensory and affective experiences. This implies that occupational therapy intervention must seek to involve the parent in treatment to the extent that the parent wishes. The parent is the primary influence on the infant's emotional life. The ways in which the parents interact with their child, modulate their emotional tone, and structure their physical environment will be of major significance.

2. The family's daily routines set the stage for providing the variety and richness of experiences that the infant needs. Therapy should seek to enhance these daily life activities rather than solely concentrating on the therapy session per se.

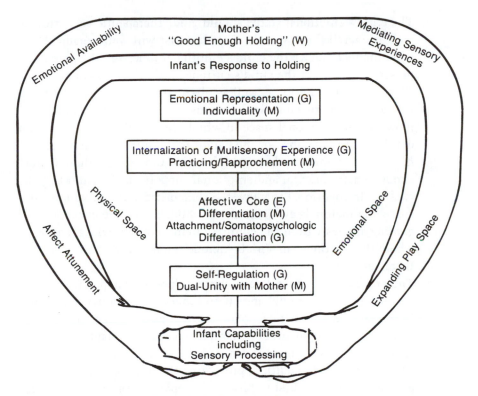

Figure 6-1 Linking psychoanalytic theory with infant research. "Good Enough Holding" in transaction with infant's capabilities provides the space for the infant's emotional growth. W = Winnicott, M = Mahler, G = Greenspan, E = Emde

3. Along with hands-on treatment and parent education, therapeutic intervention should acknowledge and support the parent's observations of the child's behaviors. The therapist enables the parent to interpret behaviors and problem solve ways of enhancing their interactions.

4. In addition to using standard and nonstandard tools to assess development and sensory processing, the therapist should plan to observe and assess the infant's emotional development. The developmental levels suggested by Greenspan's developmental-structuralist approach (1988) is one method. Emotional development must be evaluated in light of the child's developmental age as well as chronologic/corrected age and be put into the context of sensory integrative, neuromotor, or other developmental problems.

5. The child's emotional status should guide therapeutic activities as well as overall therapy goals. The therapist will want to adjust handling techniques, the child's emotional tone, and the parents' presence to support the child's current level of development. Through trial and error as well as observation of parent–infant interaction, the therapist looks for just the right amount of physical and emotional space in which the child's sense of self can develop. If the therapist or the parent is too intrusive, they are *holding* too tightly; if they *hold* the child too loosely, there is not enough environmental and emotional support for the child to explore. In traditional therapy, the therapist grades the amount of space and materials available to the child. This same concept of *grading* applies within the context of emotional development, where the treatment materials include the parent and therapist.

6. The process of emotional development does not happen in a vacuum but in an interchange with other aspects of development. In this way, traditional occupational therapy goals can support emotional development. For example, facilitating adaptive responses to environmental demands helps to organize an infant's emotional state. In addition, promoting the development of a body percept allows the child to physically separate from the parent and may support his emotional separation and emerging sense of self as an individual.

7. Just as sensory integrative therapy seeks to foster those processes that *support* skill development rather than *teach* skills, applying information about the child's sense of self in therapy should seek to foster that process rather than to teach the child to separate from his parent.

8. Therapy should seek to engage parent and child in mutually positive interactions. Interactive styles may be modified to accommodate the child's sensory processing difficulties, so as to support the infant's development of consistent, positive, internal working models of his parent.

9. The timing and rhythm of therapeutic activities must incorporate the dynamic cycling of parent–infant interactions. Through encouragement, information, and modeling of behaviors, the therapist seeks to promote the conversation-like patterns of mother–infant interactions and to enable the infant and parent to interpret each other's social signals.

10. Therapists must focus on their own internal affective state, and type and timing of expression, as well as physical distance from

the infant. Therapists seek to modulate their emotional tone in response to the infant's cues. The focus should be on engagement (rather than just handling), reciprocity, and establishing a shared meaning of experience using all forms of communication.

Clinical Applications

Following are descriptions of two children, Bryan and Alex, who were referred to occupational therapy for early intervention. These examples are intended to demonstrate how the therapist might integrate knowledge about early emotional development and its possible relationship to sensory integrative theory into the occupational therapy treatment plan for children and parents.

Bryan: Affect Attunement

Bryan was delivered at 31 weeks' gestation with a birthweight of 1000 g. During his stay in the neonatal intensive care unit, his medical problems included respiratory distress syndrome, apnea, retinopathy of prematurity, and hyperbilirubinemia. Mr. and Mrs. R., his parents, were both 33 years old, high school graduates, and worked outside the home. Bryan had a 4-year-old brother at home who did not have any health problems.

At 4 weeks' corrected age, Bryan was evaluated by occupational therapy using Brazelton's Neonatal Behavioral Assessment Scale, which provides information on an infant's ability to organize his behaviors in response to environmental input. While his visual and auditory orienting skills and motor skills were age-appropriate, Bryan showed poor regulation of his states of arousal. He was slow to rouse. When he did rouse, he quickly moved to a crying state and made few attempts to console himself. He had difficulty maintaining a quiet-alert state and in order to do so, he needed facilitation from the examiner. When he was alert, his orienting responses were noted to be somewhat delayed. Bryan's mother was present for the evaluation and independently commented on his apparent difficulty to maintain an alert, responsive state. He appeared to be overwhelmed by the sensory demands of interaction and of being handled; he coped by sleeping or crying. Together, Mrs. R. and the therapist discussed Bryan's strengths and his way of dealing with his world. They problem solved ways for modulating the amount of sensory input directed toward Bryan, thereby promoting periods of alert responsiveness. At this time, Bryan was in the regulation stage of Greenspan's model, working to modulate his states of arousal and not consistently available for interaction with his parents.

Mrs. R. brought Bryan for his first visit in the high-risk infant follow-up program when he was 4.5 months' corrected age. At the outset, she reported that the family was doing well. Bryan's brother was enjoying preschool. His father was involved in family activities after work and weekends. As Bryan's developmental assessment progressed, his mother shared with the therapist that she had not yet made plans to go back to work because Bryan was a very difficult infant and she did not feel right sending him to day-care.

Bryan's age equivalent scores on the Bayley Scales of Infant Development (Bayley, 1969) were 3 months. While his resting muscle tone was low, he showed increased extensor tone when active. He showed several fairly strong primitive reflexes. His head control was poor in all positions and he showed few antigravity movements. His movements were jerky and poorly controlled. He tended to fist both hands. Bryan did show nice visual and auditory responses but did not yet reach or engage in midline play. He vocalized in vowel sounds and showed interest, excitement, and frustration in his voice.

Clinical observations based on sensory integrative theory were that Bryan was very hypersensitive to changes in his position and in the environment. He became fussy, his movements became disorganized, and he startled easily. Once upset, he was difficult to console. When he was at his best, he showed direct eye contact and engaged in brief social exchanges. However, it was difficult to elicit these periods.

From this description of Bryan, it is apparent that he would benefit from direct therapeutic intervention based on traditional occupational therapy approaches for his developmental delays and abnormal movement patterns. There was, however, another area of concern for Bryan and his mother: Did his poor sensory processing abilities affect his affective experience? When asked about her concerns, she reported, "Bryan doesn't use his arms. He doesn't seem involved. He's not responsive. He is not like his brother was at this age." Bryan and his mother had not been able to engage in the reciprocal interaction and mutual regulation that is so important to the development of his sense of affectivity. Mrs. R. was not able to interpret his brief, difficult-to-elicit social signaling. They had no basis from which to begin to match their internal feeling states, to reach affective attunement. She did realize that Bryan was a highly sensitive boy but had not been able to help him modulate sensory information. He did not yet have his own methods of self-organization. Mrs. R. was able to recognize how she felt in response to Bryan's behaviors and had identified that she was becoming less and less emotionally available to him; however, she was not able to mobilize her inner resources to change the situation.

Intervention programming for this mother and child did indeed consist of traditional occupational therapy modalities and counseling for psychosocial support. However, another aspect of occupational therapy involved fostering

Mrs. R.'s observation of Bryan's strengths and sensitivities. She learned to adapt Bryan's environment in order to watch for overwhelming sensory input while giving him just the right amount and combination of stimulation to engage him. She observed how he responded to her when she modulated her handling and voice and play behaviors, and identified how she felt at these times. Through this mother–therapist mutual process, Mrs. R. began to see times when Bryan did respond in a positive way to her. She also realized that when Bryan shut out the therapist, it was related to his hypersensitivity, not to his dislike of the therapist. The traditional therapy approaches complemented this, Bryan began to more purposefully engage in interaction with his world as his body's movement patterns allowed.

At 10 months' corrected age, Bryan continued to be somewhat developmentally delayed; however, his movement patterns were more appropriate. He was increasingly able to engage in a social interchange without becoming overwhelmed. He continued to have times when he was unable to cope with the sensory demands of the physical and social world; however, his mother had learned ways to help him cope. She recognized his scared facial expressions (see Figure 6-2) and responded in a way that facilitated his coping and his emotional availability. She did not push him if he needed some distance from her (see Figure 6-3), but continued to be emotionally present for him when

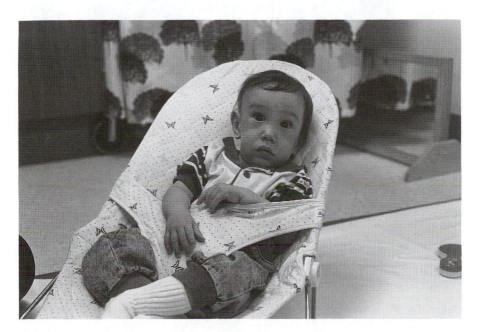

Figure 6-2 Bryan often appeared threatened or frightened, even by low-level sources of sensory stimulation

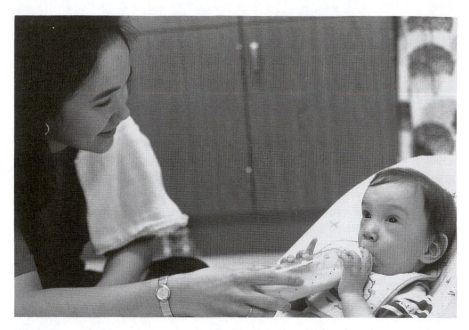

Figure 6-3 Mother modulates her affective tone and mediates her infant's sensory experience

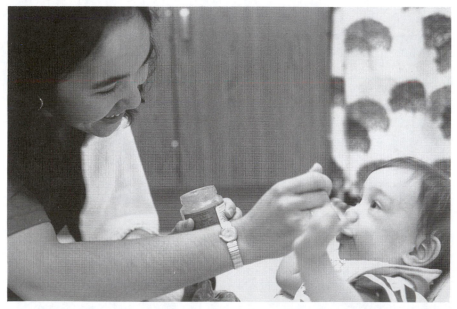

Figure 6-4 Mediating sensory input and matching internal feeling states supports a continuing positive relationship between mother and infant

he turned back to her (Figure 6-4). She not only accommodated her physical presence but also modulated her affective tone so as to bring out his strengths and interests. Now, together, they were better able to meet the next emotional challenge.

Alex: Emerging Sense of Self

At birth, Alex had meconium aspiration syndrome with subsequent respiratory distress syndrome and persistent pulmonary hypertension of the newborn. He developed severe bronchopulmonary dysplasia and also had difficulties with gastroesophageal reflux (GER). Due to his significant respiratory problems, his low pulmonary reserve for feeding, and his GER, Alex received a feeding gastrostomy prior to being discharged from the neonatal intensive care unit. Over the first several months at home, Alex was fed solely continuous feedings via gastrostomy and had significant problems with frequent reflux. He was rehospitalized several times for pneumonia.

Alex received in-home early intervention services for significant developmental delays. Once his medical status was more stable, an early interventionist began working with Alex on transitioning from tube to oral feedings, although reflux continued to be an issue.

When he was 16 months old, Alex and his parents, Mr. and Mrs. M., moved to a different part of the country and reestablished Alex's early intervention services. He received early intervention for his developmental delays in his home twice a week. In addition, he came to a center-based program for occupational therapy to work with him and his parents on transitioning from tube to oral feedings.

Alex gagged and cried when he saw a bottle, a spoon, baby food, or a bib. He was unable to inhibit his gagging and would begin to wheeze and turn cyanotic. At times he appeared to be on the verge of a bronchospasm. If he heard the word *mouth* or *teeth* he would tightly close his mouth. In general, he kept his tongue retracted and showed little movement of it. At times, he had reflux several times a day. He was still fed via gastrostomy but now in bolus form.

Alex was noted to have very low muscle tone with poor postural stability. His vocalizations were only throaty sounds. He had not yet developed even approximations of words. In addition, he was noted to be tactually and auditorally defensive as well as gravitationally insecure. Alex had difficulty coping with strangers and new situations.

Occupational therapy intervention included a variety of approaches. Keeping in mind that Alex was receiving developmental intervention at home, these intervention approaches were geared specifically to Alex's feeding abilities and to complement his in-home program. Behavior-shaping techniques were used to desensitize Alex to items that he associated with eating. Developmental activities were provided to promote increased proximal stability, movement, and communication. Since Alex's oral hypersensitivity appeared to be based in part on irregular sensory modulation, activities to promote more efficient sensory processing rather than just oral desensitization were introduced. Close contact was maintained with Alex's pulmonologist and gastroenterologist.

Alex's sensory processing irregularities, along with his motor, adaptive, and communication delays, significantly affected his emotional development. When he first came to occupational therapy, Alex needed to be in constant physical contact with one of his parents. Most often, his mother was present. His mother's presence was not just for physical support due to his poor sitting balance as the therapist could have given him that kind of support. But it was for his mother's emotional holding. If Mrs. M. tried to put Alex down on the mat without her contact, he became very distressed and unable to interact with anyone including her. He needed her firm holding to help him remain gravitationally secure and open to the environment's demands. So, at first, all activities were done in Mrs. M.'s lap. As he became accustomed to the therapist and the treatment room, he allowed his mother to put him on the mat but he still required physical contact.

As time passed, Alex made developmental gains in all areas and became better able to modulate his responses to sensory input. Alex was also able to move away from his mother, although he still needed her to be nearby. While it was evident that he looked forward to coming to therapy and genuinely liked the therapist, he could not go with the therapist to the other side of the room and leave his mother.

Finally at 26 months, Alex's sense of self as a separate person began to emerge. Emotional maturation occurred for him a few months after he made gains in the sensory processing, motor planning, and cognitive domains. Evidence of this was seen as he left his mother to briefly play in another room with a group of toddlers. In occupational therapy, he left his mother to explore in another part of the room. He actively organized the therapy equipment so that he could be in front of a mirror to practice such acts as taking a bite of food or climbing onto the swing while watching himself in the mirror. When the tasks were more demanding, such as coping with the sensory challenge of a new food texture or riding the swing in a different way, he drew his mother in closer and incorporated her into the activity (see Figure 6-5).

Alex's parents were able to slowly enlarge their holding to allow him just the right amount of physical and emotional space in which to play. Importantly, they were aware of his difficulties in sensory processing and, therefore, mediated his experiences of the world while encouraging him to move out a little further. When Alex needed close physical contact with one of them, they were available to provide the momentary comfort that he needed (see Figure 6-6). Their availability allowed Alex to separate after emotional refueling and to continue this *practicing* phase of his emotional development.

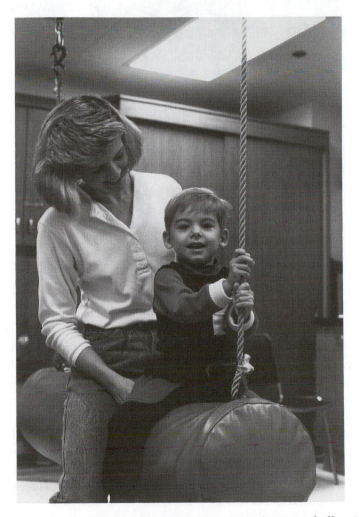

Figure 6-5 Drawing mother in for emotional support during a challenging activity

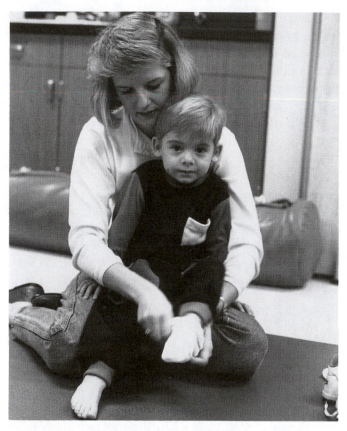

Figure 6-6 Emotional refueling when the environmental demand is stressful

Summary

While occupational therapists in early intervention acknowledge the importance of early emotional experience, little has been written in the occupational therapy literature regarding this aspect of the infant's and toddler's development. Yet, if occupational therapy is concerned with facilitating meaningful activity and skill development as the basis of occupational role acquisition, this realm must be included in intervention.

The integration of psychodynamic theories, recent empirical research regarding infant capabilities, and sensory integration theory provides one model upon which therapists may base their intervention (see Figure 6-1). The mother engaging in good enough holding of her infant provides emotional availability, mediation of sensory experiences in response to her child's reactions, and an expanding physical/emotional space to him. This process continually interacts with the infant's unique sensory processing abilities, self-regulatory abilities, temperament, and affective state. This continuous transaction provides the context in which the infant's affective core and his sense of self as a separate individual emerges (Sameroff, 1982, 1989). The child with irregularities in sensory processing may be on a different path, but with a parent who can provide for him all that *good enough holding* implies, he may still successfully negotiate his early emotional milestones.

When an infant's emotional development is affected by difficulties in sensory processing, the therapist should question the impact of this on his social-emotional development and adapt therapeutic activities accordingly. Occupational therapy intervention should be based on an understanding of this very significant aspect of the child's life and should seek to facilitate parent–child and therapist–child activities that enhance it.

References

Ayres, A.J. (1972). *Sensory integration and learning disorders.* Los Angeles: Western Psychological Services.

Ayres, A.J. (1979). *Sensory integration and the child.* Los Angeles: Western Psychological Services.

Barrett, K.C., & Campos, J.J. (1987). Perspectives on emotional development II: A functionalist approach to emotions. In J.D. Osofsky (Ed.), *Handbook of infant development.* 2nd ed. (pp. 555–578). New York: Wiley.

Bates, J.E. (1987). Temperament in infancy. In J.D. Osofsky (Ed.), *Handbook of infant development.* 2nd ed. (pp. 1101–1149). New York: Wiley.

Bayley, N. (1969). *Bayley scales of infant development.* New York: The Psychological Corp.

Bowlby, J. (1969). *Attachment and loss: Volume I attachment.* New York: Basic Books.

Bowlby, J. (1988a). *A secure base: Parent–child attachment and healthy human development.* New York: Basic Books.

Bowlby, J. (1988b). Developmental psychiatry comes of age. *American Journal of Psychiatry, 145,* 1–10.

Brazelton, T.B. (1982). Joint regulation of neonate–parent behavior. In E.Z. Tronick (Ed.), *Social interchange in infancy: Affect, cognition, and communication.* Baltimore: University Park Press.

Brazelton, T.B., & Cramer, B.G. (1990). *The earliest relationship.* Reading, MA: Addison-Wesley.

Brazelton, T.B., Koslowski, B., & Main, M. (1974). The origins of reciprocity: The early infant–mother interaction. In M. Lewis & L. Rosenblum (Eds.), *The effect of the infant on its caregiver* (pp. 49–76). New York: Wiley & Sons.

Brazelton, T.B., Tronick, E., Adamson, L., Als, H., & Wise, S. (1975). Early mother–infant reciprocity. In M.A. Hofer (Ed.), *Parent-infant interaction.* Amsterdam: Elsevier.

Bretherton, I. (1987). New perspectives on attachment relations: Security, communication, and internal working models. In J.D. Osofsky (Ed.), *Handbook of infant development*. 2nd ed. New York: Wiley.

Call, J.D. (1984). From early patterns of communication to the grammar of experience and syntax in infancy. In J. Call, E. Galenson, & R. Tyson (Eds.), *Frontiers of infant psychiatry*, Vol 2. New York: Basic Books.

Campos, J.J., Campos, R.G., & Barrett, K.C. (1989). Emergent themes in the study of emotional development and emotion regulation. *Developmental Psychology, 259*(3), 394–402.

Campos, J.J., & Stenberg, C.R. (1981). Perception, appraisal, and emotion: The onset of social referencing. In M.E. Lamb & L.R. Sherrod (Eds.), *Infant social cognition: Empirical and theoretical considerations*. Hillsdale, NJ: Lawrence Erlbaum.

Clark, F., Mailloux, Z., & Parham, D. (1989). Sensory integration and children with learning disabilities. In P.N. Pratt & A.S. Allen (Eds.), *Occupational therapy for children* (pp. 457–509). St. Louis, MO: C.V. Mosby Co.

Cohn, J.F., & Tronick, E.Z. (1988). Mother–infant face to face interaction: Influence is bidirectional and unrelated to periodic cycles in either partner's behavior. *Developmental Psychology, 24*(3), 386–392.

Crockenberg, S.B. (1981). Infant irritability, mother responsiveness, social support influences on the security of infant–mother attachment. *Child Development, 52*, 857–865.

Emde, R.N. (1980). Emotional availability: A reciprocal reward system for infants and parents with implications for prevention of psychosocial disorders. In P.M. Taylor (Ed.), *Parent–infant relationships*. New York: Grune and Stratton.

Emde, R.N. (1988). Reflections on mothering and on reexperiencing the early relationship experience. *Infant Mental Health Journal, 9*(1), 4–9.

Emde, R.N. (1989). The infants' relationship experience: Developmental and affective aspects. In A.J. Sameroff & R.N. Emde (Eds.), *Relationship disturbances in early childhood*. New York: Basic Books.

Fox, N. (1989). Psychophysiological correlates of emotional reactivity during the first year of life. *Developmental Psychology, 225*(3), 364–372.

Fox, N., & Davidson, R. (1988). Patterns of brain electrical activity during facial signs of emotion in ten month old infants. *Developmental Psychology, 24*(2), 230–236.

Fraiberg, S. (1980). *Clinical studies in infant mental health*. New York: Basic Books.

Gianino, A., & Tronick, E.Z. (1988). The mutual regulation model: The infant's self and interactive regulation and coping and defensive capacities. In T.M. Field, P.M. McCabe, & R. Schneiderman (Eds.), *Stress and coping across development*. Hillsdale, NJ: Lawrence Erlbaum.

Goldsmith, H.H., Buss, A.H., Plomin, R., Rothbart, M.K., Thomas, A., Chess, S., Hinde, R.A., & McCall, R.B. (1987). Roundtable: What is temperament? Four approaches. *Child Development, 58,* 505–529.

Greenspan, S.I. (1981). *Psychopathology and adaptation in infancy and early childhood: Principles of clinical diagnosis and preventive intervention.* New York: International Universities Press.

Greenspan, S.I. (1988). Fostering emotional and social development in infants with disabilities. *Zero to Three, 9*(1), 8–18.

Greenspan, S.I., & Greenspan, N.T. (1985). *First feelings: Milestones in the emotional development of your baby and child from birth to age four.* New York: Viking Press.

Greenspan, S.I., & Greenspan, N.T. (1989). *The essential partnership.* New York: Penguin Books.

Greenspan, S.I., & Lieberman, A.F. (1980). Infants, mothers, and their interactions: A quantitative clinical approach to developmental assessment. In S.I. Greenspan & G.H. Pollack (Eds.), *The course of life: Psychoanalytic contributions toward understanding personality development,* Vol. 1. Washington DC: DHHS Publication No. 80-786.

Greenspan, S.I., & Lourie, R.S. (1981). Developmental structuralist approach to the classification of adaptive and pathologic personality organizations: Infancy and early childhood. *American Journal of Psychiatry, 138*(6), 725–735.

Harlow, H.F. (1961). The development of affectional patterns in infant monkeys. In B.M. Foss (Ed.), *Determinants of infant behavior.* London: Methuen.

Isabella, R.A., Belsky, J., & von Eye, A. (1989). Origins of infant–mother attachment: An examination of interactive synchrony during the infant's first year. *Developmental Psychology, 25*(1), 12–21.

Izard, C.E. (1982). Measuring emotions in human development. In C.E. Izard (Ed.), *Measuring emotions in infants and children.* New York: Cambridge University Press.

Izard, C., & Malatesta, C. (1987). Perspectives on emotional development I: Differential emotions theory of early emotional development. In J.D. Osofsky (Ed.), *Handbook of infant development.* New York: Wiley.

Kagan, J., Reznick, J.S., & Snidman, N. (1987). The physiology and psychology of behavioral inhibition in children. *Child Development, 58,* 1459–1473.

Klinnert, M.D., Campos, J.J., Sorce, J.F., Emde, R., & Svejda, M. (1982). Emotions as behaviors regulators: Social referencing in infancy. In R. Plutchik & H. Kellerman (Eds.), *Emotions in early development, Vol. 2.* New York: Academic Press.

Kopp, C.B. (1989). Regulation of distress and negative emotions: A developmental view. *Developmental Psychology, 25*(3), 343–392.

Lester, B., Hoffman, J., & Brazelton, T.B. (1985). The rhythmic structure of mother–infant interaction in term and pre-term infants. *Child Development, 56,* 15–57.

Mahler, M.S. (1986). On the first three subphases of the separation-individuation process. In P. Buckley (Ed.), *Essential papers on object relations* (pp. 222–232). New York: New York University Press.

Mahler, M.S., Pine, F., & Bergman, A. (1975). *The psychological birth of the human infant.* New York: Basic Books.

Malatesta, C., Culver, C., Tesman, J., & Shepard, B. (1989). The development of emotion expression during the first two years of life. *Monographs of the Society for Research in Child Development, 54,* 1–2.

Minde, K., & Minde, R. (1986). *Infant psychiatry.* Beverly Hills: Sage Publications.

Rose, S.A., & Ruff, H.A. (1987). Cross-modal abilities in human infants. In J.D. Osofsky (Ed.), *Handbook of infant development.* New York: Wiley.

Sameroff, A.J. (1982). Development and the dialectic: The need for a systems approach. In A.W. Collins (Ed.), *The Minnesota symposium on child psychology: The concept of development,* Vol. 15. Hillsdale, NJ: Lawrence Erlbaum.

Sameroff, A.J. (1989). Principles of development and psychopathology. In A.J. Sameroff & R.N. Emde (Eds.), *Relationship disturbances in early childhood.* New York: Basic Books.

Stern, D.N. (1984). Affect attunement. In J. Call, E. Galenson, & R. Tyson (Eds.), *Frontiers of infant psychiatry,* Vol. 2. New York: Basic Books.

Stern, D.N. (1985). *The interpersonal world of the infant.* New York: Basic Books.

Stern, D.N., Barnett, R.K., & Spieka, S. (1983). Early transmission of affect: Some research issues. In J. Call, E. Galenson, & R. Tyson (Eds.), *Frontiers of infant psychiatry.* New York: Basic Books.

Termine, N.T., & Izard, C.E. (1988). Infants responses to their mothers' expressions of joy and sadness. *Developmental Psychology, 24*(2), 223–229.

Teti, D.M., & Nakagawa, M. (1990). Assessing attachment in infancy: The strange situation and alternate systems. In E.D. Gibbs & D.M. Teti (Eds.), *Interdisciplinary assessment of infants.* Baltimore: Paul H. Brookes Publishing Co.

Thomas, A., & Chess, S. (1977). *Temperament and development.* New York: Brunner/Mazel.

Tyson, P. (1984). Developmental lines and infant assessment. In J. Call, E. Galenson, & R. Tyson (Eds.), *Frontiers of infant psychiatry,* Vol. 2. New York: Basic Books.

Williamson, G.G., & Zeitlin, S. (1990). Assessment of coping and temperament: Contributions to adaptive functioning. In E.D. Gibbs & D.M. Teti

(Eds.), *Interdisciplinary assessment of infants: A guide for early intervention professionals* (pp. 215–226). Baltimore: Paul H. Brookes Publishing Co.

Winnicott, D.W. (1964). *The child, the family, and the outside world.* London: Penguin Press.

Winnicott, D.W. (1971). *Playing and reality.* New York: Tavistock Publications.

Winnicott, D.W. (1986). The theory of the parent–infant relationship. In P. Buckley (Ed.), *Essential papers on object relations.* New York: New York University Press.

7

□ □ □
□ □ □
□ □ □

Play: The Life Role of the Infant and Young Child

Janice Posatery Burke, MA, OTR, FAOTA

To the young child, play is life itself. Play fills mind and body, mentality, emotionality, and physical being. A child engrossed in play is inventive, free, and happy. Through the variety and depth of play, the child learns and grows. It is serious business; it is [his/her] world. For the adult, play is seen as recreation, something which only takes place in leisure time. Somehow the adult has learned to believe that play should only occur at a time when one is not working. (Evans, 1974, p. 267)

Play is a phenomenon that has intrigued many researchers, scholars, educators, parents, business persons, and inventors. As a society, we spend many hundreds of dollars investing in it, researching it, nurturing it, shaping it, and worrying about it. Literature tells us that play is powerful, has structure and a biology; it is make believe, imaginative, and symbolic; it may vary in form from free play to stereotypical play to gender- and cultural-specific play. The purpose of this chapter is to carve out the occupation-related nature of this multidimensional behavior so that occupational therapy intervention designed for infants, young children, and their families will have a strong base for creating occupation-forming behaviors.

The first part of the chapter addresses the theoretical and conceptual relationships of play and the domain of occupational therapy. It concludes by establishing a play-based perspective for this therapy. The second part of the chapter addresses assessment and intervention strategies designed for babies, young children, and their parents using an occupation-oriented family-centered care orientation.

Theoretical Perspectives of Play and Occupation

Addressing the Needs of Young Children

For some occupational therapists who work with young children and their families, the topic of play may often take on secondary importance in their intervention priorities. In such cases, the therapist may focus primarily on the atypical physical signs that are present in the child or on the more obvious dysfunctional patterns or behaviors that are emerging. With this perspective, the therapist uses play, or more precisely, toys, as motivators or modalities to encourage the child to move in a certain way or to calm, or to distract the child in order to apply a given type of intervention that the child might otherwise resist or protest. For example, the therapist who is interested in facilitating a quadraped position in an infant who has hypotonia may reach for the nearest toy to engage the child's visual attention while facilitating a desired position. The advantage of such an approach is that the therapist is able to use a toy to successfully distract the child from the physical handling that is being imposed on him and, thus, is able to affect a child's physical status. This is especially helpful for a child who finds physical manipulation unpleasant and something to be avoided because the play distraction may prolong the time in which he is willing to accept the handling. The disadvantage of such an approach is that because of the therapist's image of play as a diversion, she has failed to include into the treatment a whole genre of skill development that addresses the child's ability to become actively involved or occupied with the environment, both in mind and in body. These are skills that are critical underpinnings and supports for children as they enact their daily life roles. To use toys merely as objects of diversion is to miss an opportunity to learn how to engage in and elaborate in play with objects. Like the animals in primate studies, this is a missed opportunity to open up the joy of curious behavior and the importance of how to collect and store information that may be useful at another time.

The Hidden Dimension of Play

Traditionally, society has viewed play as the work of children, but that view is considered to be far too limiting. Play is more than a job to be completed and indeed has vastly different characteristics then those stereotypically associated with work. In the first place, play has an open-endedness that is not typically found in work. Play starts and, more important, ends when the player wishes it to rather than at an appointed time or preestablished end point. Additionally, its self-initiated, self-directed, almost limitless quality offers the player a flexibility that is not typically found in work or

Table 7-1 Dimensions of Play

1. As an opportunity for the child to grow and develop; to learn about physical, social, and emotional abilities and skills

2. As a mechanism for exploring and defining one's own motivation and achievement

3. Nonserious, pressure-free opportunity to perform for the process or feeling rather than the product

4. As an imaginary world for mastery over unmanageable aspects of reality

5. Activates an individual's exploration and sense of wonder

6. As a foundation and builder of interpersonal relationships

7. As a way of learning and developing interests, skills in concentration and in problem solving, and judgment

8. Arena for learning about adolescent and adult roles, as well as role behaviors

Source: Adapted from Caplan F, Caplan T: This issue. *Theory into Practice*, 1974, *13*, 267–272.

Table 7-2 Theoretical and Developmental Explanations of Play

Vantage Point	Explanation
Psychoanalytic perspective	• Wish fulfillment • Tension reduction
Cognitive/developmental perspective	• Medium for understanding child's conceptualizations about objects • Psychological function
Anthropological perspective	• Practice for adult social function • Cultural-specific
Competence perspective	• Effectance motivation • Drive to gain mastery in the environment
Biological/motor perspective	• Fine motor • Gross motor • Skill development • Cognitive maturation
Psychological perspective	• Emotional development and expression • Frustration, anger, pleasure
Social perspective	• Competition, cooperation for social interaction • Imitation, social conduct

in self-maintenance activities. A player can do whatever he wants to do; this may include changing the play at any time, restructuring it, or restarting it as the player wishes. More appropriately, the relationship between play and work involves the foundational skills that are developed during play activity. These occupation-related skills—namely the ability to manipulate objects, to problem solve, and to attend to the task at hand—are developed in play and later depended on in work.

Through play, children learn skills to support their roles as players, one of the first roles that a human assumes. As such, play behavior lays the groundwork for physical, psychosocial, and cognitive skills that are used and further developed in later roles. Success as a player will lead to success as a friend, coplayer, day-care participant, play group member, family member, and preschool/grade school student. The unfolding of these roles and their eventual influence on later childhood roles, including the roles of team member, part-time worker, apprentice, and, ultimately, worker, is a natural evolution (Burke, 1975).

An occupation-based view of play is built on basic notions concerning the importance of an occupation to an individual. This chapter gives consideration to the occupational perspective of the infant and the young child. In order to understand the relationship between play and occupation, the various explanations of play must first be considered. From there, explanations that are compatible with the philosophy inherent in the field of occupational therapy will be selected.

Framing Play for Occupational Therapy

Authors have described play using a wide range of metaphors and analyses. For many, the definition of play is multidimensional as illustrated by Caplan and Caplan (1974) in Table 7-1. The complexity and uncertainty of conclusive knowledge about play was viewed by Reilly (1974) as similar to that of moving through a cobweb. Explained from different perspectives (e.g., philosophy, evolutionary biology) and based on varying theories (e.g., psychoanalytic, sociological, psychological), professionals may see the purpose of play in vastly different ways (Table 7-2).

Reasons That Children Play

A Psychoanalytic Explanation

In looking at the conscious and unconscious motivation behind play, Freud believed that play was motivated by wish fulfillment in an effort to gain mastery over difficult and traumatic experiences. In observing and interpreting the driving motives behind play, the psychoanalytic perspective identifies three key forces. These forces are the drive to conquer unconscious fears, to work out anxieties, and to deal with difficult thoughts. Each force creates various drive states that can be resolved through play. Based on this theoretical perspective, play therapy is used as a method to prescribe and facilitate play experiences for the child who is having difficulty with specific emotions or experiences (Erickson, 1963; Millar, 1974).

Using a play therapy approach, the therapist seeks to provide materials and actions that will help children resolve conflicts in their unconscious. The child who needs to resolve a fear of needles may benefit by acting out a hospital scene using dolls and toy medical tools including toy syringes. A child recently burned in a fire may be able to overcome her fears by playing with fire trucks, alarm whistles, and puppets. Each of these examples illustrates the objective of play therapy. It is designed to help children deal with difficult or painful experiences, memories, or thoughts so that they are able to resolve the conflict and progress in their thoughts and behavior.

A Cognitive-Developmental View

Piaget's studies in the growth of reason and the processes of thought as it develops in children serve to exemplify a cognitive developmental view of play. Through long-term observational studies of his own children, Piaget derived a set of stages that he believed all children pass through as they interact in the world of objects and people. The stages are considered to be universal; that is, insured of their appearance regardless of cultural, ethnic, or racial factors. Children are expected to proceed through a stepwise progression of thinking that, in a sense, structures their interactional abilities with people and objects. Using this perspective, child's play is explained as behavior designed to facilitate mastery of thought and reason.

Concerned with the cognitive structure of the child, Piaget described the qualitative behavioral changes that are a product of maturation, social interaction, and experience, which are observable in play, school tasks, and language.

A Motor Explanation

A motor explanation for play stresses the biological, neurological, and kinesiological structures and functions that provide ready states for an infant and young child. Bayley (1969) and Gesell et al. (1940) and their colleagues set the major milestones of infants' and children's motor development and constructed developmental evaluations to identify those stages. Their use of the term *play* is limited to observable motor behavior as reflected in measurable categories of motor performance such as fine motor, gross motor, personal/social behaviors, and language skills. In addition to classical descriptions of stage-specific motor development, other factors that impact on motor performance are noted; for example, perception and memory.

A test examiner elicits motor behavior by using toys and novel objects, enabling her to collect evidence of and interpret the child's developmental stage. This perspective is limited in that the data collected from actual play give little opportunity for the tester to reflect on less visible, yet equally critical, factors that influence a child's ability to play. These would include qualities such as initiative to play, imagination, creativity, or playfulness.

An Occupation-Based View

Occupation forms a broad, organized framework reflecting the overall philosophy of occupational therapy for building a more detailed explanation of play. Using occupation as the organizer or frame of reference allows us to incorporate the various perspectives, models, and theories that form all the parts of our professional knowledge base, such as sensory integration and neurodevelopmental, multisensory, and developmental perspectives, that address the child as a player.

Like other roles that humans assume, success in the player role means that the child will experience feelings associated with productivity, satisfactory quality of life, meaningfulness, and value. For the infant and young child, play is the central focal point for learning about and interacting in the world. (See Figure 7-1.)

An occupational therapist, using the occupation-based perspective of play, observes, assesses, interprets, and intervenes in the child's role performance as a player as well as the other roles of the child (e.g., family member, brother or sister). Thus, intervention includes analysis of the environments that the child interacts in and the human and nonhuman objects the child relates to in everyday functioning.

In order to fully understand play as occupation, therapists need to understand how play shapes occupational roles and behaviors. More specifically, the occupational therapist needs to ask: What about play makes it such an important occupational phenomenon? What is the magic of play exemplified by the sense of well-being derived from playful activity? In addition, therapists need to know: What about the play phenomena is related to what we know about occupation? Drawing on similarities and comparisons between play and occupation will contribute to our understanding of the purposefulness or utility of play. By pursuing this line of inquiry, how humans develop goal-directed qualities based on play experiences and how they derive a sense of meaning and activity can be determined. Finally, an understanding of how

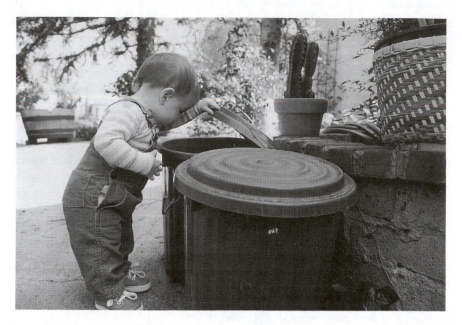

Figure 7-1 Play is the child's primary mode for learning about the world. (Photograph by Neil W. Goldstein.)

physical, cognitive, and psychosocial variations present in children with disabilities can be shaped to yield magical variations in play equal to those of the typical child (Burke, 1989).

The Occupational Therapist's View

The explanations of play and behavior that are put forth by scholars, researchers, and clinicians vary greatly in the rationales they provide for the impetus, motives, outcomes, and purposes of play. Each observation, focus, and interpretation is filtered through a knowledge base that is congruent with the specific professional discipline. For example, a physical therapist will observe and interpret play according to the child's physical abilities. Factors such as balance, muscle tone, strength, and endurance will be considered in the summary of the child's play. For the psychologist, play will be a reflection of the child's ability to relate to objects and people; in other words, a barometer of the child's self-control, anger, and happiness. A speech pathologist will observe the child's play and assess his verbal skills, auditory processing skills, and receptive and symbolic language abilities.

Even within a particular discipline, play interpretations may vary. The differences between disciplines result not from different knowledge bases but rather from the influence of a particular set of techniques and theory, or from the frame of references of the individual practitioner. For example, occupational therapists with a sensory integration perspective observe play and reflect on the child's ability to process sensory input and to maintain a state of organized behavior as a means of gauging the child's inner drive and as a way of eliciting an adaptive response. Using a neurodevelopmental perspective, the occupational therapist views play as a reflection of the child's muscular status and of symmetry, tone, and quality of the child's movement. Each frame of reference significantly influences the practitioners approach to the child. What is in question is whether the approaches that are represented in occupational therapy truly embrace the occupational nature of the child. If they do not, then it is likely that a therapist may be shortcutting their intervention mandate.

The Meaning of Play

Play has been classified and qualified by different cultures as it first emerges in young infants and later becomes more complex in the growing child, but regardless of the culture, play is a phenomenon that appears universally across the human species. Among those universal characteristics are the playful state, the motives for play, and the kind of learning that occurs in play. (See Figures 7-2 and 7-3.)

Bruner (1977) suggests that the main characteristic of play is not its content but its mode; that is, any activity can be play if the player so wishes. For example, certain tasks that one adult may take on as work, feeling the stereotypical drudgery and dullness that is associated with it, may be treated by another in a much lighter, more playful, and fun way. For some people, their spirit of playfulness is wholly retained as adults in their work lives as well as in their leisure lives. Observers of behavior at high-powered think tanks, in laboratories, and among inventors and athletes frequently highlight the quality of playfulness that surrounds creativity, problem solving, and the pursuit of excellence. The antics of workers in think tanks who shoot rubber bands at one another while seeking innovative solutions to complex problems, of toymakers who put themselves into the playful state of the would-be consumer, and of inventors and scientists who look for innovative solutions to problems by making a game about the problem all demonstrate the notion that it is not what you do that makes it play but rather how you do it. In the case of a 2-year-old child, each task that is encountered in a given day is approached in a playful way—mealtime, bath time, a trip to the food store, waiting for his mother or father to return from work. Each is approached with equal zest, exploration, curiosity, and playfulness. The child considers

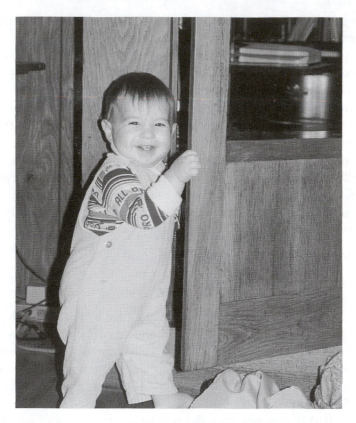

Figure 7-2 All play is characterized by its playful state. (Photograph by Neil W. Goldstein.)

the situation at hand to be an open invitation to explore and engage in interaction with people and objects.

As Bruner (1976) suggests, play is an approach to action that reflects how the person doing the activity feels about it. With playful and serious appearing at opposite ends of the continuum, individuals may demonstrate how they approach similar tasks differently. In such a circumstance, their behavior is not simply dictated by the form of activity but rather by their feeling about it. Given this definition, play is a state of mind that leads the player to act in a certain way when involved in various human and nonhuman interactions.

Robert White describes the motivation for play as a drive to have an effect on the world, to be competent. White (1959, 1971) postulated that humans engage in activity because they derive a positive feeling, or *effectance motivation*, from such behavior. This desire to interact with the environment is supported in the work of Csikszentmihalyi (1990) who suggests the notion of *the optimal experience* as a way of understanding what drives activity.

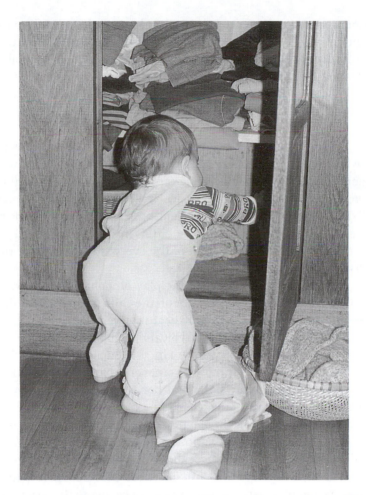

Figure 7-3 Play is motivated by a drive to have an effect on the world. (Photograph by Neil W. Goldstein.)

Defined as *flow*, he explains that "an activity that produces such experiences is so gratifying that people are willing to do it for its own sake, with little concern for what they will get out of it, even when it is difficult, or dangerous" (p. 71).

Play is more than simply having fun. Many important studies have yielded significant understanding as to the learning nature and survival value of play in primates. Primatologists such as Goodall (1986, 1990) and Suomi and Harlow (1971, 1976) have compiled and interpreted ethnographic data that give insight into the play of primates and the importance of it as a mechanism for learning behaviors necessary for adulthood. This includes acquiring behavior suitable for interacting within the given primate society such as the development of survival-oriented physical and manipulative skills needed for feeding, protecting, and building nests and shelters, and the self-control skills needed to mitigate aggressive tendencies and ensure that an animal will be included in social relationships that hold together a primate society structure.

Play in Children with Special Needs

Some important behaviors may be lost or neglected when play times are abbreviated or severely limited as is frequently the case with very sick infants and those who require long-term special programming (i.e., therapy services). For such a child there are greater agendas (i.e., therapeutic, medical/surgical) that will be sought and used for the purpose of making certain behaviors more feasible for the child. In these situations, play is a behavior that may or may not be part of the everyday repertoire of the child with a disability.

Other factors that may influence the play of a child with special needs include the physical limitations imposed on the child directly by the disability and those imposed on the child by medical intervention, as in the case of a child who is ventilator dependent. Atypical development, physical disabilities, and cognitive limitations may have a further impact on the child's ability to play. When play is limited by these internal and external factors, the ability to learn and the concomitant skills and behaviors that are by-products of playful experiences are also affected. Play experiences allow the child to manipulate objects and engage in playful actions in order to create an image of the world and the way all the various parts fit together.

Social constraints will also affect the infant player role and overall play development. One key factor that influences play development is low availability of peers and playmates. In part, this may be due to the social isolation that is experienced by individuals with disabilities and may be the result of natural discriminatory practices that are very much a part of these children's lives. People develop friendships as a part of their daily course of activity. For children with disabilities, the opportunity to interact with neighbors is significantly impaired if they do not attend the same school or are placed in different classrooms.

A disability or chronic disease may also affect the family and their given roles and behaviors. For some families, roles fail to develop; in others, they may emerge in dysfunctional patterns. This may occur due to the birth of an infant with special needs or the discovery of a disability or chronic disease during early childhood. Consider, for example, the difficulties in role development that may occur when parents have experienced a long separation from their infant or when the infant has specialized care needs that are provided by other adults. In such instances, parents may believe they have failed as parents because of the many unexpected circumstances surrounding the birth of their child (Barrera & Vella, 1987). For example, a premature delivery along with unsuccessful experience with breastfeeding and feelings of discomfort and awkwardness in handling a small or very ill infant may cause the mother to experience feelings of helplessness, hopelessness, and failure. Likewise, fathers may experience similar feelings of inefficacy and failure.

Play and Occupational Role-Based Assessment

A family-centered approach assesses the child within the given family culture, with an understanding that there are specific values and needs that are expressed within the context of the home environment and the family's role behaviors. The family-centered approach requires that therapists carefully recognize and include cultural values as they develop assessment and treatment programs.

Using an occupation-based perspective, therapists approach assessment from the standpoint of occupational role function and dysfunction. With this stance, the therapist collects assessment data along three lines of inquiry: (1) information about the child's role performance (player), (2) information about the parents' or caregivers' role enactment (parenting), and (3) information about the environmental supports and constraints to role performance. For an individual, role is an amalgamation of intraindividual, interpersonal, and external factors (Burke, 1975). In the instance of the individual child, play may be disrupted due to intraindividual factors, such as disease or disability; interpersonal factors, such as maternal deprivation, abuse, or neglect; and/ or external factors that are present in the environment. For the parent, role disruption may be due to intraindividual factors (e.g., anxiety, stress, or depression); interpersonal factors (e.g., chemical abuse or relationship problems); and/or external factors (e.g., the environment). Family-centered evaluation uses interviews, history-taking, observation, extrapolation, and analysis of play information from performance-based assessment instruments to assemble relevant information.

A family-centered care perspective implies that the family be part of the assessment and any ensuing treatment program. Given this perspective, a therapist needs to go beyond simply including a family member in the assessment as a source for information. This limited level of inclusion does not fulfill the family-centered criteria. Indeed, the therapist will need to carefully elicit information from family members directed by their concerns and work in close alliance with the family to decide on assessment strategies that best uncover relevant data.

By learning about the kinds of questions families have about their children, a therapist may also learn what kinds of information they are interested in learning from an assessment. For example, a therapist receives a referral for a 6-month-old baby who receives gastrostomy feedings. The referring public health nurse is concerned about the child's oral-motor abilities as she prepares the child to take food by mouth. On the first visit to the child's home, the therapist finds that the mother and the aunt have questions about the child's ability to see them and visually focus on objects as well as his reluctance to maintain a sitting position on his own. After the initial meeting with the child, the occupational therapist is primarily concerned about the child's lack of interest in his environment and general irritability in response to objects and to people. If the therapist in this case is to be truly family-centered in her assessment approach with this child, what does she do? Does she follow the requests of the referring nurse, does she answer the questions from the family, or does she follow her own intuition as to the primary problems? Family-centered assessment calls for open recognition of these three areas of concern, and respect for the importance of parental preference for guiding decisions that are made.

In this section a variety of assessments designed to assess role behavior will be reviewed. For the infant and toddler, instruments that address the role of player will be investigated; for the parent, assessments that focus on parent roles will be addressed; and, for the environment, tools that yield information on supports and constraints that affect role behavior will be discussed.

The Play History

Takata's "The play history" was first published in 1969, further elaborated in 1974, and later submitted to validity and reliability testing (Behnke & Fetkovich, 1984). Takata, an occupational therapist, developed this assessment tool as a result of her graduate work at the University of Southern California where she studied with Mary Reilly, the primary architect of occupational behavior. Using an interview format, the assessment seeks information on the materials, actions, people, and settings that are part of the child's everyday world. By eliciting this information from the child's parents and primary caregivers, the therapist is able to interpret findings using a taxonomy of play. The taxonomy was designed to allow the child's play to be analyzed and compared to typical developmentally derived examples of play behavior.

With experience, the interview will take 1 to 1.5 hours to complete. The interview uses a semistructured, open-ended format. A basic set of questions, which may be rearranged based on the flow of the session and the content of the information that is being given, are asked. The parent or primary caregiver is given an opportunity to answer these questions with descriptive responses rather than simply a yes or a no response. For example, when asked about the child's favorite play things, the parent describes the kind of toys the child likes as well as the kinds of things the child does with her favorite toy. The therapist questionnaire is designed to include (1) the questions to be asked, (2) the cues as to the type of information to be elicited, (3) the yield for the question, and (4) examples of probes so that adequate information to analyze the responses is collected.

Following the interview, the answers are organized and analyzed on a worksheet according to the child's assigned epoch of play. The therapist assigns the child to an epoch based on age expectations and on developmental and behavioral evidence. The therapist completes a worksheet assigning information to categories of *evidence*, or *no evidence*, or *no opportunity* to support the information that has been compiled. When a child engages in play that is expected and there are materials, actions, people, or settings to support that play, then the behavior is assigned to the *evidence* category. When there has been no mention of a particular play behavior, it is assigned to the *no evidence* category. In the event that a family does not provide materials, actions, people, or settings to promote a certain behavior, then it is assigned to the *no opportunity* category. This may be the case in situations where, for example, a child lives on a busy street and is not permitted to ride a trike, or may have skin allergies that do not allow her to experience a wide range of tactile materials. As evidence regarding the child's play behavior is analyzed, it is possible to formulate a profile of the child's strengths and weaknesses and to develop a treatment plan, or what Takata (1974) calls a *play prescription*.

In describing each epoch, Takata (1969) designed a strategy for looking at what she called *elements* of play behavior across age spans. Together with consideration of the age-appropriate materials, actions, people, and places for the child, Takata described what she called the *emphasis* of the epoch. In this way, she called attention to the key areas of skill acquisition and activity during each play epoch (Table 7-3). Additionally, Takata addressed the idea of *play style* as a way of describing individual variation in preferences, tempo, and rhythm of play, quality, and quantity of play experiences (Takata, 1969, 1974). This is an important notion that recognizes the individual differences that are uniquely human.

The Play Scale

In addition to observing the child's play history, a therapist may find it helpful to directly observe the child's play. A second play taxonomy, the Play Scale (Knox, 1974) was designed for this purpose. Like Takata, Sue Knox designed the assessment tool in conjunction with her graduate work with Mary Reilly at the University of Southern California. The assessment uses naturalistic observation to evaluate the presence of specific play behaviors within the domains of space management, material management, imitation, and participation. Observed behaviors are recorded on an observation

Table 7-3   Takata's Play Epochs

Epoch	Emphasis
Sensorimotor 0 to 2 years	Emergence of independent play Exploration play based on trial-and-error behavior
Symbolic and simple constructive 2 to 4 years	Parallel play Emergence of sharing Simple pretense and simple constructive play

Dramatic and complex constructive
    and pregame
    4 to 7 years
	Emergence of cooperative play
	Materials for constructive play
	Dramatize reality
	Skill and tool use

Games 7 to 12 years	Complex constructional play Sports and play with rules Competition and cooperation in play
Recreation 12 to 16 years	Team play Special interest and hobby groups

grid that is divided into these four categories across yearly increments. The Play Scale was also subjected to validity and reliability studies (Bledsoe & Shepherd, 1982; Harrison, 1984).

The Play Scale involves the therapist observing the children in their own environments and recording observations of play behaviors. Using a +, −, and an N.O. notation, the therapist tabulates information regarding the range of play behaviors that a child engages in during periods of play. The results of the observation are analyzed with comparisons made across the domains of play as well as across age spans. The therapist is then able to compute a play age, determine if the child is playing at age expectancy, and decide whether the play behaviors that are exhibited are relatively consistent across domains. Play that is analyzed to be below age expectation may signal an overall developmental delay. Play that is unevenly developed across the dimensions and age levels may provide evidence of particular performance dysfunction. In both cases, treatment objectives are derived from the assessment findings.

Play Observation Guide

Designed by Mulrooney & Schaaf (1990) as a further extension of their Family-Centered Care Framework (Schaaf & Mulrooney, 1989), the Play Observation Guide provides a more elaborate system for observing and analyzing the playful components of a child's environment, the family or caregiver, and the child. Each of the three categories are further analyzed according to subcategories. When considering the environment, the therapist is concerned with human and nonhuman factors; in regard to the family or caregiver, the emphasis is on routines, habits, and roles that are enacted and on values, interests, and goals that are inherent in the family. In observing a child, the emphasis is placed on performance skills, routines, habits, and roles that are enacted and on interests, motivation, and attention that are observed in interactions with objects, people, and the environment.

A Classification Grid

Linda Florey, also a part of the University of Southern California cadre of occupational behaviorists, compiled an additional classification of play and play development. Florey's guide (1971) was developed based on a review of the literature of developmental studies. In her analysis, Florey divided play into the categories of human objects and nonhuman objects, with 11 age increments beginning from birth to 6 months of age and following through to 9 to 11 years of age. The play behaviors that were considered part of the human grouping included play with parents, peers, and self. Play that was considered nonhuman fell into three types for grouping (see Table 7-4). In later work by Florey (1981), she continued with her concern for play by analyzing data from studies of play to yield another set of clinical guidelines. Useful in informal observation of child's play, Florey's work is particularly helpful to therapists when they are generating program guides or treatment plans.

Parent/Teacher Play Questionnaire

The Parent/Teacher Play Questionnaire (Schaaf, Merrill, & Kinsella, 1987) was developed in conjunction with a single case study to evaluate the changes in play behavior in a child receiving a sensory integration

Table 7-4   Florey's Classification of Play Development

Type of Play	Nonhuman Objects
Type I	Objects that change shape and form when manipulated (e.g., paints, clay, sand, and water)
Type II	Objects that change shape and form when manipulated and combined (e.g., beads, blocks, and craft and construction materials)
Type III	Toys that do not change shape or form when manipulated (e.g., balls, stuffed animals, dolls, cars, trucks, and play figures)

treatment program. The areas of consideration on the questionnaire include the child's activities during unstructured or free time, the types of choices that are made in play, the duration of play, the types of preferred play spaces, the amount and kind of interaction the child has with play peers, and the child's preference for sensory-based play experiences.

Important assessment data about play behavior are also available from performance-based testing that is completed by an occupational therapist. Using careful observation during testing and analysis of test results, a therapist will be able to extract critical information regarding infants' and young children's reactions to situations and skills that are necessary prerequisites of play. This would include consideration of the child's ability to focus his eyes on people and objects; to use his hands to reach out and swipe at objects; to be comforted, aroused, or upset by touch; and to react appropriately to sound and other sensory experiences. This information can be assembled to support a therapist's hypothesis regarding an infant or young child's successful or dysfunctional role behavior and to support evidence collected from the play assessment. Instruments such as the Miller Assessment of Preschoolers (Miller, 1982) and the Peabody Developmental Motor Scales (Folio & Fewell, 1983) are performance-based tests that provide some information about the child's play skills.

Parent or Caregiver Interview

A variety of parent questionnaires, as well as informal inquiry and rapport building assist the therapist in developing insights into the parent's view of their role acquisition, role enactment, and role satisfaction, as well as their priorities and preferences for the child's play development.

The Play Observation Guide (Mulrooney & Schaaf, 1990) outlined in the child portion of this section on assessment may be useful to guide questions and observations regarding family or caregiver skills, routines, habits, roles, interests, goals, and values. By gleaning information in these areas, the therapist may be able to help a parent find ways to identify and fulfill meaningful roles.

In addition to role acquisition, parents may find few ways to interact, have fun, and play with their child that they define as meaningful. Parent and caregiver values will significantly influence priorities for certain preferred play behaviors and the family-centered approach supports assessment that will reveal this information (Table 7-5). For example, take these three different family value priorities. One family may highly value books and reading and be concerned that their child has no interest in and no strategies for interacting with books. In another family, the father and mother may feel that roughhouse play is highly desirable. In a third family, messy play with food is considered

Table 7-5 Designing Family-Centered Play Prescriptions

What kinds of interactions do the child and family enjoy?
• Play with others
• Self-directed play
• Play initiated by someone else
• Play sustained by someone else

Who else is present in the home and how is that experienced by the child?
• Ages of other children
• Behaviors of family members
• Schedules of family members
• How and what they play with
• Involved family members
• Uninvolved family members

the perfect play for their child—its absence from their child's play repertoire may make the family feel sad and depressed, signalling that the child is abnormal and different. This type of information is best revealed in informal interviews with parents. Formal assessment is inappropriate as the intent is *not* to evaluate a family's behavior in relation to other families in order to determine whether the family is functioning within some sort of normal zone. Rather, the purpose of such information is to assess what is important to the family in order to help them as they devise ways to realize their goals.

In addition to defining family play preferences, the family should assess their own interests and willingness to participate in therapeutic programming. Do parents want recommendations for their own or a caregiver's use? Do the parents want strategies and even home treatment programs to engage their child in or would they prefer to keep their interactions with their child separate from therapeutically derived strategies? If they wish to include therapeutic activities in their interactions, then it will be essential to incorporate their play preferences into fun and meaningful therapeutic ideas for home use.

The Environment

A complete play assessment includes information about the child's environment. The environment is viewed as a catalyst in the facilitation of play behavior that will ultimately enhance the competence of the child and family members in their respective occupational roles (Schaaf & Mulrooney, 1989). Occupational therapists are able to make use of the environment to create challenges, provide organization, develop an inner drive, self satisfaction and a pattern of successful interaction in individuals with special needs (Burke & King-Thomas, 1989). Consideration of the environmental complexity, presence of novelty and variety, and the relationship of play and the play environment are all applicable to assessment and intervention at the environmental level.

Infants and young children interact most commonly in the home and day-care or preschool environment; therefore, these environments tend to be the keypoints of assessment by occupational therapists. For assessment and treatment issues, the therapist analyzes the most frequently used environments in order to determine the animate and the inanimate characteristics that are present in each setting. The goal is to assess the influence of these characteristics on the physical, mental, cognitive, and social aspects of the child's and parents' occupation (Burke & King-Thomas, 1989).

Play as a Framework for Treatment

The Infant and Young Child

With primary roles of player and family member identified as high-priority, treatment is designed to encourage successful enactment of these identified roles. As in a typical occupational therapy approach, simultaneous consideration is given to the whole child. With a family-centered approach to the player role, the child's strengths and weaknesses are weighed in relation to social, sensory, motor, cognitive, and language behaviors and are used to design activities that emphasize strengths to enhance areas of need (see Table 7-5).

The Parents or Caregivers

The playful interactions that occur, or could potentially occur, between parent and child offer a wealth of opportunity for the therapist. Using an occupation-based perspective of the parent or caregiver roles includes paying attention to the parent as a player and a nurturer within the family's culture, values, and needs. Treatment focuses on enhancing competence in these roles. By using play as the mode of interaction, the parent or caregiver helps the child to develop specific skills, to enhance her overall role performance, to develop her own role satisfaction while staying within a framework of playfulness and fun. For example, in the game of peek-a-boo, a parent is able to engage the child in an activity that facilitates tactile, social, visual, cognitive, and language development. In addition, the child learns the player role. For the parent, the game serves as a mechanism to enhance satisfactory parenting through play and to increase the parent's emotional bond with the child.

Table 7-6 Rules for Designing a Play Experience

Consider the following when designing a play experience:
- Toys that match a child's capabilities
- Toys chosen based on individual child's response as overstimulated or understimulated
- Toys to arouse and stimulate curiosity
- Age/stage appropriate materials
- Opportunities for success, to build confidence and self-esteem
- Opportunities to see others and learn from them
- Places that are playful
- Individual child preferences/styles
- Presence of novel objects

Environments

Designing environments and material and emotional experiences for the child and family provides a catalyst for facilitation of play behavior and enhances the child's and family's competence in their respective roles. Successful intervention requires examination of factors that influence the child, the family, and the environment and their fit to developmental stage guidelines and play expectations. For example, a simple environmental adaptation (e.g., an adaptive switch for a toy) can enable the child to become more successful and independent during play, and also allow the parent to interact with the child when they play together. By facilitating play with the toy, the parent successfully engages the child in the occupational role of player; facilitates the child's interaction with the environment; and promotes social, cognitive, and skill development. The parent, in turn, experiences positive feedback from the child, which leads to feelings of success and satisfaction in their role as parent.

Therapists may contribute significantly to an infant's or toddler's play development and to a parent's role development as they lend their expertise to the design of play settings and selection of play materials that stimulate play behaviors (see Table 7-6). By influencing factors such as the placement of toys and their availability, the therapist increases the likelihood that the toys will be used. Toys need to be placed where they are within easy reach of the child; for example, on floor level shelves, in shallow baskets or boxes, or on the floor. By observing how a child best obtains a toy, whether she knocks it over to get it within reach, rolls to it, or needs adult assistance, the therapist can determine best placement strategies for their accessibility.

The use of additional supports or adaptations is also critical to ensure toy use and playful interaction. For example, by adding a simple adaptive switch to a toy, a child has the potential to experience and learn from a variety of play experiences, to understand cause-and-effect relationships, to successfully and independently play, and to engage in play with a parent. Thus, this environmental adaptation facilitates the child's competence in the role of player as well as allows the child to successfully interact with the environment to promote development. The parents, through play with the child and the adaptive toy, experience positive feedback and feel successful and satisfied with their interaction.

Infants and toddlers are stimulated in their play when there is novelty in the arrangement of their environment. The use of play containers, such as baskets, boxes, and aluminum pans, present situations that arouse curiosity, exploration, and manipulation. Play spaces that have easy-to-move objects (e.g., small tables, beanbag chairs, assorted containers) are best utilized when they are frequently rearranged, added to, and taken from in an effort to keep the environment interesting.

Novelty and Variety in Toys

The use of novelty and novel objects is perhaps one of the most potent ways to influence play. Infants and toddlers are attracted to new materials to manipulate, to various arrangements of those objects in unexpected ways, and to different combinations of those objects. Cereal boxes, plastic soda bottles, assorted food containers, or other small boxes and packaging materials that are clean and safe to the touch with no sharp surfaces or edges provide an endless supply of intrinsically motivating play objects for young children. Typically, these objects remain of interest to the child as long as they remain intact. When they are lost or broken, they are replaced with other novel objects; thus, a whole new round of manipulation, exploration, and curious behavior is instigated. Novelty brings spontaneity, tapping a child's inner drive or his effectance motivation.

Along with novelty, variety has an important relationship to play. When familiar objects are found in predictable places, a child habituates to their presence. Much can be said for the positive value of rotating toys into storage and play space in regular intervals. Closets, basements, and even toy chests or storage boxes are helpful for moving certain toys out of sight.

Playfulness in Everyday Interactions

Play does not occur when time constraints, emotional or physical fatigue, and stress are present; to play, one needs freedom from pressure.

Frequently, parents and caregivers may only have limited opportunities to participate in playful interactions with their children. They may not feel that they have the physical resources they need to play. Therefore, in addition to addressing play environment and materials, the therapist and parents may wish to focus on the physical behaviors contributing to their role-restricted behavior. This may include intervention to address work simplification, body mechanics, and role balance. In a study conducted by Johnson and Deitz (1985), time spent in child care activities by mothers of children with physical disabilities was examined. When compared to their peers, mothers who cared for children with special needs spent less time in play and social interaction activities. By devising favorite times to play and materials for play, as well as directing their attention to stimulating the mood for play, parents may find themselves involved in more playful situations. One of the ways in which the playfulness state can be evoked is by removing the care and worry of how the activity is done and, instead, enjoying it for what it is. Toys that include the elements of surprise and spontaneity will also increase the potential for smiling and laughing.

Finding Ideas for Play

Ideas for play are everywhere. Opportunities to observe infants and toddlers in their daily situations at parks, in their play spaces, and out with their parents in shopping malls and restaurants can allow parents and caregivers to collect ideas on play. Many of the trade books written for parents and preschool teachers will also provide ideas that can appropriately be adapted for younger audiences (Table 7-7). The housewares section of a store

Table 7-7 Sample Play Materials and Games for the Developing Infant and Toddler

0 to 4 months
  Colorful mobiles
  Dangling toys
  Musical carousels
  Finger play
  Games moving arms and legs
  Rattles
  Rubber or plastic rings
  Vocal play as in talking to baby
  Large black and white or brightly colored simple pictures

(continued)

Table 7-7   *Continued*

4 to 8 months
  Plastic measuring spoons
  Pots and pans
  Yarn pom-poms
  Cereal for finger feeding
  Nonbreakable mirror
  Colorful plastic cups
  Textured balls
  Squeeze toys
  Balls
  Stacking toys
  Nesting toys
  Take-apart toys and play materials
  Water play
  Peek-a-boo type games

9 to 12 months
  Soft toys
  Bathtub play with toys that float
  Toys to fill and empty
  Large beads, spools for stringing
  Cloth or cardboard books
  Beanbags
  Playground exploration

1 to 2 years
  Chasing and hiding games
  Imitation play
  Play phone
  Soft toys
  Bathtub play with squeezing and pouring toys
  Toys to hammer
  Climbing on one step
  Pull toys
  Wooden and large cardboard blocks
  Toys with screw tops or plastic nuts and bolts
  Dropping shape toys or disks through slot in box
  Low sliding boards
  Sand play
  Water play
  Large crayons
  Books
  Sound-producing toys (horns, drums, toy record player)

2 to 3 years
  Toy materials for imaginative/imitative play
  Dolls

Table 7-7 *Continued*

Dress up clothes
Household toys (small broom, toy kitchen, realistic moving objects like toy
  blender)
Water play with sponges, containers, doll clothes, soap, straws, or bubble blowers
Play-Doh
Paints—finger paints, tempura paints
Puzzles—simple shape
Little toys (cars, trains, animals, and people)
Cutting with children's scissors
Playgrounds for climbing
Large balls to kick and throw
Wagons and wheelbarrows
Wheel toys with pedals (Big Wheels, trikes, cars)
Sand play with sand toys and shovels
Walking on balance beams
Roughhouse play
Short field trips (zoo, pony rides, carnival)

or the family's kitchen cabinets are readily available resources of inexpensive play objects. Therapists in early intervention programs or community programs for young children often maintain lists of their favorite toys and play activities.

Table 7-8 Questions to Be Answered Through the Study of Play

Clinic-Based Questions
- Are we able to teach play?
- What kinds of play encourage development?
- In what kinds of settings should play be taught?

Theory and Research Questions
- What is the function of play?
- How are playmate preferences developed?
- What kinds of sex differences are present in play?
- What kinds of play signals do children use to indicate their interest in playing
  with others?
- What behaviors or characteristics result from individual play deprivation?
- What is play in adulthood?
- What rhythms and patterns do children use in play? (approach/withdrawal, brief
  contact, rough and tumble)

Summary

As ways of interacting in play with children are reflected upon and refined, the true nature of play will undoubtedly be discovered. In these ways, the answers to the set of questions in Table 7-8 can be uncovered. What are the signposts that indicate a person is playing? How can the pleasure of the play experience be incorporated into unconnected behaviors traditionally thought to lack a quality of play, behaviors such as work? These and other similar inquiries found in Table 7-8 will lead to a rich and full understanding of this unique, satisfying, and totally involving activity known as play (Burke, 1989).

Suggested Readings

American Occupational Therapy Association (AOTA). (1986). *Play: A skill for life.* Rockville, MD: Author.

Burtt, K.G., & Kalkstein, K. (1981). *Smart toys for babies from birth to two.* New York: Harper & Row Publishers.

Gordon, I.J. (1970). *Baby learning through baby play.* New York: St. Martin's Press.

Hagstrom, J., & Morrill, J. (1979). *Games babies play.* New York: A & W Visual Library.

Leach, P. (1977). *Your baby and child.* New York: A.A. Knopf.

Lear, R. (1977). *Play helps: Toys and activities for handicapped children.* London: Heinemann Health Books.

Levy, J. (1973). *The baby exercise book.* New York: Random House.

Linderman, C.E. (1979). *Teachables from trashables: Homemade toys that teach.* St. Paul, MN: Toys 'n Things Training and Resource Center. (Distributed by Gryphon House, P.O. Box 217, Mount Rainier, MD 20822.)

Marzollo, J., & Lloyd, J. (1972). *Learning through play.* New York: Harper & Row Publishers.

Newton, E., & Newton, J. (1979). *Toys and play things: In development and remediation.* New York: Pantheon Books.

Riddick, B. (1982). *Toys and play for the young handicapped child.* London: Croom Helm.

Taetzsch, S., & Taetzsch, L. (1974). *Preschool games and activities.* Belmont, CA: Tearon Teacher Aids, Pitman Learning, Inc.

References

Barrera, M.E., & Vella, D.M. (1987). Disabled and nondisabled infants' interactions with their mothers. *American Journal of Occupational Therapy, 41,* 169–172.

Bayley, N. (1969). *Bayley scales of infant development.* New York: The Psychological Corporation.

Behnke, C.J., & Fetkovich, M.M. (1984). Examining the reliability and validity of The Play History. *American Journal of Occupational Therapy, 38,* 94–100.

Bledsoe, N., & Shepherd, J. (1982). A study of reliability and validity of a preschool play scale. *American Journal of Occupational Therapy, 36,* 783–788.

Bruner, J. (1976). Nature and uses of immaturity. In J. Bruner, A. Jolly, & K. Sylva (Eds.), *Play—Its role in development and evolution.* New York: Basic Books.

Bruner, J. (1977). Introduction. In B. Tizard & D. Harvey (Eds.), *Biology of play.* Philadelphia: J.B. Lippincott Co.

Burke, J.P. (1975). A model of occupational behavior: The evolution of role, personal causation and socialization. Unpublished master's thesis, University of Southern California.

Burke, J.P. (1989). Variations in childhood occupations: Play in the presence of chronic disability. Wilma West Lecture, Occupational Science Symposium II: Co-occupations of Infants and Mothers. University of Southern California, Los Angeles.

Burke, J.P. & King-Thomas, L. (1989). The environment of the child: Assessment consideration, treatment/intervention implications. *AOTA practice symposium guide.* Rockville, MD: AOTA.

Caplan, F., & Caplan, T. (1974). This issue. *Theory into Practice 13,* 267–272.

Csikszentmihalyi, M. (1990). *Flow: The psychology of optimal experience.* New York: Harper & Row.

Erickson, E. (1963). *Childhood and society.* New York: Norton.

Evans, M.W. (1974). Play is life itself. The value of play for learning. *Theory into Practice. 13,* 267–272.

Florey, L.L. (1971). An approach to play and play development. *American Journal of Occupational Therapy, 25,* 275–280.

Florey, L.L. (1981). Studies of play: Implications for growth, development and for clinical practice. *American Journal of Occupational Therapy, 35,* 519–524.

Folio, R., & Fewell, R. (1983). *Peabody Developmental Motor Scales* (Revised Edition). Allen, TX: DLM Publishing.

Gesell, A., Halverson, H.M., Thompson, H., Ilg, F.L., Castner, B.M., Ames, L.B., & Amatruda, C.S. (1940). *The first five years of life.* New York: Harper & Brothers.

Goodall, J. (1986). *The chimpanzees of Gombe.* Cambridge, MA: Belknap Press of Harvard University Press.

Goodall, J. (1990). *Through a window.* Boston: Houghton Mifflin.

Harrison, H. (1984). Examining the reliability and validity of the preschool play scale with a disabled population. Unpublished master's thesis, Virginia Commonwealth University, Richmond, Virginia.

Johnson, C.B., & Deitz, J.C. (1985). Time use of mothers with preschool children: A pilot study. *American Journal of Occupational Therapy, 39,* 578–583.

Knox, S. (1974). A play scale. In M. Reilly (Ed.), *Play as exploratory learning: Studies in curiosity behavior.* Beverly Hills: Sage Publications.

Millar, S. (1974). *The psychology of play.* New York: Jacob Aronson.

Miller, L.J. (1982). *Miller assessment for preschoolers : Manual.* Littleton, CO: The Foundation for Knowledge in Development.

Moos, R. (1974). *Family environment scale.* Palo Alto, CA: Consulting Psychologists Press.

Mulrooney, L., & Schaaf, R. (1990). Play observation guide. Unpublished Assessment. Philadelphia: Thomas Jefferson University.

Reilly, M. (1974). Defining a cobweb. In M. Reilly (Ed.), *Play as exploratory learning: Studies in curiosity behavior.* Beverly Hills: Sage Publications.

Schaaf, R., Merrill, S., & Kinsella, N. (1987). Sensory integration and play behavior: A case study of the effectiveness of occupational therapy, using a sensory integrative approach. *Occupational Therapy in Health Care,* 4(2), 61–75.

Schaaf, R., & Mulrooney, L. (1989). Occupational therapy in early intervention: A family centered approach. *American Journal of Occupational Therapy, 43*(11), 745–754.

Suomi, S., & Harlow, H. (1971). Monkeys at play. *Natural History Journal of American Museum of Natural History, 80,* 72–75.

Suomi, S., & Harlow, H. (1976). Monkeys without play. In J. Bruner, A. Jolly, & K. Sylva (Eds.), *Play—its role in development and evolution.* New York: Basic Books.

Takata, N. (1969). The play history. *American Journal of Occupational Therapy, 23,* 314–318.

Takata, N. (1974). Play as a prescription. In M. Reilly (Ed.), *Play as exploratory learning: Studies in curiosity behavior.* Beverly Hills: Sage Publications.

White, R.W. (1959). Motivation reconsidered: The concept of competence. *Psychological Review, 66,* 297–323.

White, R.W. (1971). The urge towards competence. *American Journal of Occupational Therapy, 25,* 271–274.

Acknowledgment
With special thanks to my colleague and friend, Roseann C. Schaaf, MEd, OTR/L, who assisted in the design of this chapter (especially part 2) and who made available her library of papers and lecture materials.

8

□ □ □
□ □ □
□ □ □

Feeding and Oral-Motor Skills

Robin P. Glass, MS, OTR
Lynn S. Wolf, MOT, OTR

For most newborns and young children, feeding is an effortless function that is eagerly engaged in many times a day. The majority of children grow and thrive without assistance from the medical community. However, infants and toddlers who are at risk for developmental difficulties or who have been diagnosed with abnormalities may also have dysfunction in their feeding abilities. These problems might include poor intake, excessive time needed to feed, unusual feeding characteristics (e.g., abnormal oral-motor patterns or inappropriate progression of feeding skills), and physiological compromise associated with feeding. Although feeding dysfunction is often seen along with other medical or developmental problems, it may also be found in otherwise healthy infants and young children.

Feeding performance in the young child is intimately related to family functioning and family dynamics. Feeding provides an opportunity for early bonding and its success strengthens maternal confidence. Conversely, feeding dysfunction can erode maternal confidence, causing stress that may alter the mother–child relationship, and interfere with bonding. Alternately, dysfunction in family dynamics has the potential to exacerbate existing feeding difficulties or, at times, can be the primary etiology of a feeding problem.

Occupational therapists working in early intervention programs have the knowledge and the skills to make unique contributions to the treatment and management of feeding dysfunction in infants and young children, particularly within the context of the family unit. A background in neuromotor control, in the medical aspects of disease and disability, and in general child development must be combined with a solid foundation in human interaction and behavior in order to effectively manage feeding problems in this population.

This chapter reviews the developmental aspects of feeding and considers general concepts in the evaluation of feeding. Functional problems in feeding are discussed along with treatment strategies. Finally, nonoral methods of feeding are presented and discussed in relationship to oral feeding.

Developmental Aspects of Feeding

For infants and toddlers, changes occur in feeding as oral-motor skills become more sophisticated, as maturational changes take place in the relationship between breathing and swallowing, and as anatomic growth occurs. For these reasons, the young child, when compared to adults, has functional differences in feeding abilities. Knowledge of functional anatomy and the normal developmental sequence of feeding-related skills is needed as a foundation for providing high-quality early intervention services in this practice arena.

Anatomy

The structures that are involved in feeding, swallowing, and breathing are physically close in proximity and frequently share overlapping functions. The feeding structures provide a conduit for moving food to the stomach and include the mouth, pharynx, and esophagus. The breathing structures provide a conduit for air moving to and from the lungs and include the nose, mouth, pharynx, larynx, and trachea. This combined physical and functional arrangement often underlies the feeding disorders encountered in infants and in toddlers.

Schematically, this area can be thought of as beginning with two distinct channels—the oral and the nasal cavities. These two channels combine into one channel in the pharynx. They diverge again into two channels at the level of the larynx or trachea and the esophagus. Valve-like structures, such as the soft palate and epiglottis, serve to seal off areas of this system so that food and air are directed along the appropriate channel (Morris, 1982).

Anatomic Maturation

With growth, changes occur in the size and anatomic relationship of the oral, pharyngeal, and laryngeal structures. These changes are rapid during the first 12 to 18 months of life, then progress slows throughout the remainder of childhood resulting in less functional impact. One role of these structures is to provide stability for the functions of feeding, swallowing, and breathing. With anatomic changes, the manner by which stability is achieved also changes.

Methods of Achieving Stability

In early infancy, stability of the oral and pharyngeal area is achieved by the close physical proximity of the oral, laryngeal, and pharyngeal structures (Bosma, 1967). The larynx is located high in the throat, under the base of the tongue. The tongue fills the oral cavity and abuts the alveolar ridges and lips. There is a large amount of subcutaneous fat, including the sucking or fat pads, that provide the firm consistency and puffy shape to the infant's face and cheeks. These tissues, in combination with the anatomical configuration, form an exoskeleton that provides *positional stability* for oral and pharyngeal function (Bosma, 1972).

As the infant matures, the oral cavity enlarges, elongates, and the fatty tissue diminishes. *Postural stability*, through muscular contraction and the development of more rigid connective tissue, develops to provide the stability for the highly specialized movements of the lips, cheeks, tongue, and jaw, which are involved in chewing or in cup drinking (Bosma, 1967, 1972).

Changes in Size of Oral and Pharyngeal Cavities

In the newborn period, the mouth is a potential cavity as it is filled by the tongue with close approximation of the lips and cheeks (Bosma, 1980; Schechter, 1990). As the infant grows, the oral cavity enlarges and there is a downward elongation of the pharyngeal region. The larger oral cavity allows greater mobility of the lips, tongue, and cheeks and, therefore, the emergence of a wider variety of oral skills. As the pharynx elongates, the hyoid must develop greater mobility to achieve continued protection of the airway (Bosma & Donner, 1980). This pharyngeal elongation occurs around 4 to 6 months of age. If the functional abilities of the hyoid and larynx do not match the new anatomical configuration, swallowing difficulties may suddenly become apparent.

Relationship of Breathing and Swallowing During Feeding

For many years, professionals held the view that infant sucking and swallowing could occur simultaneously with breathing. It was believed that, due to anatomic differences in the infant, liquid flowed down the lateral food channels and passed safely around the open larynx. As recently as 1975, this issue was yet unresolved (Johnson & Salisbury, 1975).

More recent investigations (Thach & Menon, 1985; Wilson, Thach, Brouillette, & Abu-Osba, 1981) demonstrate that respiration is always interrupted during swallowing, and that swallowing and breathing do not occur simultaneously in the infant. Therefore, precise coordination between breathing and swallowing must occur during feeding. Most of the time, swallowing appears to take precedence over breathing since it is a protective mechanism that clears the airway of foreign material before inspiration occurs.

Since swallowing interrupts breathing, changes in the respiratory pattern can occur in response to the extensive swallowing that accompanies feeding. Swallowing generally interrupts the breathing cycle for 0.5 to 1.0 second. Since infants normally suck and swallow at a rate of 1 cycle per second and breathe 40 to 50 breaths per minute (bpm), this pattern allows enough time for the infant to maintain an appropriate respiratory rate during repetitive swallowing.

Difficulties can arise when the infant has a high resting respiratory rate (above 60 bpm). In this case, the respiratory rate is effectively reduced during repetitive swallowing. The size of the bolus, speed with which the bolus travels, and number of swallows needed to clear the bolus will affect the manner in which the respiratory pattern is altered to accommodate swallowing. Fluid flowing rapidly and continuously will increase the rate of swallowing, leaving less time available for breathing (Mathew, 1988a). Again, the respiratory rate is effectively reduced. Any aspect of feeding that reduces the respiratory rate and interferes with the infant meeting his own respiratory needs can lead to fatigue, inefficient feeding, transient hypoxia, or incoordination between swallowing and breathing.

With solids or semisolids taken by spoon or through finger feeding, swallowing is less frequent than in bottle feeding. Therefore, in these situations swallowing has potentially less impact on respiration than during nipple feeding. The coordination between breathing and swallowing, however, is still a factor once these foods are introduced. Solids require more bolus preparation, and the formation and propulsion of the bolus into the pharynx must be accurately timed with swallowing. Deficits in oral-motor control may result in an ill-timed release of food into the pharynx or release of the bolus in a piecemeal fashion. In either case, food may be present in the pharynx during inhalation, increasing the risk of aspiration.

Respiratory mechanisms support feeding and swallowing in other ways. Respiration provides oxygen to the blood for the physiologic work needed for effective and efficient feeding. Respiratory protective mechanisms, such as the cough and gag, will also clear the pharynx and larynx of food that has not been handled properly.

Oral-Motor and Self-Feeding Components

As in other aspects of development, feeding evolves in a step-wise fashion. Skills progress from stereotyped and reflexive to adaptive, varied, and volitionally controlled. Oral movements progress from mass, patterned activity to refined and isolated activity, with independent control of the various oral structures.

Knowledge of the small steps in this normal progression of oral-motor and feeding development is necessary for effective evaluation and treatment of pediatric feeding problems. It allows the therapist to identify strengths, as well as delays, in feeding skills. Understanding the normal developmental sequence helps the therapist set appropriate goals and develop treatment plans that respect the typical developmental progression. Table 8-1 outlines the developmental sequence for the components of oral-motor and self-feeding skills.

Special Features of Infant Feeding

For young infants, the primary method of obtaining nutrition is by sucking. This is in contrast to the older child who may use a spoon, his fingers, or a cup. Nutritive sucking is a more complex process than is commonly realized. First, precise coordination must occur between rapid sequences of sucking, swallowing, and breathing. In addition to the motoric interplay between these three functions, there is a maturational component. These functions mature independently and at varying rates. If a developmental lag is present in one system, the function of the other two systems may be altered or impaired.

Sucking Characteristics

While sucking develops at 15 to 18 weeks' gestation (Humphrey, 1964; Ianniruberto & Tajani, 1981), the well-coordinated, efficient sucking needed for feeding does not generally develop until 34 to 35 weeks' gestation (Casaer, Daniels, Devlieger, DeCock, & Effermont, 1982; Hack, Estabrook, & Robertson, 1985). Sucking can be characterized by its type (nutritive vs. nonnutritive), rate (sucks/second), rhythm, burst/pause pattern, and force of suction or compression. Feeding efficiency is a combination of these characteristics. Infants who are good feeders tend to have sucking patterns that are faster and stronger, as well as more stable and rhythmic. These infants will spend more time actively sucking than pausing when compared to poor feeders (Braun & Palmer, 1985).

Motoric Components

The movement components of sucking have been investigated radiologically and with ultrasound (Ardran, Kemp, & Lind, 1958a; Weber, Woolridge, & Baum, 1986). As sucking is initiated, the tongue forms a central groove or trough along the median raphe. This central groove stabilizes the nipple and channels the flow of liquid. The medial portion of the tongue

Table 8-1 Developmental Sequence of Oral-Motor and Self-Feeding Skills

Age	Reflexes	Jaw/Cheeks	Lips	Tongue	Swallowing	Self-feeding
12 to 14 weeks' gestation					Swallowing begins	
15 to 18 weeks' gestation				Emergence of sucking movements		
27 to 28 weeks' gestation				Disorganized, random nonnutritive sucking (NNS) pattern		
32 weeks' gestation				NNS: Burst/pause sucking pattern emerging—no stable rhythm		
34 weeks' gestation				NNS: Stable sucking rhythm	Some coordination between suck and swallow	
34 to 35 weeks' gestation					Adequate coordination between suck and swallow	

Age	Reflexes	Jaw/Cheeks	Lips	Tongue	Suck/Swallow	Hand
Term to 1 month	Palmonental Babkin Rooting Gag Phasic bite	Fat pad present Primary jaw movement downward during sucking	Upper lip exerts more pressure than lower in sucking No lateral lip closure Lips closed at rest	Fills oral cavity Provides compression and suction during sucking	Suck/swallow sequence 1:1 at start of feed; 2–3:1 toward end of feed Air swallowing common	Hand-to-mouth activity
1 to 2 months	Same	Fat pad thinning	Lateral borders close on nipple			Expects feeding at regular intervals
3 to 4 months	Palmonental, babkin, and phasic bite disappearing	Buccal cavity begins to develop	Smacks lips Protrudes lips to surround nipple	Tongue protrudes in anticipation of feeding or if nipple touches lip Ejects food voluntarily	Visual recognition of nipple Pats bottle or breast Can voluntarily inhibit suck to look or listen	
5 to 6 months	Rooting begins to diminish Gag elicited farther back in mouth	Buccal cavity developed Up and down munching and biting Inner cheeks draw inward during eating Positions mouth for spoon	Draws in lower lip when spoon removed Upper lip active in cleaning food from spoon Purses lips at corners	Tongue moves in up and down manner with pureed foods, no lateralization Tongue quiet in anticipation of food Tongue protrudes prior to swallow	Choking rare on breast or bottle One sip at a time from cup No gagging on pureed food	Begins finger feeding Plays with spoon

(continued)

Table 8-1 *Continued*

Age	Reflexes	Jaw/Cheeks	Lips	Tongue	Swallowing	Self-feeding
7 to 8 months	Mature gag	Munching continues Jaw closes on solid then sucks it Jaw held closed while a piece of soft solid is broken off	Blows raspberries Upper lip moves downward and forward to actively clean spoon	Tongue begins lateral shift when food is at side of mouth	Does not gag on ground foods or soft semisolids	Feeds self cracker May hold own bottle
9 months		Munches with diagonal movements as food is transferred from center to sides Voluntary biting on food and objects	Lips active with jaw during chewing Briefly closes lips on cup rim	Lateral movements to transfer food from center to sides of mouth	On cup—takes 1–3 sucks before stopping to swallow or breathe	More precise finger feeding Reaches for spoon, may insert crudely in mouth
12 months		Controlled, sustained bite on soft cookie Begins rotary chewing movements	Lips closed during swallow with no food or liquid loss Lower lip is drawn inward to be cleaned by upper gums	Lateralizes from center to sides Licks food off lower lip Intermittent tongue tip elevation	May take majority of liquids from cup Takes 4–5 continuous swallows Swallows ground, mashed, or chopped table foods without gagging	Finger feeds independently Holds and lifts cups but has spillage Brings spoon to mouth but inverts spoon prior to mouth Fills spoon poorly

Age					
15 to 18 months	Rotary chewing smooth and well coordinated Begins to bite on cup rim for external stabilization Cheeks draw inward to assist with food placement Chews meats	Upper lip draws inward to clean food Lower lip cleans upper lip Lateral lip flexibility	Tongue licks lower lip Elevated tongue intermittently or consistently	During cup drinking, swallowing follows sucking without pause Able to sequence at least 3 sip/swallows without pause Able to sequence at least 1 oz. without major pause Swallows solid foods with no loss of food or saliva	Drinks from cup with two hands and replaces on table Feeds self messily with spoon, inverting spoon within mouth
24 months	Internal jaw stabilization on cup through co-contraction Cheeks act with tongue in chewing in a "squish-push" action Circular rotary chewing	Lips contain food and saliva within mouth during chewing	Tongue used in free sweeping movements to clean upper and lower lips Transfers food from one side to the other side	Lengthy sip/swallow sequences during cup drinking	Holds cup with one hand with voluntary cup release Feeds self from bowl with moderate spillage Fills spoon without use of fingers Brings spoon to mouth without inversion

moves in a rhythmic anterior to posterior peristaltic wave during active sucking (Bosma, Hepburn, Josell, & Baker, 1990). The lips and tongue tip seal the
anterior aspect of the mouth, while the cheeks provide support laterally. The
soft palate rests against the posterior aspect of the tongue, thus fully sealing
the oral cavity.

Pressure Components

Both *compression* (positive pressure) and *suction* (negative pressure) are used in removing liquid from the breast or bottle (Sameroff, 1968).
At the beginning of the sucking cycle, the tongue tip squeezes or compresses
the nipple, creating positive pressure to express liquid. Then, the posterior
portion of the tongue moves downward in a piston-like action, the jaw lowers
slightly, and the oral cavity is enlarged. With the lips sealed, enlarging the
oral cavity creates negative intraoral pressure, or suction, to draw liquid into
the mouth. The relative role of suction and compression appears to vary
between infants and with differing feeding conditions.

Sucking Types

Two types of sucking have been identified, nutritive sucking
(NS) and nonnutritive sucking (NNS) (Wolff, 1968). Nutritive sucking occurs
when a flow of liquid is present, and is the process by which infants obtain
nutrients. Nonnutritive sucking occurs in the absence of liquid flow and may
be used to satisfy the infant's basic sucking urge or as a behavioral state
regulatory mechanism. Table 8-2 compares the differences between nutritive
and nonnutritive sucking. Both NS and NNS occur in a regular pattern of
bursts punctuated by pauses. The NNS pattern is quite stable with respect

Table 8-2   Comparison of Nutritive and Nonnutritive Sucking

Characteristic	Nutritive Sucking	Nonnutritive Sucking
Rate	1 suck per second, during the sucking burst	2 sucks per second
Burst/pause pattern	Initial continuous sucking; gradually increasing pauses toward end of feed	Stable number of sucks per burst (4–13 sucks) and duration of pauses (3–10 secs)
Suck to swallow ratio	1 : 1 at start of feed; 2–3 : 1 toward end of feed	Multiple sucks to 1 swallow

to the number of sucks per burst, rate of sucking, and duration of pauses. In NS there is a temporal organization to the burst/pause pattern over the course of a feeding. The mature infant begins feeding with a long period of continuous sucking, with infrequent, brief pauses. As the feeding progresses, these bursts shorten and the duration of pauses gradually increases (Mathew et al., 1985).

Comparison of Breast- and Bottle Feeding

Studies of in vivo breast- and bottle feeding have identified similarities and differences (Ardran, Kemp, & Lind, 1958a, 1958b; Smith, Erenberg, & Nowak, 1988). The infant who is breast-feeding needs to elongate and shape the human breast to position it correctly in the mouth. This latch-on is accomplished by creating negative intraoral pressure (suction). Suction is also needed to maintain the nipple shape and position throughout the feeding. In contrast, the manufactured nipple is a predetermined shape and is positioned in the baby's mouth by the feeder. Once the baby has latched on to the breast or had an artificial nipple placed in the mouth, the sucking mechanics are similar, though the role of suction and compression may vary. Efficiency in bottle feeding is dependent on creating adequate suction, with compression playing a minor role. In breast-feeding, however, compression or positive pressure may play a greater role than suction in expressing milk from the ducts.

Maturation of Sucking and Feeding in the Preterm Infant

Development of Sucking Patterns

Disorganized, short, nonnutritive sucking bursts are demonstrated by infants between 29 and 30 weeks' gestation (Wolff, 1968). Coordination between sucking and swallowing is reported at 32 weeks (Klaus & Fanaroff, 1978), with feeding occasionally introduced between 32 and 34 weeks (Brake, Fifer, Alfasir, & Fleischman, 1988; Casaer, Daniels, Devlieger, DeCock, & Effermont, 1982). Clinical experience suggests, however, that coordination is more fully developed and oral feeding is more likely to be successful at 34 weeks or later. Around this time, the burst/pause pattern becomes more stable and begins to resemble that of the term infant, though with shorter bursts and longer pauses. By 36 weeks, the sucking pattern closely approximates that of a term infant (Casaer, Daniels, Devlieger, DeCock, & Effermont, 1982).

Feeding in premature infants from 36 weeks to term is more likely to be limited by the preterm infant's respiratory control than by the sucking mechanics. Since gestational age can be inaccurate by 1 or 2 weeks, gestational ages can provide a guide for introducing feeding, but should not be used to establish specific expectations.

Respiratory Control During Feeding

Changes in respiratory control during feeding at various gestational ages has been described by Shivpuri, Martin, Carlo, and Fanaroff, (1983). Premature infants between 36 and 38 weeks demonstrate a decrease in respiratory rate and tidal volume during the continuous sucking phase with a return to baseline of these parameters during the intermittent sucking phase. Oxygen saturation also dips during the continuous sucking phase but returns to baseline before the end of the feeding (Mathew, Clark, & Pronske, 1985). This pattern is similar to term infants. In contrast, premature babies at 34 to 35 weeks' gestation show the same dips in respiratory rate, tidal volume, and oxygen saturation, but they may take a longer time after the intermittent phase to return to baseline.

The presence of these respiratory dips and recoveries during feeding suggests that inadequate recovery mechanisms could lead to problems such as apnea, oxygen desaturation, and hypoxia during feeding. Mathew and colleagues have found that apnea and cyanosis *are* relatively common occurrences, in both preterm *and* term infants, although they are more frequently seen in premature infants (Mathew, Clark, & Pronske, 1985). With maturation, this apnea and cyanosis appear to resolve in the absence of underlying pathology. Respiratory diseases, such as those common in premature infants, will also limit recovery mechanisms, making apnea, cyanosis, and oxygen desaturation during feeding more likely.

General Principles in Evaluation and Treatment of Pediatric Feeding Problems

Evaluation

Areas of Evaluation

The evaluation of feeding in the infant and toddler must focus on two broad areas. The first is developmental. The relative maturity versus immaturity of feeding skills must be considered individually, as well as in relation to other developmental areas. An overview of the development of oral-motor skills is presented in Table 8-1. While the maturation of many motor skills is determined using evaluation tools with normative standards, no such tool is currently available for the evaluation of the development of pediatric feeding. Checklists are available (Wolf & Glass, 1992; Furuno et al., 1984; Jelm, 1990; Morris & Klein, 1987), but require that the therapist have a thorough knowledge of the developmental feeding progression, including normal expectations for the premature infant.

The second area of focus in the evaluation is *performance factors*. Normal versus abnormal functions must be considered in the context of the following areas of performance:

1. neuromotor performance, including the influence of muscle tone, reflex activity, and motor control on overall posture, position, and oral-motor skill
2. sensory responses
3. swallowing ability
4. physiologic support for feeding
5. structural integrity
6. behavior and interaction during feeding

To include each area in a feeding evaluation, the clinician may need to use multiple observation forms and checklists, or in many cases, independently determine the methods and parameters for evaluation. A global approach to the evaluation of each of these areas, including functional problems that may be observed, are described in subsequent sections of this chapter.

The Evaluation Process

The specific feeding evaluation of the infant or toddler should be seen as one step in a larger problem solving process, rather than an isolated evaluation. A comprehensive evaluation is often multidisciplinary. Potential team members and their roles are listed in Table 8-3. For the therapist, the steps in the feeding evaluation should include the following.

Gathering Information

This includes background information from chart review and discussions with physicians or nurses involved in the child's care. The parent or caregiver should also be interviewed to determine specific concerns regarding feeding, current feeding methods, and observations that have been made during feeding.

Planning the Feeding Observation

Information gathered in the preliminary history is compiled to plan what equipment will be needed during the feeding observation. For example, feeding tools (e.g., special nipples, spoons, and cups) as well as the food types and textures are selected. The need for equipment to monitor physiologic status is determined. The sequence of observation for various skills may also be planned.

Table 8-3   Potential Members of a Feeding Team and Possible Roles

Potential Team Members	Role of Assessment Process
Parents	Provide historical and current information on the feeding problem. Careful history and parental reporting can help to narrow the focus of the evaluation.
Occupational/physical/ speech therapists	Any one of these therapists may be the primary feeding specialist and carry out the feeding evaluation. Occupational and physical therapists may also evaluate general motor components and position during feeding. Speech therapists may relate oral-motor findings during feeding to speech and language.
Nutritionist	Able to determine optimal nutritional needs. Can suggest dietary modifications to achieve best caloric intake.
Social worker	Assesses parent resources. May help parents clarify their feelings about the child's feeding problems and treatment.
Nurses	Includes hospital nurses, clinic nurses, community nurses, and clinical nurse specialists. The nurse may initially help to identify the feeding problem. Nurses may also provide support for treatment/management strategies that are implemented.
Primary physician	May initially identify the feeding problem. Often coordinates the feeding evaluation process.
Gastrointestinal specialist	Provides assessment of gastroesophageal and gastrointestinal anatomy and function, including assessment of GE reflux and GI motility.
Pulmonary specialist	Provides detailed evaluation of pulmonary function, including assessment of work of breathing and, in some cases, respiratory control.
Otolaryngologist (ear, nose and throat)	Identifies structural abnormalities in the nose, pharynx, larynx, and trachea.
Radiologist	Often involved in conducting studies of feeding-related functions using fluoroscopy, ultrasound, and nuclear medicine scans.
Neurologist	Helps to identify neurologic basis or feeding problems, such as CNS damage or cranial nerve dysfunction.

Feeding Observation

1. General observations: Baseline physiologic status is noted. Posture, movement, and developmental skill should be observed briefly if these characteristics are not known to the feeding specialist.
2. Naturalistic observation: The typical feeding situation should be observed. It is most effective if a primary caretaker can be observed feeding the infant. If this is not possible, the therapist should try to duplicate characteristics of the child's standard feeding situation (i.e., foods, tools, and position) and observe the child's baseline responses.
3. Elicited observations: The therapist or feeder modifies the feeding session to elicit behaviors or feeding skills that have not occurred spontaneously. The interplay of naturalistic observation and elicited responses will vary for each child, depending on the type of feeding problems.

Treatment Exploration

Based on the information that has been gathered and the observations of feeding, hypotheses are developed to explain the observed problems. These hypotheses can be explored by altering aspects of the feeding, such as the food texture, feeding tools, position, or feeding techniques, and by monitoring changes in performance. This information may suggest strategies useful for treatment, as well as clarify the underlying basis of the feeding problem.

Synthesizing Information

The information gathered during the feeding evaluation must then be synthesized into a cohesive and rational plan. It should allow the therapist to answer the following questions, which are key to developing appropriate feeding strategies.

1. What is the child's level of function? In particular, how adequately and safely can the child's nutritional needs be met through oral feeding?
2. What factors interfere with feeding function? Do developmental factors or abnormal function affect one or more of the performance areas?
3. How well does the child's feeding performance match the caregiver's concerns or expectations?
4. Is additional information necessary? Must other tests or consultations be undertaken to provide adequate information to develop a treatment/management plan?

5. Which treatment techniques, if any, appear to improve oral feeding function?

Communicating Results

With multiple health professionals and family members involved in this process, care must be taken to effectively communicate results and suggestions for further testing or treatment techniques. While multidisciplinary meetings are ideal, they are not always possible. Written documentation is necessary, but verbal communication is encouraged. Communicating in person or by phone allows immediate feedback to and from parents or team members. The overall problem solving process becomes faster and potentially more effective.

Treatment

The goal of the evaluation process is to develop a comprehensive understanding of the underlying causes of the feeding problem. This is the key to a successful treatment program. Just as documenting the delays in gross motor development does not explain *why* the child is delayed, simply identifying a set of feeding problems does not explain why they are occurring, whether they are related, or their significance. It is the clinician's knowledge of feeding and related processes, combined with thoughtful interpretation of the evaluation, that can lead to an understanding of the underlying causes of the feeding problem. This understanding of the problem, along with knowledge of the resources available to the child, provides the basis for developing a relevant and effective feeding plan. Basic criteria for the feeding plan are as follows.

1. The feeding methods must be safe. They should not endanger or compromise the child's health.
2. The feeding methods should be successful in promoting appropriate weight gain. Caloric intake should be adequate. Energy expenditure to obtain the required calories should not be excessive.
3. The feeding plan must meet the needs of the family. It should reflect their resources, particularly in terms of time and skill. It should address both their concerns and expectations, and if possible prioritize feeding goals based on the family's preference.

Specific techniques and strategies that can lead to improvement of oral feeding are developed within these criteria. These may be treatment techniques or management strategies. Treatment techniques reflect an attempt to change or to improve the underlying problem; for example, the provision of jaw support to reduce excessive jaw movement. Management strategies acknowledge inability to change the basic underlying feeding problem at the present time, but provide a method of circumventing the problem to allow adequate nutrition and growth. Both treatment and management techniques may be included as part of a feeding plan. For example, a premature infant who does not have the energy to nipple all required feedings is given every other feeding by nasogastric tube. The infant's nutrition is managed by providing adequate caloric intake, while supporting the infant's emerging skills in feeding.

The treatment and management techniques that can be used in a feeding plan are limitless, with ideas available from numerous resources (Connor, Williamson, & Siepp, 1978; Furuno et al., 1984; Logemann, 1983; Morris 1982; Morris & Klein, 1987; Mueller, 1972, 1975; VandenBerg, 1990; Wilson, 1977). Based on the belief that treatment techniques are most effective when the rationale for their use is well understood, subsequent sections of this chapter include guiding principles of treatment. While selected techniques are described, it is hoped that an understanding of the guiding principles of treatment will allow appropriate selection of techniques from other sources as well as creative development of new treatment techniques.

Neuromotor Components of Feeding

Neuromotor factors are often a leading contributor to the feeding problems seen by occupational therapists who work in early intervention programs. They are also the most widely discussed aspect of feeding dysfunction in therapy literature. Since this chapter seeks to provide a comprehensive view of all aspects of feeding dysfunction, only a broad overview of the role of the neuromotor components is possible. The reader is referred to additional references for further information in this area (Bly 1983; Connor, Williamson, & Siepp, 1978; Finnie, 1975; Morris & Klein, 1987).

Evaluation

The evaluation of neuromotor control includes assessment of muscle tone, reflex activity, and specific motor skills. Total body movement and posture as well as oral-motor control must be considered when assessing neuromotor factors as they relate to feeding.

Total Body Movement and Position

Motoric maturation and quality of movement should be assessed, particularly as they influence control of the head and trunk. Abnormalities in muscle tone, retained primitive postural reflexes, or stereotyped movement patterns should be identified. Their effects on the feeding process can then be delineated. Control of the shoulder girdle, forearm, and hand need to be considered when the child is expected to engage in self-feeding.

Neuromotor dysfunction can have a significant impact on the feeding posture, therefore, the feeding position should be carefully evaluated. Whether in the mother's arms or in a chair or other positioning device, the characteristics of the typical feeding position would include

1. neutral alignment of the head and neck (or slight neck flexion)
2. midline orientation
3. symmetric trunk position
4. hip flexion, though the degree will vary with the child's age
5. symmetric arm position with the shoulders relaxed and forward

The body angle during feeding will be dependent on the level of head control present. Infants and those with limited head, neck, and trunk control are fed in a semireclined position. Older children who have adequate postural control are in an upright position for feeding.

Oral-Motor Control

The assessment of oral-motor control includes facial muscle tone, oral reflex activity, and functional oral-motor skills. While oral reflexes are often evaluated for their presence or absence, it is more important to consider their contribution or interference with feeding function. Table 8-1 provides further information on expectations for primitive reflexes, while protective reflexes are described in more detail later in the chapter. The child's skill in complex activities, such as sucking or chewing, is based on the movement characteristics of each oral structure—the tongue, jaw, lips, and cheeks—as well as their coordinated function. Both the resting position and movement patterns of each structure must be evaluated. The expectations for movement will vary based on developmental age and feeding activity (e.g., cup versus spoon), and are most effectively observed during these feeding activities. Evaluation should include observation of all feeding activities in the child's repertoire or of all those appropriate for the child's developmental level. Normal function includes a number of basic characteristics.

Tongue

At rest it should appear soft, flat, and of moderate thickness. A slight central groove should be noted running in the anterior-posterior direction. The tip should be rounded and rest in the bottom of the mouth. The expected range of tongue movements will vary with age as described in Table 8-1.

Jaw

At rest, the upper and lower jaw should be in neutral alignment, allowing the lips to oppose easily. Movement is typically well-graded and in small ranges, providing support to other oral structures. Ungraded movement in larger ranges can normally be expected during acquisition of a new skill, such as chewing or cup drinking.

Lips

At rest, the lips should be relaxed and of moderate thickness. During feeding they should be able to purse and generate enough tension to seal the nipple during sucking, close on a spoon, or stabilize the edge of a cup. They should have sufficient mobility to draw in and clean the upper or lower lip with the other lip when developmentally appropriate.

Cheeks

At rest, the cheeks should be soft, but provide slight resistance to pressure. With movement they should become slightly firmer. They should be firm enough to provide lateral support, yet supple enough to pull inward or pouch outward depending on the characteristics of the bolus.

Atypical Development/Functional Problems

Total Body Movement and Position

Abnormal muscle tone and motor control not only leads to delays in functional motor skills, but may also alter the relationship of the head to the neck and affect trunk control, thereby adversely affecting the feeding position. Retained primitive reflexes and abnormal muscle tone may compromise postural alignment and upper extremity control needed for self-feeding. There are some specific problems that may impact feeding.

Hypertonic Muscle Tone

Hypertonicity can result in postures dominated by flexor or extensor patterns of movement, with excessive extension more commonly noted. Increased tone can be present at rest, though it is generally most pronounced with movement.

In relationship to feeding, hypertonicity, which is expressed as strong extensor tone, typically leads to neck hyperextension. This abnormal head/neck alignment can result in abnormal movements of the tongue, lips, and jaw that interfere with oral control for feeding. Extensor hypertonicity of the hips makes it difficult to maintain hip flexion. Independent sitting for feeding may not be possible, and even passive positioning with hip flexion may be

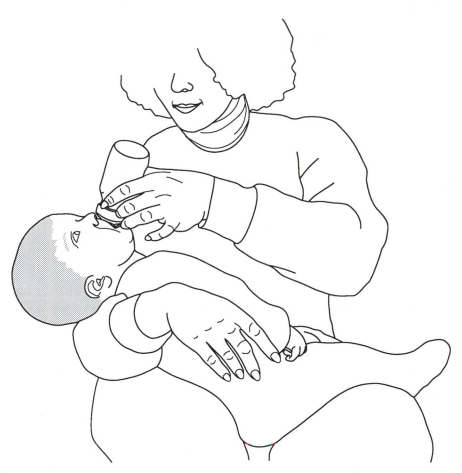

Figure 8-1 Neck hyperextension during feeding—Infant [From FEEDING AND SWALLOWING DISORDERS IN INFANCY by Lynn S. Wolf and Robin P. Glass, copyright 1992, by Therapy Skill Builders, a division of Communication Skill Builders, Inc., PO Box 42050, Tucson, AZ. Reprinted with permission.]

difficult. In the hypertonic child, it is often very difficult to achieve appropriate head and neck alignment with the hips in extension. The scapula may also be adducted, retracting the arms and positioning the hands away from the midline. This may compromise hand-to-mouth skills for self-feeding. Figures 8-1 and 8-2 illustrate neck hyperextension in an infant and a child.

Hypotonic Muscle Tone

When hypotonicity is present, the child has difficulty opposing the force of gravity to achieve an upright posture. As the child is held or sits upright for feeding, excessive truncal flexion may be observed. The head may passively flex forward, potentially interfering with the patency of the airway.

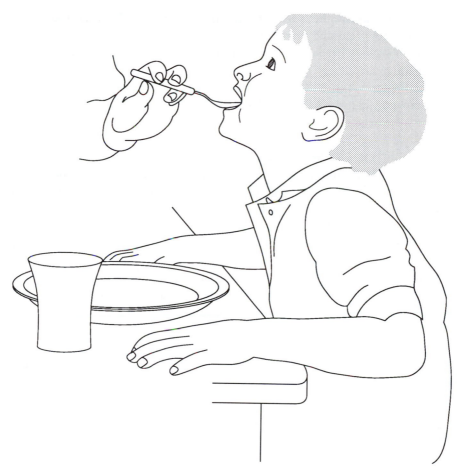

Figure 8-2 Neck hyperextension during feeding—Child

In the face of hypotonic muscle tone, the child may respond with compensatory strategies to increase stability, particularly in more upright positions. The neck may be hyperextended and shoulders elevated to achieve head control. The scapula may adduct and the arms may retract in an effort to obtain head and trunk stability. These postures are then similar to those described for hypertonicity. While the impact on feeding is similar, the underlying mechanism is different.

Influence of Primitive or Abnormal Reflexes

Influence of the tonic labyrinthine reflex often leads to increased extension of the head and trunk in the semireclined feeding position used by the child with poor head and trunk control. Excessive trunk and neck extension are commonly seen, and result in the same type of problems described for hypertonic muscle tone.

When the asymmetric tonic neck reflex (ATNR) is abnormally strong or inappropriately retained, the child may have asymmetries of head and neck movements as well as asymmetric oral movement. Hand-to-mouth skills for self-feeding may also be impaired. When the child turns the head toward the self-feeding arm, the ATNR could cause the arm to extend, moving it away from the mouth. If the ATNR limits midline head positioning and the child is fed with the head turned to the side, swallowing may be difficult or impaired.

Oral-Motor Control

The infant may exhibit numerous abnormal oral movement patterns that create functional problems. Poor oral-motor control may be associated with abnormal muscle tone in the oral structures, inappropriate feeding positions, and structural anomalies. A child with difficulties in upper extremity control who engages in self-feeding may also demonstrate associated reactions in the oral area that interfere with oral-motor function. While it is possible to see impairment in a single aspect of oral-motor control, more frequently several oral-motor problems are seen in association. Specific abnormal oral problems of the tongue, lips, and jaw are discussed.

Tongue Retraction

The tongue is held posteriorly in the mouth with the tip well behind the alveolar ridges. A retracted tongue often appears very thick and bunched. It is most often associated with abnormalities in muscle tone or position, particularly increased extensor tone. When associated with structural problems such as micrognathia, the tongue may be sufficiently retracted to intermittently obstruct the pharyngeal airway, possibly compromising respiration. More typically, the consequence of tongue retraction is limitation of normal tongue movement. Anterior-posterior and lateral movements may be impaired.

Tongue Tip Elevation

The tip of the tongue is elevated and in contact with the upper alveolar ridge. This position may be maintained with a fair degree of strength, often in an attempt to maintain stability in the oral area. It can interfere with nipple or spoon insertion, and may limit the development of isolated tongue movements.

Tongue Thrust

This is a rhythmic, in-and-out pattern of tongue movement with the emphasis on the out component. The tongue may also be humped and bunched. This pattern is frequently seen in association with overall abnormal extensor tone, but may also develop in compensation for tongue retraction. It is a stereotyped movement pattern that inhibits the development of more mature and varied tongue movements.

Tonic Biting

Tonic biting is an abnormal response to touch/pressure on the gums or teeth that results in a strong, forceful closing of the jaw. Due to the force and tension generated, reopening of the mouth may be extremely difficult. Jaw clenching may resemble tonic biting and may develop in an attempt to develop jaw stability, but is not elicited by tactile input to the gums. This pattern interferes with all aspects of feeding.

Jaw Thrust

This is a forceful downward movement of the lower jaw. The jaw may appear to jut forward. A jaw thrust is frequently seen in conjunction with very strong extensor tone. It may occur as food is presented or during oral manipulation of the food, and it can impair control of the lips and tongue.

Jaw Instability

Jaw instability is characterized by ungraded or excessive jaw movement. It is frequently associated with hypotonia or weakness. The mouth may hang open and the child may have difficulty with adequate mouth closure on a spoon or a cup. The infant may show excessive jaw movement during sucking, which leads to an inefficient or weak suck. Jaw clenching may be noted as a compensation for jaw instability.

Lip Retraction

Both lips are pulled backwards revealing the teeth or gums. They may form a tight horizontal line above the mouth. Lip retraction is frequently seen as a component of overall extensor tone particularly if head, neck, and arm extension or retraction are present during feeding. To overcome the strong pull away from the middle, some children will respond by excessively pursing their lips. Either pattern makes lip seal to contain foods within the mouth or clearance of the spoon extremely difficult.

Lip/Cheek Instability

This pattern usually accompanies overall hypotonia. The lips may lack sufficient tone to sustain approximation and, thus, fail to keep food and saliva in the mouth. During sucking, cheek instability can contribute to poor placement of the nipple in the mouth and a decrease in the amount of negative pressure generated. The child may have difficulty with lateral placement and containment of food during chewing if the cheeks do not provide sufficient support.

Lip/Cheek Immobility
The lips and cheeks can be immobile due to a lack of adequate muscle tension for movement from hypotonia or from being rigidly held in a particular position secondary to hypertonia. The resultant immobility limits the variety of lip and cheek movements necessary for all aspects of feeding.

Guiding Principles of Treatment

1. Alignment: Proper alignment of the body and the head are crucial to optimal feeding performance. Abnormal alignment of body structures can influence the function of all the oral structures. For example, neck and head extension can lead to tongue retraction or thrusting during feeding.
2. Provide proximal stability: Controlled extremity movement requires a stable base. The movements of the tongue and lips for feeding are distal movements, requiring stability of many proximal structures, particularly the jaw. For the mandible to be stable, head and neck stability built upon trunk stability is required.
3. Facilitate appropriate movement patterns: Once proper alignment and stability have been achieved and postural tone is normalized, the therapist or caregiver facilitates appropriate oral movement patterns. Simultaneous application of inhibitory and facilitory techniques elicit the desired movement patterns.

To achieve proper alignment, stability, and appropriate movement patterns, preparation of the child by using neurodevelopmental handling techniques prior to feeding may be beneficial in some cases. This will be particularly true when postural and motoric abnormalities are the result of CNS disturbances. If the underlying feeding problem is rooted in factors such as stress, immaturity, or various medical conditions, feeding may not be enhanced by these techniques. Therefore, the decision to use preparatory handling activities prior to feeding should be a consciously considered treatment decision that is part of the overall treatment plan and based on the etiology of the oral-motor abnormalities.

Examples of Treatment Techniques

Positioning
Modifications of physical handling or adaptations to seating should be made to allow neutral shoulder and neck position, midline orientation of arms and head, flexed hips, and a straight trunk at an angle appropriate for the child's age and skill. Finnie (1975) and Morris and Klein (1987) provide many examples of positions that can be effectively used.

Providing Head and Jaw Support

The feeding therapist can support the head and stabilize the jaw using her hand and arm as described by Mueller (1975) and by Morris (1982). By controlling the jaw and head position, improvement in jaw, tongue, and lip movement may result. Abnormal head/neck extension or jaw and tongue thrust may also be inhibited. Morris and Klein (1987) and Mueller (1975) provide details of this technique for the toddler, while Wolf and Glass (1992) describe it for the infant. Figures 8-3 and 8-4 show examples of this technique for an infant and a young child.

Facilitation of Appropriate Tongue Movement

A tongue that is retracted may benefit from firm pressure and downward stroking in the midline from the back to the front. For a tongue thrust or a protracted tongue, firm downward and inward pressure with a finger, spoon, or firm nipple may encourage the tongue to remain centered within the mouth.

Alteration of Facial Tone

Oral-facial hypotonia may respond to firm tapping directly to the lips, cheeks, and tongue. Quick stretch over the masseter and buccinator

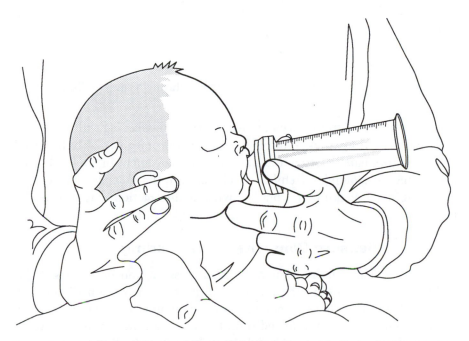

Figure 8-3 Head/jaw support—Infant [From FEEDING AND SWALLOWING DISORDERS IN INFANCY by Lynn S. Wolf and Robin P. Glass, copyright 1992, by Therapy Skill Builders, a division of Communication Skill Builders, Inc., PO Box 42050, Tucson, AZ. Reprinted with permission.]

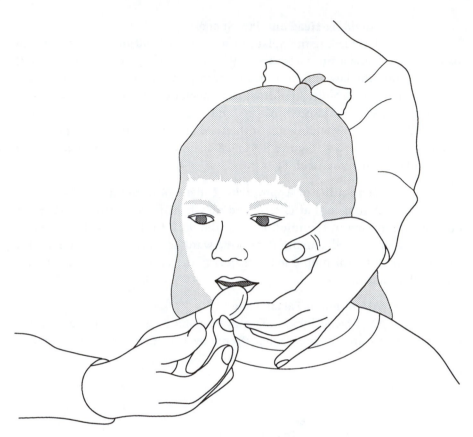

Figure 8-4 Providing head/neck and jaw support during feeding—Child

muscles may also improve facial tone and, thus, the feeding skills (Leonard, Trykowski, & Kirkpatrick, 1980). Hypertonia in the oral area may be improved by preparatory handling to normalize tone and movement in the head, neck, and shoulders. Holding the child's cheek between the therapist's fingers and providing rapid shaking or vibration with slight traction may also reduce facial tone.

Sensory Components of Feeding

The sensory systems—touch/pressure, movement/vestibular, auditory, and visual—are the primary means by which the baby interacts with and learns from the environment. Sensory input is derived from multiple channels—eyes, ears, mouth, and skin. In particular, the sensation of touch (both orally and over the entire body) plays a key role in feeding. When sensory perception or registration is abnormal, feeding problems may result. Sensory-based feeding problems can have their etiology in a variety of factors.

Immaturity or Chronic Illness

An infant born prematurely enters the extrauterine environment with an immature central nervous system (CNS) that is ill-equipped to deal with the demands of the environment, particularly those of the typical NICU. Due to CNS immaturity, the infant may be overly sensitive to stimuli and unable to filter or inhibit incoming stimuli. The response may be hyperresponsivity to sensory input. Conversely, in order to deal with the demands of the environment, other infants shut-down or tune-out as a coping strategy.

Infants or children who are chronically ill may be at the mercy of their physiologic status. With all of their resources harnessed toward simple survival, they may not have sufficient reserve to deal with increased sensory demands. This may lower their tolerance to tactile or sensory input.

Unpleasant Oral-Tactile Experiences

Many children who go on to develop abnormal responses to oral-tactile stimuli have had frequent unpleasant or traumatic experiences in the oral-facial area as part of their medical treatment. These children may have experienced intubation for mechanical ventilation (with frequent taping and retaping of the tubing); endotracheal, oral, or nasal suctioning; or the repeated insertion of nasogastric or orogastric tubes for feeding. Medical restrictions may also have limited normal oral-tactile comforting, such as hand-to-mouth behavior.

Thus, these children experience a period of relative deprivation of normal oral-tactile activity and pleasure, combined with a period of aversive oral stimuli. They may, therefore, learn a pattern of defensiveness in response to all stimulation in and around the oral area. This defensive response tends to persist well beyond the end of the medical procedures and manifests in oral hypersensitivity and feeding aversion (Morris & Klein, 1987).

Delayed Introduction of Oral Feeding

When a baby is born prematurely or is chronically ill, the introduction of oral feeding may be substantially delayed. When feeding is attempted at a later date, the child may have difficulty acquiring the appropriate oral-motor skills or manifest oral hypersensitivity. Some authors feel (Illingworth & Lister, 1964) that delay in introduction of feeding beyond the critical or sensitive period, when the child is most receptive to learning, makes acquiring feeding skills at a later time difficult, if not impossible. Not only may the onset of all oral feeding be delayed, but the normal progression through the various food textures and types may also be delayed or lengthened. Depending on the severity of the child's early medical difficulties, the parents may be reluctant to move the child to the next developmentally appropriate feeding level. If resistance is encountered when the parent does attempt to move the child forward, the parent may be more likely to acquiesce for fear of a medical setback.

Neurologic Impairment
With abnormal neurological function, any aspect of sensory processing may be deficient. Perception, as well as registration of sensory stimuli, may be inadequate. Hypersensitive or hyposensitive responses may result.

Evaluation of Sensory Components of Feeding

In order to be a successful eater, a child must be able to adapt to the changing tactile properties of the food bolus, as well as to the tools of feeding (i.e., breast, nipple, spoon, and cup). Appropriate responses to this tactile input allow the child to make the correct or adaptive motoric response. Assessment of the sensory components of feeding can occur (1) through casual observation of the child's response to feeding and oral-tactile stimuli throughout the feeding assessment or (2) through structured application of selected oral-tactile stimuli to evaluate the child's response.

Structured Oral-Tactile Evaluation
When the latter method of evaluation is chosen, the feeding therapist should consider and select

1. the area of the face or mouth to stimulate first
2. the type of tactile input to apply
3. the order in which the stimuli is applied, generally progressing from the easiest to tolerate or least threatening to the most difficult or most aversive

Area of Face
Tolerance of tactile input is generally greatest when it is applied furthest from the face. Therefore, to grade the child's response to tactile stimuli, initial presentation of stimuli should be distal to the mouth, perhaps even beginning on the arms or neck. It can then progress to the cheeks, outer lips, and finally inside the mouth to the gums and tongue. The point at which a gag reflex is observed when stimulating inside the mouth may give an indication of whether the child's responsivity is commensurate with his developmental level.

Type of Tactile Input

The type of tactile stimulation can also be graded. Most children tolerate firm pressure more easily than light pressure. Response to vibratory input is variable. By using items with differing textures (smooth, soft, rough, prickly), the therapist can determine those most easily tolerated. All food textures that are currently in the child's diet should be assessed. If possible, the next highest level should also be attempted. Grading generally moves from liquid to pureed, to chunky but uniform, to crunchy and harder chewing foods. A variety of tastes (such as sweet, sour, spicy, and bland) and temperatures might also be evaluated.

Atypical Development/Functional Problems

Some specific examples of functional problems that are associated with somatosensory problems are listed as follows:

Tactile Hypersensitivity

The child's responses to oral-tactile stimulation are exaggerated or out of proportion to the magnitude of the stimulus. For example, a 1-year-old is hungry, but bats his mother's hand away each time she tries to bring a spoonful of food toward his mouth. This response is out of proportion to the stimuli, perhaps because the infant has an abnormal perception of the spoon (hypersensitivity), or because the infant has poor regulation of his response to that stimuli.

Oral Aversion

Aversive responses may include components of the hypersensitive response, but they are more negative and generally include a behavioral component. Thus, an infant or toddler may cry, grimace, arch away, or keep the mouth closed when asked to feed (hypersensitive responses), but if the feeder persists, the infant may begin to gag. If the caregiver does not attend to the child's gagging, the infant may actually vomit. Tantrums can occur in response to tastes or even to the visual presentation of foods or utensils. Aversive and hypersensitive responses may occur not only in response to touch, but also to taste, temperature, texture, or odor.

Tactile Hyposensitivity

In this case, a large amount of stimulation is required to elicit a response; the responses are slow or only partially complete. For example, the 2-year-old with Down syndrome who drools is hyposensitive to saliva on the lips and fails to control it, unless asked to close his mouth and swallow (increased stimulation). With diminished oral-sensory awareness, the quality of oral-motor control may suffer, though functional feeding is generally possible. Swallowing disorders may also be seen in children with oral hyposensitivity, as bolus formation is poor or the swallowing reflex is not initiated appropriately. Abnormal sensory registration or perception can contribute to oral hyposensitivity.

Oral Dyspraxia
A child may have difficulty planning and executing the fine oral movements required for eating or speech. Inadequate registration or interpretation of oral-tactile and proprioceptive input may lead to dyspraxia.

Guiding Principles of Treatment

1. Promote normal oral-sensory experiences. Minimize the presence of potentially aversive tactile stimuli.
2. Modulate tactile input. When oral-tactile input is provided, the stimuli must be graded with attention to the type of stimuli, amount of pressure, or location of stimuli.
3. Build a trusting relationship with the child. From a base of trust, the child may be better able to handle the stress of imposed sensory input. The therapist should respect the child's drive for independence and allow the child to direct the flow of treatment as often as possible.
4. Oral-tactile sensory treatment does not need to occur exclusively at mealtimes. Many play and care activities provide wonderful opportunities for the provision of added oral-tactile sensory input.

Examples of Treatment Techniques

Minimize Aversive Oral-Tactile Stimuli
Attempts should be made to eliminate aversive tactile facial experiences. If the child is nonorally fed, the use of an indwelling nasogastric tube is preferable to intermittent insertion of the nasal-gastric (NG) tube, which results in repeated noxious stimulation. If nonoral feeding will continue for a lengthy period of time, a gastrostomy tube would be preferable to remove noxious stimuli from the oral area. If an NG tube is taped in place, efforts should be made to use extremely soft taping materials, which require less frequent retaping, and which allow better movement of the facial musculature beneath the tape. Oral suctioning should be minimized, and if possible, elimi-

nated. Pain from gastroesophageal reflux should be treated medically to avoid association of the pain with eating.

Environmental modifications should be used to decrease overall environmental overstimulation. Als (1986) describes examples appropriate for infants, including containment via nesting or bundling, shielding from excessive visual or auditory input, and grouping of procedures to decrease intermittent sensory overload.

Grade Tactile Input

The key to treatment of oral-sensory disturbances is the provision of graded sensory input. Treatment should begin at the level at which the child is comfortable, then slowly build to a point just below the threshold for elicitation of a hypersensitive-aversive response. To make progress, the feeding therapist must work on the narrow margin just at the edge of the child's tolerance. The therapist must be willing to risk sometimes inadvertently crossing over the child's threshold in order to allow the child to progress.

Touch/Pressure

This type of sensory input is known to have an overall integrating effect on the CNS. The therapist can provide firm pressure or rub the face or lips using her hands, textured toys, rubber or cloth animals, or clothing. Mueller (1975) has described a technique of firmly rubbing the gums or tongue to decrease hypersensitive responses. This technique can occur as a preparation for eating or occur periodically throughout the day. Using one finger, the therapist can walk backwards on the tongue to the point just prior to the elicitation of a gag reflex. This point is often indicated by an eye blink.

Vibration

Small, hand-held vibrators can be used to provide input to even small babies on the face, lips, or inside of the mouth and tongue. Since vibration tends to be carried along an entirely different neural pathway than light touch or touch/pressure, this type of sensory input is often more easily accepted by the hypersensitive child.

Bathing and Dressing

These activities provide many opportunities for oral-tactile input. During dressing, the child's face or extremities can be firmly rubbed with clothes. After bathing, extra time can be spent rubbing the face or the body firmly with a towel. During the bath, water can be dripped onto the child's face, or a washcloth saturated with clean water or juice can be given to the child to suck on.

Physiologic Support for Feeding

Feeding is a complex process that not only requires the support of basic physiologic functions, in particular the respiratory system, but it can also affect the function of these systems. This is most clearly apparent in the infant who is nipple feeding. The intricate coordination between sucking, swallowing, and breathing not only requires precise timing, but also requires considerable energy expenditure, making feeding the infant's primary work. It is by engaging in this work that feeding has an impact on the cardiorespiratory system. This concept of the interrelated nature of feeding and physiologic function is crucial to understanding infant feeding; however, it can also apply to children of all ages who have certain types of feeding difficulties.

Evaluation

Physiological Response to Feeding

Since feeding is work, it requires energy, which is generated by using oxygen to burn nutrients or calories. Therefore, the body's cardiovascular and behavioral responses to that work can be evaluated in a manner similar to assessing the body's response to other forms of exercise. Baseline measures are needed to establish the underlying physiological support for feeding. Responses must also be measured during and after feeding to determine the impact of feeding on the child's basic physiological systems.

Heart Rate and Respiratory Rate

Assessment of these parameters can occur by periodic manual counts or by a cardiorespiratory monitor. This monitor not only gives a numerical readout of heart rate and respiratory rate but also gives a visual picture that can detect brief changes in either parameter. High baseline heart rate or respiratory rate indicate that considerable physiological work is required to maintain homeostasis. As a result, the infant has less reserve for additional work such as feeding. Large increases in heart rate or respiratory rate during feeding suggest that the work of feeding is accomplished at a high physiological cost to the child. High respiratory rates (tachypnea) during feeding can put the infant who is nipple feeding at risk for aspiration, as rapid breathing may leave less time available for safe swallowing. Apnea during feeding may lead to progressive hypoxia or oxygen deficit. A significant drop in heart rate (bradycardia) during feeding can also lead to hypoxia and may be a potential life threatening event.

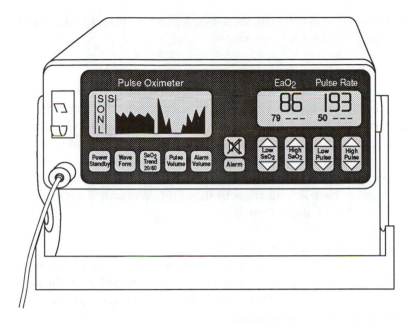

Figure 8-5 Pulse oximeter [From FEEDING AND SWALLOWING DISORDERS IN IN-FANCY by Lynn S. Wolf and Robin P. Glass, copyright 1992, by Therapy Skill Builders, a division of Communication Skill Builders, Inc., PO Box 42050, Tucson, AZ. Reprinted with permission.]

Oxygen Saturation

This is expressed as the percentage of oxygen being carried by the blood and, thus, is available to the tissues for work. It can be measured with noninvasive methods such as pulse oximetry (Figure 8-5). Low baseline values suggest that the amount of oxygen available in the blood may be inadequate for the increased work of feeding. Decreases during feeding, or oxygen desaturation, indicate that feeding is in some way compromising the infant's ability to maintain an adequate oxygen supply in the blood.

Color

Skin color can be an indication of oxygen saturation, as it reflects the amount of oxygen carried by the blood to the skin. The areas around the mouth and eyes are particularly sensitive to changes in oxygen saturation, often becoming gray or bluish when oxygen saturation is poor. While a general-ized pale or grayish color can result from poor oxygen saturation, it can also be a reflection of poor blood perfusion to the skin. Skin color should be monitored but is not a reliable method of assessing oxygen saturation, as profound desaturation can occur in the absence of any appreciable change in color. If poor color or color change during feeding is observed, however, further evaluation by oximetry is warranted.

Quality of Respiration

The effort used in breathing, often called the work of breathing, is assessed in several ways. Observations of increased respiratory effort include nasal flaring and sternal, substernal, or intercostal retractions. The respiratory pattern should be observed, noting whether respirations are smooth or uneven, and the frequency and length of respiratory pauses. Respiratory sounds such as stridor, grunting, or wheezing can also provide information on respiratory effort. Signs of fatigue or changes in the child's endurance over the course of the feeding should also be noted.

Protective Mechanisms

Since the pharynx serves as the passage for both food and air, mechanisms to protect the respiratory system from aspiration during feeding are located in this region (Mathew, 1988a). The primary protective mechanisms are the cough and gag.

Cough

If food passes the epiglottis and enters the larynx, receptors are stimulated and a cough is triggered. This response thus protects the upper airways from foreign material by expelling it before it can enter the larynx. The strength of the cough should be observed to determine if it is strong enough to clear foods of the various weights and consistencies that are in the child's diet.

Gag

The gag reflex protects the child from swallowing a bolus that is too large to safely enter the esophagus. It also protects the respiratory system by forcing such a bolus back into the mouth where it cannot obstruct the entrance to the larynx. It is triggered by a large bolus or foreign object in the oral pharynx (or the mouth in young infants). Determining whether the gag response is intact is particularly important when introducing solid foods that require chewing. It is less important for nipple feeding since the size of the bolus is controlled.

Atypical Development/Functional Problems

In the medically compromised child, inadequate physiological support for feeding can be manifest in many ways. Some of the more common difficulties are as follows.

Acute Compromise During Feeding

This might include dramatic color change, bradycardia, apnea, or falling oxygen saturation. If problems of this magnitude are present, immediate attention should be given to determining the underlying cause and developing techniques that will alleviate the problem. Consideration should be given to terminating routine feeding during this process. Possible causes for these responses during feeding might include gastroesophageal reflux, hyperactive vagal responses from stimulation to chemo- or baroreceptors, or inadequate oxygen supply, possibly due to lung damage from disorders such as respiratory distress syndrome. Many other medical problems can also result in acute compromise during feeding (see Wolf and Glass [1992]).

Fatigue or Low Endurance

A child who is not able to sustain the work needed for feeding may stop before taking in adequate calories. Sometimes the child's fatigue may be apparent. The respiratory rate may increase significantly during or after feeding, the child may sweat or become diaphoretic, or the work of breathing may become greater. At other times, the child may simply stop eating before taking in an adequate volume of food, though outwardly she may not appear fatigued. In these cases, the child may have experienced partial relief of hunger, lowering the drive to eat in relation to the need for rest, even though their overall intake may be inadequate for growth.

The basis for low endurance may be respiratory, cardiac, or muscular. Conditions involving muscular weakness can result in muscle fatigue that limits the duration of activities such as feeding. Weight gain may be marginal because a child with a chronic illness may have increased caloric needs but may be unable to take in adequate calories due to fatigue during feeding. If a child is working extremely hard to feed, she may, in fact, burn more calories in the work of feeding than she does in taking in food.

Poor Coordination of Swallowing and Breathing

During swallowing, efforts to breathe must cease or aspiration may result. In infants, the rapid sequencing of sucking and swallowing necessitates remarkably precise coordination of swallowing and breathing. Inadequate coordination can result in coughing, choking, and, at times, prolonged apnea or bradycardia (marked slowing of the heart rate). In neonates, such problems may reflect immaturity of brain stem control of respiration. This is commonly seen in premature infants. When respiratory compromise is present, incoordination between swallowing and breathing can also result. The child's need to breathe overrides the suppression of respiration during swallowing.

In the older child who is feeding by spoon and by cup, swallows are more discrete and less frequent. Apnea and bradycardia, therefore, are less common, although coughing and choking may be noted when the coordination of swallowing and breathing is deficient. Neuromuscular incoordination or significant respiratory compromise are often at the root of the problem.

Inadequate Protective Mechanisms

If the protective cough is not functioning adequately and the swallowing mechanism is dysfunctional, aspiration of food may occur without visible external evidence. This is termed silent aspiration. In such cases, there may be a history of recurrent pneumonia or other respiratory illnesses. When frequent and unexplained exacerbations of respiratory disease occur (sometimes referred to as reactive airway disease), the possibility of silent aspiration should be considered. While aspiration with swallowing of food (descending aspiration) can be evaluated, the possibility of ascending aspiration in conjunction with gastroesophageal reflux may also need to be explored (Orenstein & Orenstein, 1988). Based on the role the gag mechanism plays in protecting the airway, inadequate function may be of little consequence for the infant who is taking a full liquid diet. Lack of a gag response, however, is an indicator of poor neurological function, so it is not without significance. Inadequate function of the gag, in the older child eating solid foods that require chewing, can lead to obstruction of the airway from poorly chewed food that is not able to be cleared from the pharynx. The relationship between frequent gag and aversive responses is not clear. It seems that one may follow or precede the other.

Guiding Principles of Treatment

1. Minimize acute compromise: If acute physiological compromise is noted during feeding, the underlying problems should be determined and addressed before continuing with a normal feeding routine.
2. Provide adequate physiological support: A child of any age may need additional support for physiological functions during feeding to enhance endurance, minimize fatigue, and reduce the possibility of additional physiological compromise during feeding.
3. Develop appropriate expectations: For a child with poor physiological support for the feeding process, the expectations for oral feeding should be carefully considered and may need to be reduced. In these children, oral feeding may come at the expense of needed weight gain or by risking further physiological compromise.

Examples of Treatment Techniques

Provide Adequate Medical Support

As feeding is the major work of an infant, those with resolving respiratory problems may need additional respiratory support. This could include using supplemental oxygen during feeding or giving nebulizer treatments just prior to feeding. When infants are being weaned from supplemental oxygen, oximetry measurements should be made during feeding. Medication schedules may also need to be coordinated to provide the maximum respiratory benefits at feeding times.

Positioning

Feeding positions can support physiological function. Avoiding flexion of the head and neck assists in maintaining a fully open airway. The trunk position should allow maximal thorax excursion with minimal effort; it should be elongated and well supported.

External Pacing

For infants having difficulty coordinating sucking, swallowing, and breathing, external pacing methods may be used. The bottle is removed, or the suction broken, after 3 to 5 sucks, allowing the infant adequate time to pause and breathe. When the sucking rhythm is very disorganized, providing a strong external rhythm through movement, touch, or music may be useful in minimizing coughing and choking (Wolf & Glass, 1992).

Utilize Supplemental Feeding Methods

The child with problems of endurance, particularly if weight gain is poor, often benefits from using nonoral supplemental feeding methods (see the final section of this chapter). These methods provide tools that help work *toward* oral feeding. The results of supplemental feeding—weight gain, growth, and the reduction of pressure on oral feeding—support improvement in feeding skills. Often, supplemental feeding methods can be used in conjunction with oral feeding, further enhancing oral skill. If that is not possible, ongoing therapy can focus on maintaining oral-motor skills and pleasure from oral experiences. With adequate nutrition and thus growth, the child's overall endurance may improve.

Modifying the Characteristics of the Food

One technique might be to increase the caloric density for an infant with marginal intake due to poor endurance. This provides additional calories in the same total food volume, thus requiring less energy to eat it. For older children on spoon foods, high calorie puddings may be used to increase calories (Pipes, 1985). Additionally, using thicker foods may help some children who are having difficulty in coordinating their swallowing and breathing, as the child has slightly more control over initiating the swallowing process with thicker foods than with thin liquids.

Swallowing Function in Feeding

Swallowing, or deglutition, is a complex motor sequence that involves the coordination of all the oral, pharyngeal, and esophageal structures with the respiratory system. Precise coordination of breathing and swallowing is essential since these two systems share physical space within the pharynx. It is this duality of function within the mouth and the pharynx that underlies some of the difficulties in swallowing observed in infants and young children.

Phases of Swallowing

Swallowing is generally divided into segments or phases to describe the sequence of events. Most typically, it is divided into three phases: (1) the oral phase, (2) the pharyngeal phase, and (3) the esophageal phase (Donner, Bosma, & Robertson, 1985; Logemann, 1983; Miller, 1986).

Oral Phase

The primary functions of the oral phase are to process food into appropriate size particles for travel through the pharynx and the esophagus, and to transfer food from the front of the mouth to the pharynx in preparation for the initiation of the swallowing reflex (Miller, 1986). In early infancy, this phase consists exclusively of sucking but with maturity includes removing food from a spoon, biting, chewing, and drinking from a cup or a straw. An important function of the oral phase is the consolidation of the food into a cohesive bolus that is retained in the mouth until it is released into the pharynx as the swallowing reflex is triggered. By retaining the bolus in the mouth for the appropriate length of time, the oral phase establishes correct timing and coordination of the swallowing mechanism.

Pharyngeal Phase

The pharyngeal phase, which lasts approximately 1 second, begins as the swallow is triggered by sensory stimulation of the bolus to the faucial arches, soft palate, pharyngeal walls, and posterior aspect of the tongue (Logemann, 1983). The pharyngeal phase appears to have three functional components: (1) the closure of the nasal, laryngeal, and oral openings to direct the flow of the bolus and prevent leakage into inappropriate spaces; (2) the opening of the upper esophageal sphincter (UES); and (3) the creation of pressure gradients within the pharynx that assist with bolus propulsion into the esophagus.

The muscle activity that occurs during the pharyngeal phase is in a preset, time-locked sequence. If the duration of the phase is lengthened, the time that the muscles activate is lengthened but the sequence remains unchanged (Donner, Bosma, & Robertson, 1985). This muscle sequence begins with a leading complex that raises the hyoid (to aid in full protection of the larynx), and contracts the posterior pharyngeal wall (Doty, 1968). The sequence ends with the bolus in the esophagus and the pharyngeal structures returning to baseline. The complex events that comprise the pharyngeal phase are outlined in Figure 8-6.

During this phase of swallowing, the bolus is propelled not only by active contraction of the pharyngeal musculature, but also by changing pressure gradients within the mouth, pharynx, and esophagus (Kennedy & Kent, 1988). The mouth, pharynx, and esophagus are chambers with a series of valves that close off particular portions of the system. Closing these valves physically channels food, prevents aspiration, and also creates pressure gradients that aid in propelling the bolus (Cumming & Reilly, 1972).

Esophageal Phase

The final phase of swallowing is the esophageal phase, which begins with the opening of the upper esophageal sphincter (UES) and ends when the bolus enters the stomach through the lower esophageal sphincter (LES). This phase involves the relaxation of the upper and lower sphincters, and peristaltic action (Code & Schlegel, 1986).

The cricopharyngeus muscle serves as the UES and at baseline is tonically contracted. When stimulated during swallow, it relaxes to allow passage of the bolus. It then contracts to prevent reflux of the bolus back into the pharynx (Miller, 1987). The LES is not a specific muscle group but rather is a zone of increased pressure approximately 3 cm in length. This zone of pressure combined with the anatomical placement of the LES below the level of the diaphragm, creates pressure gradients that make it difficult, in normal circumstances, for the contents of the stomach to climb retrograde up the esophagus.

Control of Swallowing

Initiation of swallowing is dependent upon sensory feedback, primarily from the faucial arches, but also from the uvula, soft palate, posterior tongue, and the pharynx. These afferent messages are carried along cranial nerves V (trigeminal), IX (glossopharyngeal), and X (vagus). The initiation of swallowing is not automatic, even if a bolus has reached the faucial arches. The threshold for elicitation of the swallowing reflex can be altered by input

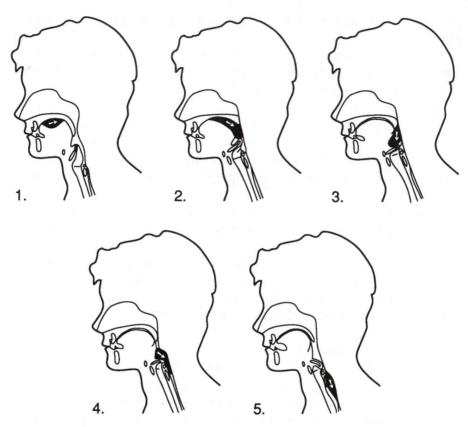

Figure 8-6 Steps in the pharyngeal phase of swallowing: (1) The initiation of the swallow occurs as the bolus is propelled backward by the tongue. Opposition of the tongue and soft palate prevent premature leakage of the bolus into the pharynx before the swallow is initiated; (2) As the swallow is initiated, the soft palate elevates and the posterior pharyngeal wall constricts to close the nasal cavity; (3) The larynx elevates and the epiglottis folds downward to cover the open airway. The true and false vocal folds also contract to provide additional airway protection. The bolus moves through the pharynx by the combined action of pharyngeal peristalsis and changing pressure gradients within the pharynx; (4) The bolus moves past the closed airway. The cricopharyngeus muscle relaxes and opens, allowing the bolus to pass into the esophagus; and (5) Once the bolus is totally within the esophagus, the cricopharyngeus tonically closes to prevent reflux back into the pharynx. Peristalsis carries the bolus to the stomach. [Source: From FEEDING AND SWALLOWING DISORDERS IN INFANCY by Lynn S. Wolf and Robin P. Glass, copyright 1992, by Therapy Skill Builders, a division of Communication Skill Builders, Inc., PO Box 42050, Tucson, AZ. Reprinted with permission.]

from higher cortical or hypothalamic regions as well as by peripheral stimuli, such as cold (Miller, 1986). The amount of reflexive versus voluntary control of the swallowing mechanism has been debated. Traditionally, swallowing has been considered to be a reflexive, stimulus-response activity. The complexity of the neural control of swallowing and the interaction of the swallowing mechanism at all levels of the nervous system, however, suggest that this view is too simplistic. Currently, it is felt that each phase of swallowing has varying degrees of reflexive and voluntary control. This leads to differences in the variability and repeatability of motor sequences in each phase (Kennedy & Kent, 1988). Voluntary control is greatest during the oral phase, as the oral structures respond to the changing properties of the bolus in terms of size, texture, temperature, or taste. However, the motor sequence that unfolds during the pharyngeal phase, after the swallowing reflex is initiated, appears to be preset.

Evaluation of Swallowing Function

Occupational therapists currently have several methods available to evaluate swallowing. Clinical evaluation of swallowing can always be undertaken, and requires only the therapist's clinical skill and simple feeding equipment. With technical equipment and trained personnel available, more detailed evaluation can be done radiologically or with ultrasound. The most comprehensive evaluation of swallowing includes both clinical and technical components.

Clinical Swallowing Evaluation

Swallowing History
To obtain an accurate clinical evaluation of swallowing, an in-depth history of functions related to swallowing is crucial. Interpretation of clinical observations may be impacted by the history of swallowing functions. Specific information that should be gathered includes

1. feeders' impressions of swallowing functions
2. amount of coughing and choking that the child does during feeding
3. specific food textures or tastes that elicit coughing, choking, or other problems noted by the feeder
4. timing of the problem within the feeding session
5. timing of the problem in relation to an individual bolus
6. incidence of respiratory illnesses
7. methods that have been used to try to correct the problem, and their effects

Clinical Observation

During the clinical evaluation, direct observations can be made of certain aspects of the oral phase of swallowing. Only inferences can be made about the function of the pharyngeal and esophageal phases, as these phases are not clinically observable. Swallowing function should be observed for all textures currently in the child's diet. Detailed observations of the child's oral-motor control should contain particular attention to

1. the ability to form a bolus, move the bolus posteriorly, and retain the bolus in the mouth prior to swallowing
2. the ability to completely clear the mouth after swallowing a single bolus
3. the ability to alter the size of the bolus, if needed, to prepare for swallowing

A baseline assessment of the child's respiratory control should occur along with observation of the coordination between swallowing and breathing. More detailed information regarding assessment of respiratory control can be found in the section on physiological support for feeding.

Clinical Signs of Swallowing Dysfunction

A variety of clinical signs can indicate swallowing dysfunction. These are outlined in Table 8-4. Excessive drooling, constant upper airway noise that sounds like the child is breathing through secretions, or the need for intermittent upper airway suctioning to clear secretions suggest that swallowing is dysfunctional in the child's management of saliva. At times, these findings are associated with very limited swallowing function. If the noisy, wet-sounding breathing occurs primarily with feeding, difficulty in swallowing is associated with the feeding process and the clearing of each bolus.

Table 8-4   Clinical Signs of Swallowing Dysfunction

---

1. Coughing or choking during swallowing

2. Inability to handle own oral secretions

3. Noisy, wet upper airway sounds after individual swallows, or increasing noisiness over course of feeding

4. Multiple swallows to clear a single bolus

5. Apnea during swallowing

6. History of frequent upper respiratory infections (URIs) or pneumonias

---

Source: From FEEDING AND SWALLOWING DISORDERS IN INFANCY by Lynn S. Wolf and Robin P. Glass, copyright 1992, by Therapy Skill Builders, a division of Communication Skill Builders, Inc., PO Box 42050, Tucson, AZ. Reprinted with permission.

Multiple swallows to clear a single bolus can indicate a problem in pharyngeal clearance. Apnea, or long pauses in breathing after swallowing, may also indicate inadequate clearance or aspiration. Coughing or choking during the swallow can be an indication of aspiration of a portion or all of the bolus. If there is a history of frequent upper respiratory infections (URIs), even in the absence of choking during feedings, aspiration during swallowing should be considered. As each of these findings can have alternate explanations, their interpretation must be made in relation to the full feeding observation and history.

Radiologic Evaluation of Swallowing

The videofluoroscopic swallowing study (VFSS), or modified barium swallow, is a more definitive method of evaluating swallowing function (Figure 8-7) (Warren & Fox, 1987). This radiologic procedure is structured to simulate the child's typical feeding situation, including position and food types and textures. Special devices may be needed to allow appropriate positioning using the X-ray equipment. All food textures currently in the child's diet should be evaluated, starting with the most typical and most easily managed foods progressing to the most problematic foods. All foods must be mixed with barium. Swallowing function is observed during real-time fluoroscopy (X-ray) and the study is recorded on videotape for later review. As a relatively small sample of feeding is observed, swallowing dysfunction may be present, but not seen during the sample that is studied (Donner, 1985; Kramer, 1985).

Videofluoroscopy is generally most useful if preceded by a clinical evaluation of swallowing. This allows the therapist to accomplish three things that can help improve the effectiveness of the VFSS. First, the therapist can assess baseline feeding behaviors to determine whether the behaviors observed during the VFSS are typical. Second, the therapist can determine typical food textures and the child's response. This helps in ordering their presentation during VFSS. The therapist may also develop other ideas for structuring the study, such as the position of the child, to best observe the feeding problems. Third, the therapist can formulate hypotheses regarding techniques that might improve feeding and swallowing. For example, the therapist might wonder if altering the head position or food texture would improve swallowing function. These techniques could be tried during the VFSS, and the results observed.

Atypical Development/Functional Problems

Common patterns of swallowing dysfunction that are seen in infants and toddlers are described. These patterns are specifically identified by the VFSS (Logemann, 1983).

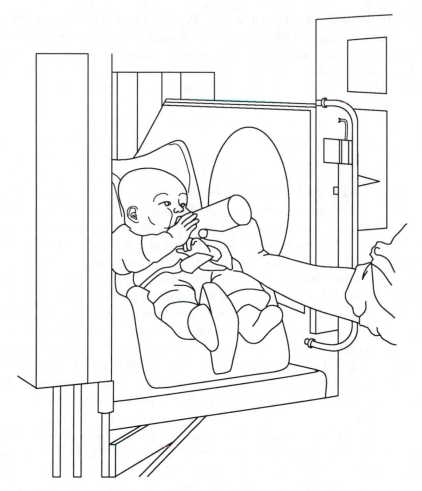

Figure 8-7 Child having a VFSS [From FEEDING AND SWALLOWING DISORDERS IN INFANCY by Lynn S. Wolf and Robin P. Glass, copyright 1992, by Therapy Skill Builders, a division of Communication Skill Builders, Inc., PO Box 42050, Tucson, AZ. Reprinted with permission.]

Aspiration (or Risk of Aspiration) Before the Swallow

A delay in initiating the swallow or inadequate oral control, allowing premature spilling of the bolus into the pharynx, permits food to fall into the pharynx during respiration when the larynx is open. Even if aspiration in not seen during the VFSS, the presence of food in the pharynx prior to swallow presents a high-risk situation.

Aspiration During the Swallow

Aspiration during the swallow is generally secondary to reduced or inadequate laryngeal elevation and closure. In this position, the larynx is not adequately protected. Food may seep under the epiglottis and into the airway.

Aspiration (or Risk of Aspiration) After the Swallow

When there is residue of foods or liquids in the pharynx after the swallow, it may be inhaled during respiration. This is generally secondary to poor pharyngeal clearance mechanisms, but can also be due to reduced laryngeal elevation or dysfunction of the cricopharyngeus muscle. Again, aspiration may not be observed during VFSS, but when food is not cleared properly, there is risk of aspiration.

Guiding Principles of Treatment

1. The exact nature of the swallowing problem must be clearly understood before appropriate intervention can occur. The multiple techniques described for treating various swallowing problems are effective only when applied appropriately. If applied without a full understanding of the child's swallowing problem, however, they can be harmful to the child. At times, they might lead to greater swallowing dysfunction during feeding. At other times, they may encourage continued oral feeding in a child who is aspirating.
2. Treatment procedures must be safe for the child. That is, they must not place the child at additional risk of aspiration or of damage to the respiratory system.

Examples of Treatment Techniques

Improve Initiation of Swallowing

Thermal stimulation while feeding can be provided by giving the child liquids and solids chilled in the freezer. Children can be given water popsicles to suck on prior to swallowing their most difficult food type. For infants, a hollow pacifier can be filled with water then frozen. Hypothetically, sucking on this frozen pacifier may chill the infants saliva, improving the timing of the swallowing reflex.

Improve Bolus Formation

The tongue plays a crucial role in bolus formation and propulsion; therefore, treatment techniques should focus on aspects of tongue control. Treatment suggestions and further references can be found in the section on neuromotor components of feeding. In addition, some food textures support bolus organization more than others (i.e., thicker foods), so diet modifications may help minimize the problem. Providing the child with one bolus at a time, followed by a pause to organize the swallow, is also useful.

Managing Aspiration During the Swallow
Since the larynx moves upward during the swallow to close the airway, forward head flexion may improve laryngeal movement and closure by preelevating the larynx or decreasing the distance the larynx must elevate. Particularly in young infants, hyperflexion of neck, which could collapse the airway, must be avoided. Giving thicker foods may allow the bolus to remain in a more cohesive mass or move more slowly through the hypopharynx allowing the larynx sufficient time to elevate and close the airway.

Reduced Pharyngeal Peristalsis
This problem is difficult to treat as it is generally not possible to alter pharyngeal peristalsis. If the residue is more pronounced with solids than liquids, following each bolus of solids with a sip of liquids may assist in flushing the hypopharynx. Providing dry swallows by using a pacifier after each bolus may improve clearance.

Structural Considerations

Evaluation

There are numerous structural problems that may interfere with feeding in infants and in children. Some examples include tracheoesophageal fistulas, laryngeal clefts, macroglossia, tracheal stenosis, laryngomalacia, and tracheomalacia. Most of these problems are relatively rare and many therapists will never encounter them. This section will address two defects that are more commonly seen—clefts of the lip and palate, and micrognathia.

Clefts of the Lip and Palate
These congenital defects result from failed fusion of the upper lip or of the palate during embryonic development. The cleft lip and cleft palate may be seen individually or together. They may be unilateral or bilateral. The bilateral cleft lip and palate is usually considered the most severe defect. A cleft lip is often surgically repaired in the first few months of life. Repair of a cleft palate generally occurs between 12 and 18 months of age (Shah & Wong, 1980).

Feeding problems resulting from clefts are most evident in the infant period. They result from an inability to generate suction and are specific to bottle and breast-feeding. If feeding difficulties persist for the older child, they may be the result of secondary problems such as inappropriate tongue movement, aversive oral stimulation in infancy, or neuromotor dysfunction unrelated to the cleft. For the older child, these problems should be evaluated as described in other sections. Evaluation of the infant with cleft lip or palate should include (Clarren, Anderson, & Wolf, 1987) the following.

1. Negative pressure suction: The degree of negative pressure suction that the infant is able to generate must be determined. This is the force that pulls the examiner's finger or a nipple into the mouth; it should be differentiated from the positive pressure exerted by the tongue and jaw to compress the nipple. When negative pressure suction is weak or absent, the infant may have difficulty holding the nipple in the mouth and extracting fluid efficiently. The amount of positive pressure compression on the nipple can also be assessed, as this force will remove some fluid.

2. Tongue movements: The tongue should be in the midline, cup around the nipple (central groove), and produce rhythmic pressure on the nipple. The infant's ability to hold the nipple in the center of the mouth should be noted, particularly if there is a large bilateral cleft palate.

Micrognathia

This term refers to a small or posteriorly placed mandible. On visual observation, the chin appears small and recessed. In the mouth, the tongue is often of normal size, but posteriorly positioned in relation to the oral cavity and pharyngeal airway. Micrognathia, seen in conjunction with a cleft palate, is referred to as the Pierre-Robin malformation sequence (Figure 8-8) (Lewis & Pashayan, 1980). With micrognathia, feeding problems are typically encountered in infancy during bottle and breast-feeding. These problems generally resolve with the rapid mandibular growth that occurs during the first months of life. Feeding also becomes easier as the child moves to spoon and finger feeding, with their reduced demands on the coordination of breathing and swallowing. Infant feeding evaluation should focus on the following components.

1. Respiration: The posteriorly placed tongue associated with micrognathia may obstruct the pharyngeal airway and compromise respiration. The rate of respirations, the pattern of respirations (including evidence of obstruction), and signs of increased work of breathing should be observed closely at rest and during feeding. The effect of position changes should be considered. Monitoring oxygen saturations is strongly recommended to determine the significance of intermittent obstruction.

2. Tongue position and movement: Note how far back the tongue

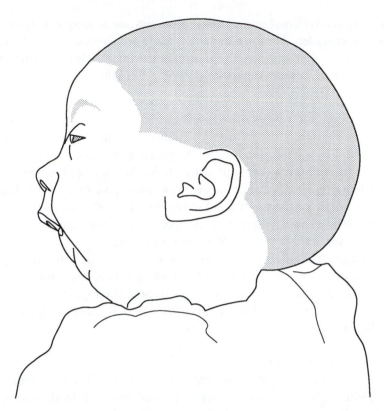

Figure 8-8 Micrognathia [From FEEDING AND SWALLOWING DISORDERS IN IN-
FANCY by Lynn S. Wolf and Robin P. Glass, copyright 1992, by Therapy Skill Builders,
a division of Communication Skill Builders, Inc., PO Box 42050, Tucson, AZ. Reprinted
with permission.]

characteristically sits, how far forward it is able to move, and what
sucking movements are generated.
3. Suction: When a cleft palate is also present, the generation of
   suction should be evaluated as previously described.

Functional Problems

Limited Suction
    Typically, in cleft lip and cleft palate, the primary functional
feeding problem is the inability to generate negative intraoral pressure. Thus,
there is inadequate suction to draw fluid from a nipple during bottle feeding
or to draw the breast into the mouth and maintain its position during breast-
feeding. To generate negative pressure suction, the oral cavity must be sealed
and then enlarge slightly. When a cleft lip is present, it may be difficult

to maintain an anterior seal on the nipple. If there is a cleft palate, it is no longer possible to effectively seal the oral cavity from the nasal cavity, though some infants seal the small clefts intermittently with their tongue. While small amounts of fluid may be expelled from a bottle by compression of the nipple by the tongue or by intermittent suction, feeding is very inefficient and requires considerable time and caloric expenditure (Clarren, Anderson, & Wolf, 1987).

Airway Obstruction

This is the most significant problem for infants with micrognathia, and it may become worse during feeding. The infant is frequently semireclined and gravity pulls the already retroplaced tongue into the pharyngeal airway. This can lead to severe difficulty in the coordination of swallowing and breathing, resulting in coughing and oxygen desaturation. At worst, it can lead to total airway obstruction, apnea, and bradycardia. Interestingly, in some infants, respiration is optimal during sucking as the tongue moves forward to hold the nipple. However, as the nipple is removed for burping or if the infant falls asleep and stops sucking, airway obstruction may be noted.

Abnormal Tongue Movement During Sucking

With micrognathia, the posterior position of the tongue often limits the contact between the tongue and the nipple. The nipple may not sit in the central groove of the tongue; therefore, sucking is inefficient.

Guiding Principles of Treatment

1. Cleft lip: Establish an anterior seal around the nipple or compensate for the reduction of suction.
2. Cleft palate: Minimize the impact of reduced intraoral suction. Possibilities include obstructing the cleft by using an obturator or assisting with milk delivery to the mouth by a squeeze bottle or other similar device. Use of normal oral-motor patterns should also be promoted with midline nipple orientation, encouragement of normal sucking mechanics during feeding, and therapeutic oral-motor activities if needed.
3. Micrognathia: Maintain a stable airway during feeding. This may be possible with positioning, although special respiratory or surgical management are often required. *If a stable airway can not be maintained in a position that allows feeding, the child should not be fed orally.* Maximal contact between the tongue and the nipple should also be established by facilitating forward tongue movement or by nipple selection. If there is also cleft palate, those treatment principles must be applied.

4. Feeding must be efficient to be effective: Most children with these structural problems are able to feed orally, within a reasonable time period with appropriate feeding modifications. If an efficient oral feeding method cannot be found (i.e., for an infant, a full required volume should be taken in 30 to 40 minutes at 3 to 4 hour intervals), supplementary nonoral feedings, discussed later in this chapter, should be considered.

Examples of Treatment Techniques

Squeeze Bottles

These can be used when the child does not generate adequate negative intraoral pressure. By squeezing these soft plastic bottles, milk flow from compression of the tongue against the nipple is enhanced. They encourage normal sucking patterns; with minimal practice, the feeder can match the baby's sucking rhythm. The type of nipple used with a squeeze bottle should be carefully considered.

Feeding Position

Using an upright position to feed a child with a cleft palate allows gravity to assist in reducing the possibility that fluid or soft foods will enter the nasal cavity through the cleft. For the child with micrognathia (without a cleft palate), feeding may be possible in a prone or semiprone position. Gravity may assist in keeping the tongue forward and the airway open. A special angled-neck bottle may be needed for adequate milk flow in this position.

Nipple Type

When a squeeze bottle is used, a nipple with a conventional hole rather than a crosscut nipple is recommended. Using a crosscut nipple, the hole size varies with the amount of nipple compression. In conjunction with the feeder squeezing the bottle, a crosscut nipple can lead to an uneven flow of liquid. Excessively large, homemade nipple holes should also be avoided, as milk flow will be triggered by minimal oral movement. Flow can then be difficult to control, possibly leading to the use of abnormal oral-motor patterns.

For the child with micrognathia and a recessed tongue, a long straight nipple may make the best contact with the tongue and allow for the most effective sucking. For a child with a narrow midline cleft palate, however, a straight narrow nipple might be pushed into the cleft during sucking. A wider nipple might allow compression of the nipple against intact segments of the palate and expression of some milk. A nipple with a broad base is suggested for the infant with a cleft lip, as the nipple can assist in occluding the cleft.

Behavioral and Interactional Aspects of Feeding

The process of feeding is multidimensional, having a substantial impact on all aspects of a child's development. Competency in physical, social, and emotional skills can be developed out of early feeding experiences. Unfortunately, many oral-motor and feeding intervention programs emphasize the mechanical aspects of oral control and have not focused on the dynamic relationship between the parent and the child (Morris, 1978). For this reason, occupational therapists working in the area of early feeding difficulties need an understanding of the behavioral, social, and interactional components of the feeding process (Humphry, 1987, 1991).

Parental Considerations

Eating is one of the infant's first avenues for interaction with the environment. Regularity of parental response to the baby's hunger cues leads to development of the foundations of cause-and-effect behavior and the development of a basic sense of trust. Feeding provides the medium for a wealth of early sensory and play experiences (Day, 1982). Parents frequently do not set aside a specific play time with their infants, but rather provide interaction over the course of the day through caregiving activities (Humphry, 1987). Since eating occurs frequently in early infancy, it encompasses a large percentage of the time a parent spends with an infant.

Feeding is also a milieu for the expression of parental feelings and attitudes about the adequacy of their parenting. The act of providing nutrition for children is intimately tied to the culturally defined role of the parent, most often the mother (Cronin, 1987). If there are feeding difficulties, the parent may internalize these as a reflection of inadequate parenting skills. This perception may lead to anxiety and depression; thus, further eroding parental confidence. In turn, this may accentuate feeding difficulties or impede the remediation process.

Child Considerations

Characteristics of temperament and personality can be reflected in both feeding and eating styles. Chess, Thomas, and Birch (1965) were the first to identify characteristics of temperament, which are reflected in all aspects of a child's behavior. They outlined nine temperamental qualities influencing behavior: activity level, regularity, adaptability, approach/withdrawal, physical sensitivity, intensity of reaction, distractibility, positive or negative mood, and persistence. For each characteristic, a child's behavior can be rated high or low on that attribute. Not only will a child's basic temperament influence the development of feeding-related behaviors, but it will also affect the type of intervention strategies that are most effective in resolving the problem.

Als (1986) has adapted a similar concept to the behavior of premature infants. Within her synactive model of neonatal behavioral organization, a baby's behavior is viewed as a reflection of the interaction between the environment and the inherent function of the baby's autonomic, motoric, state, regulatory, and attentional/interactive subsystems. Behavioral cues by the baby will reflect the degree of stability and self-regulation versus stress and disorganization of any subsystem.

Considerations in Parent–Child Interaction

Clear behavioral cues from the baby are more likely to elicit parental behaviors that meet the infant's needs and enhance stability. Disorganized infant cues frequently lead to caretaker responses that increase stress and cause further disorganization for the infant. While there is an interplay between the infant and the parent, ultimately effective parental interpretation of the infant's cues is necessary for the baby to make the most adaptive response.

Children with difficult temperaments learn to feed successfully and overcome feeding problems. At times, however, there may be a mismatch between characteristics of the infant's temperament and that of the parent, or the infant's temperament and the environmental roadblocks with which the child must cope. For example, the infant who has high adaptability and low physical sensitivity may exhibit fewer behavioral sequelae from endotracheal intubation than the infant with the opposite temperament. The parent with low activity level and intensity of reaction may have considerable difficulty feeding a toddler with high activity level and intensity of reactions, particularly if a feeding problem is also present.

Finally, feeding is an area for the expression of control by both the parent and the child. Eating is one of the first areas in which a baby can develop independence from his parents. Through self-feeding and the nonverbal expression of food preferences, the baby begins the process of differentiation and independence. Behavioral problems around feeding, such as food refusals, tantrums or limited intake, may be expressions of a child's emerging independence that has been thwarted in other areas. For the child with a disability, these feeding-related behavioral problems may be efforts to gain control by a child who otherwise feels powerless. Pipes (1985) underscores this point by stating "developmentally delayed children experience the same responses to parental anxiety about their food intake as any child, and in a like manner, can control their parents by their acceptance or rejection of food" (p. 174). Likewise, parents who feel threatened by their child's emerging independence, or who are less skilled in appropriate limit setting, may use feeding as a time to exercise their own control and authority.

The behavioral aspects of any feeding interaction, therefore, will be an amalgamation of the baby's own temperamental characteristics, physical abil-

ities, and environmental considerations, combined with the parent's temperament, values, stresses, resources, and parenting skill.

Evaluation of Behavioral Components

Standard Evaluation

Systematic observation of the relationship between the child
and primary feeder is an essential part of a comprehensive feeding evaluation.
Unfortunately, occupational therapists are faced with a lack of appropriate
evaluation tools (Humphry, 1987). Two structured evaluation tools that are
available might be considered. Denton (1986) has described suggestions for
observation of mother–infant interaction during feeding of infants with non-
organic failure to thrive that could form the basis of a standard behavioral
observation of feeding. The NCAST (Nursing Child Assessment Satellite
Training) Feeding Scale is a fully developed, reliable, and valid observational
assessment of feeding interaction. Special training is required to establish
examiner reliability (Barnard, 1978).

Informal Evaluation

At a minimum, throughout the parent interview and feeding
observation, the occupational therapist should make informal observations
of the parent–infant interaction. The child's behavior and temperament
should be addressed. It might be considered in relation to the characteristics
described by Chess, Thomas, and Birch (1965) or Als (1986). The parents'
goals for feeding should be clarified. The parents' style of interaction and
responses to the child should also be observed. Information on the level of
parental stress regarding feeding and other areas, resources, and supports
should also be gathered. These factors may influence parents' interactions
with the child.

Videotaping the feeding session may be useful in identifying parent and
child behaviors that influence the feeding problem. Reviewing this tape with
the parent may be a useful teaching tool in the therapeutic process.

Atypical Development/Functional Problems

Child Problems

1. Limited adaptability: When faced with changes in routine or new
   experiences, the child becomes disorganized and responds negatively. Best performance is achieved when the environment is
   highly structured or predictable.
2. Behavioral cues or nonverbal communication lacks clarity: The
   child may be very subtle in providing cues, making him difficult to
   read. The child may also use similar behaviors to mean different
   things.

Caretaker Problems

1. Difficulty reading behavioral cues or nonverbal communication: If the caregiver is unable to correctly interpret the infant's or child's behavior, it is unlikely that she will respond appropriately to the child's needs.
2. Limited parenting skills: The range and repertoire of responses to the child's behavior may be limited. The approach to problem solving may be dogmatic, or they may view problems as having limited possibilities for solutions.
3. High level of stress or limited resources or support: Parental stress and pressure can compromise parent–child interactions in all situations.
4. Inappropriate expectations for feeding: This may reflect a lack of understanding of the feeding problem or can reflect unresolved anger or denial in regard to the child's disability.

Feeding Dyad Difficulties

1. Feeding as a battleground in the struggle for control: The parent or the infant may be using feeding-related behaviors to exert control over their environment. The parent may have unrealistic expectations for the level of the child's independence or dependence.
2. Mismatch between child and feeder: This can be a mismatch in personality or temperament, or can result from the caregiver misreading or misinterpreting the child's cues.

Guiding Principles of Treatment

1. Treatment to modify behavioral or interactional difficulties must be based on respect for the basic characteristics and values of both the parent and the child.
2. Both the parent and the child need to be empowered with the appropriate level of control and independence.
3. Providing information and educating caretakers can be a powerful tool in facilitating change. Education might focus on infant behavioral cues, social-emotional development, further understanding of the specific feeding problem, or increased understanding of behavioral interactions.
4. Utilize behavior modification techniques to increase the child's cooperation and compliance.
5. Modify the environment to foster optimal interaction.

Examples of Treatment Techniques

Environmental Modification

For the parents, this may mean assisting with time management, babysitting, or possibly counseling so they have enough emotional energy and time to carry out treatment recommendations. For the baby, this may mean limiting visual distractions, providing age-appropriate seating or physical support.

Reinforcement of Appropriate Behaviors with Rewards

For older children, tangible, verbal, or nonverbal rewards such as praise, toys, hugs, or preferred foods should be incorporated into all treatment sessions. Initially, reinforcement for appropriate behaviors should occur immediately following each behavior. As the behavior becomes more consistent, an intermittent reward schedule will become more effective to maintain the behavior.

Modeling Appropriate Behavioral Interaction

During all sessions, the therapist should model the type of interaction they would like to see performed by the parent. Since differences may exist between the therapist's and parents' basic personality, an attempt should be made to model behaviors that match the parents' capabilities.

Videotaping Treatment Sessions

This may assist parents in becoming conscious of their own behavior and the behavior of their child. If appropriate interaction is modeled by the therapist, the parent may also use the tape as a later reminder.

Nonoral Feeding Methods

The ultimate goal of any feeding or feeding-related program must be optimal nutrition for the child. Meeting nutritional requirements supports overall growth, promotes appropriate development, and provides the background for stable health or medical improvement. A downward spiral may develop, however, when there are problems in the feeding process. Feeding dysfunction may lead to poor intake or excessive energy expenditure for feeding. Nutrition is then not optimal, and growth as well as medical and developmental status may suffer. In turn, these factors may further compromise feeding performance and limit the possibility of improvement. For example, an infant with a heart defect may have poor endurance for feeding, and frequently demonstrate inadequate intake. However, weight gain and growth, which could improve endurance, may be necessary before heart surgery.

Table 8-5 Types of Feeding Tubes

Type of Feeding Tube	Insertion/Destination	Strengths	Limitations
Nasogastric tube (NG)	Nose/stomach	No surgical placement required; Oral feeding possible with tube in place	Insertion and presence in nose or throat is uncomfortable and may be aversive; May trigger vagally mediated bradycardia; May be cosmetically unacceptable for long-term use
Orogastric tube (OG)	Mouth/stomach	No surgical placement	Same as NG, plus difficult to feed orally with tube in place
Duodenal tube	Nose/duodenum	No surgical placement; Bypasses stomach, so decreases risk of GE reflux	Same as NG, though softer, so may have fewer hypersensitive responses; Must use continuous drip feeding; Difficult to place and maintain in correct position
Gastrostomy (standard, percutaneous, button)	Surgically placed in stomach	No aversive oral-facial stimuli; Despite surgical placement, can be removed easily when no longer needed; Sits beneath clothing, cosmetically acceptable	Requires surgical placement; Site needs daily care and possibly trip to medical facility if tube falls out; Potential risk for increased GE reflux after tube placed
Jejunostomy	Tube surgically placed in jejunum, possibly in association with gastrostomy	Same as gastrostomy; Bypasses stomach, so reduces risk of GE reflux	Requires surgical placement; Site needs daily care, requires trip to hospital if tube falls out; Requires continuous drip feedings

Source: From FEEDING AND SWALLOWING DISORDERS IN INFANCY by Lynn S. Wolf and Robin P. Glass, copyright 1992, by Therapy Skill Builders, a division of Communication Skill Builders, Inc., PO Box 42050, Tucson, AZ. Reprinted with permission.

In planning treatment for feeding problems, the first goal is to determine if techniques, which improve the quality or quantity of the oral feeding performance, can be identified. In some cases, intake may still be inadequate, energy expense too high, or oral feeding unsafe. In such cases, nonoral tube feeding methods should be considered. While parents and health professionals may see the use of tube feeding as an indication of the infant's failure at oral feeding, the appropriate use of tube feeding methods can be considered a tool to improve nutrition for the child. Better nutrition leads to growth, developmental changes, and possibly, medical improvement, all of which can support positive changes in oral feeding.

Nasogastric, orogastric, and duodenal tubes; gastrostomies; and jejunostomies are the most common methods of nonoral feeding. While nutritional improvement may be possible using tube feeding methods, there are also potential disadvantages that must be considered (Nelson & Hallgren, 1989). Table 8-5 describes the strengths and weaknesses of the various types of feeding tubes. Not only must the type of tube be matched to the child's needs, but the most appropriate feeding schedule must be determined. Table 8-6 identifies various schedules that are possible when these nonoral feeding methods are used.

Transition from Tube to Oral Feeding

Although tube feeding can be a tremendous support to oral feeding, as well as to the child's health, it should not be an isolated management strategy. If tube feedings are instituted without giving thought to later oral feedings, health professionals may be faced with the dilemma of how to

Table 8-6   Options in Using Tube Feeding

Amount of Feeding by Tube	*Examples:*
1. Tube-oral combination	Alternate feedings—tube, oral, tube, oral
	Oral feeds during day, tube feeds at night
	Oral feed to endurance limit, giving balance by tube
2. Total tube feeding	
Methods of Tube Feeding	*Description:*
1. Bolus	At each feeding time, the full amount required is given over 10 to 20 minutes
2. Continuous drip	Formula is infused continuously over a long period of time (10 to 24 hours per day) at a set rate

move a child with minimal skills back to oral feeding months or years later (Monahan & Shapiro, 1988). When tube feeding is used most effectively, it is part of a comprehensive feeding plan (Morris & Klein, 1987; 1989). In this situation, consideration is given to the eventual transition back to full oral feeding at the time tube feeding is introduced. Pertinent principles include the following.

1. Establish the level of oral feeding that is safe and within the child's functional capabilities. Routinely carry out this level of oral feeding. It may be as much as taking half of the feedings orally, or as little as receiving a teaspoon of food or liquid per day. Perseverance in this area may be the greatest predictor of positive outcomes in the eventual return to oral feeding. If it appears, however, that even a minimal level of oral feeding is unsafe, *no* oral feeding should be done.

2. Minimize aversive oral-tactile experiences, including prolonged use of NG tubes and oral suctioning. Tolerance and enjoyment of oral-tactile input should be promoted. Oral exploration should be encouraged.

3. Existing oral-motor skills must be maintained and other developmentally and medically appropriate skills should be encouraged through therapeutic activities.

4. If possible, a link should be established between pleasant oral activity and the satiation of hunger.

Based on the medical condition and developmental status of the child receiving tube feedings, the prognosis for returning to oral feeding will vary. In most cases, steady progress will lead to a gradual, or sometimes sudden, return to oral feeding. The length of time it will take a child to reach this goal, however, is extremely variable.

There are some children for whom the goal of returning to full oral feeding, or in some cases *any* oral feeding, is not realistic. In these cases, the limiting factors are generally medical considerations that are beyond the ability of a feeding specialist to control or modify. Oral therapy for these children focuses on maintaining existing oral-motor skills, developing additional oral skills appropriate for language, encouraging pleasurable oral experiences, and ensuring that oral hygiene is tolerated and practiced.

In the process of developing oral feeding abilities in the nonorally fed child, there may be times when the family or medical professionals feel that the child has reached a plateau or that progress is not as rapid as desired. At this point, an effort may be made to make a major push toward the goal of oral feeding. For this child, before a large effort is made to transition to oral feeding, a number of questions must be considered. These fall into the categories of child readiness and parent readiness.

Questions to Determine Child Readiness

1. Is the underlying problem that led to the need for tube feeding resolved? Will the child's current medical condition and weight allow aggressive work toward oral feeding?
2. Are the child's oral-motor skills adequate for increased oral feeding?
3. Is swallowing function safe?

Questions to Determine Parent Readiness

1. Do the parents or caregivers understand that this may be a lengthy process and progress may be made in very small steps?
2. Do the parents or caregivers understand that such a program will require considerable repetition and consistency, and that much of it will need to be carried out at home?
3. Do the parents or caregivers have the time and the emotional resources available to undertake this effort?

If the child and the parents both appear to be ready to undertake this process, two approaches are possible. The traditional approach is slow and steady (Morris & Klein, 1987). Initially, the focus is on manipulating the tube feeding schedule to normalize hunger-satiation cycles. A program of normalizing responses to the oral-tactile and taste components of feeding is generally required. Activities to improve oral-motor skills may be required for some children. Additionally, behavioral management strategies are usually needed, as children on prolonged tube feedings have often learned to manipulate many aspects of the feeding process. The second approach to making the transition from tube feeding is the rapid introduction of oral feeding (Blackman & Nelson, 1985). After a team evaluation, the child is admitted to a hospital or other 24-hour care facility for 2 to 3 weeks. Strict behavioral protocols are followed, with trained staff members gradually giving the child more food orally. As the child progresses, the parents are included in the feeding process. Since there is an element of force-feeding involved in this program, it is more controversial and does not meet the needs of many families. However, the relatively quick changes that are possible do appeal to some families.

Summary

Traditionally, in feeding evaluation and in treatment programs, the occupational therapist has primarily focused on the oral-motor aspects of feeding dysfunction. With increasing awareness of the complex nature of the feeding process, therapists need to move toward comprehensive approaches to the feeding problems of infants and toddlers. A thorough evaluation and accurate interpretation form the basis for an effective treatment program.

This evaluation must move beyond the oral motor aspects of feeding to include swallowing function, sensory components, physiologic support for feeding, and interpersonal dynamics. Interpretation must reflect a full understanding of the interplay between the child's medical diagnosis and the clinical signs and symptoms of feeding dysfunction. This foundation allows the therapist to select strategies that form a comprehensive plan and, thus, provide exemplary service to both children and their families.

References

Als, H. (1986). A synactive model of neonatal behavioral organization: Framework for the assessment of neurobehavioral development in the premature infant and for support of infants and parents in the neonatal intensive care environment. *Physical and Occupational Therapy in Pediatrics, 6,* 3–53.

Ardran, G.M., Kemp, F.H., & Lind, J. (1958a). A cineradiographic study of bottle feeding. *British Journal of Radiology, 31,* 11–22.

Ardran, G.M., Kemp, F.H., & Lind, J. (1958b). A cineradiographic study of breast feeding. *British Journal of Radiology, 31,* 156–162.

Barnard, K. (1978). *Nursing Child Assessment Satellite Training-Feeding Scale.* Seattle: School of Nursing, University of Washington.

Blackman, J.A., & Nelson, C.L.A. (1985). Reinstituting oral feedings in children fed by gastrostomy tube. *Clinical Pediatrics, 24,* 434–438.

Bly, L. (1983). *The components of normal movement during the first year of life and abnormal motor development.* Chicago, IL: Neuro-Developmental Treatment Association.

Bosma, J.F. (1967). Human infant oral function. In J.F. Bosma (Ed.), *Oral sensation and perception* (pp. 98–110). Springfield, IL: Charles C Thomas.

Bosma, J.F. (1972). Form and function in the infant's mouth and pharynx. In J.F. Bosma (Ed.), *Oral sensation and perception: The mouth of the infant* (pp. 3–29). Springfield, IL: Charles C Thomas.

Bosma, J.F. (1980). Physiology of the mouth. In M.M. Paparella & D.A. Shumrick (Eds.), *Otolaryngology* (pp. 319–331). Philadelphia: W.B. Saunders.

Bosma, J.F., & Donner, M.V. (1980). Physiology of the pharynx. In M.M. Paparella & D.A. Shumrick (Eds.), *Otolaryngology* (pp. 332–344). Philadelphia: W.B. Saunders.

Bosma, J.F., Hepburn, L.G, Josell, S.D., & Baker, K. (1990). Ultrasound demonstration of tongue motions during suckle feeding. *Developmental Medicine and Child Neurology, 32,* 223–229.

Brake, S.C., Fifer, W.P., Alfasi, G., & Fleischman, A. (1988). The first nutritive sucking responses of premature newborns. *Infant Behavior and Development, 11,* 1–9.

Braun, M.A., & Palmer, M.M. (1985). A pilot study of oral-motor development dysfunction in "at risk" infants. *Physical and Occupational Therapy in Pediatrics, 5,* 13–25.

Casaer, P., Daniels, H., Devlieger, H., DeCock, P., & Effermont, E. (1982). Feeding behavior in preterm neonates. *Early Human Development, 7,* 331–346.

Chess, S., Thomas, A., & Birch, H.G. (1965). *Your child as a person.* New York: Viking Press.

Clarren, S.K., Anderson, B., & Wolf, L.S. (1987). Feeding infants with cleft lip, cleft palate, or cleft lip and palate. *Cleft Palate Journal, 24,* 244–249.

Code, C.F., & Schlegel, J.F. (1986). Motor action of the esophagus and its sphincters. In C.F. Code (Ed.), *Handbook of physiology. Alimentary canal* (pp. 1821–1839). Washington, DC: American Physiology Society.

Connor, F.P., Williamson, G.G., & Siepp, J.M. (1978). *Program guide for infants and toddlers with neuromotor and other developmental disabilities.* New York: Teachers College Press.

Cronin, A. (1987). Incorporating social/behavioral aspects of eating dysfunction into oral-motor programs. In *Problem with eating: Intervention for children and adults with developmental disabilities* (pp. 51–64). Rockville, MD: American Occupational Therapy Association.

Cumming, W.A., & Reilly, B.J. (1972). Fatigue aspiration. *Radiology, 105,* 387–390.

Day, D. (1982). Mother–infant activities as providers of sensory stimulation. *American Journal of Occupational Therapy, 40,* 352–358.

Denton, R. (1986). An occupational therapy protocol for assessing infants and toddlers who fail to thrive. *American Journal of Occupational Therapy, 40,* 352–358.

Donner, M.W. (1985). Radiologic evaluation of swallowing. *American Review of Respiratory Diseases, 131,* Suppl. S20–S23.

Donner, M.W., Bosma, J.L., & Robertson, D.L. (1985). Anatomy and physiology of the pharynx. *Gastrointestinal Radiology, 10,* 196–212.

Doty, R.W. (1968). Neural organization of deglutition. In C.F. Code (Ed.), *Handbook of physiology. Alimentary canal, Vol. 4* (pp. 1861–1902). Washington, DC: American Physiological Society.

Finnie, N.R. (1975). *Handling the young cerebral palsied child at home.* New York: E.P. Dutton.

Furuno, S., O'Reilly, K., Hosaka, C.M., Inatsuka, T.T, Allman, T.A., & Zeisloft, B. (1984). *Hawaii Early Learning Profile (HELP).* Palo Alto, CA: VORT Corporation.

Hack, M., Estabrook, M.M., & Robertson, S.S. (1985). Development of sucking rhythms in preterm infants. *Early Human Development, 11,* 133–140.

Humphrey, T. (1964). Some correlations between the appearance of human fetal reflexes and the development of the nervous system. *Progress in Brain Research, 4,* 93–135.

Humphry, R. (1987). Feeding problems and the mother–infant relationship. In *Problem with eating: Intervention for children and adults with developmental disabilities* (pp. 27–39). Rockville, MD: American Occupational Therapy Association.

Humphry, R. (1991). Impact of feeding problems on the parent–infant relationship. *Infants and Young Children, 3*(3), 30–38.

Ianniruberto, A., & Tajani, E. (1981). Ultrasonographic study of fetal movements. *Seminars in Perinatology, 5,* 175–181.

Illingworth, R.S., & Lister, J. (1964). The critical or sensitive period, with special reference to feeding problems in infants and children. *Journal of Pediatrics, 65,* 839–848.

Jelm, J. (1990). *Oral-Motor/Feeding Rating Scale.* Tucson, AZ: Therapy Skill Builders.

Johnson, P., & Salisbury, D.M. (1975). Breathing and sucking during feeding in the newborn. *Ciba Foundation Symposiums, 33,* 119–135.

Kennedy, J.G., & Kent, R.D. (1988). Physiological substrates of normal deglutition. *Dysphagia, 3,* 24–37.

Klaus, M., & Fanaroff, A.A. (1978). *Care of the high risk neonate.* Philadelphia: W.B. Saunders.

Kramer, S.S. (1985). Special swallowing problems in children. *Gastrointestinal Radiology, 10,* 241–250.

Leonard, E.L., Trykowski, L.E., & Kirkpatrick, B.V. (1980). Nutritive sucking in high risk neonates after perioral stimulation. *Physical Therapy, 60,* 299–302.

Lewis, M.B., & Pashayan, H.M. (1980). Management of infants with Robin Anomaly. *Clinical Pediatrics, 19,* 519–528.

Logemann, J.A. (1983). *Evaluation and treatment of swallowing disorders.* Boston: College-Hill Press.

Mathew, O.P. (1988a). Regulation of breathing pattern during feeding: Role of suck, swallow and nutrients. In O.P. Mathew & G. Sant'Ambrogio (Eds.), *Respiratory Function of the Upper Airway* (pp. 535–560). New York: Marcel Dekker, Inc.

Mathew, O.P. (1988b). Respiratory control during nipple feeding in preterm infants. *Pediatric Pulmonology, 5,* 220–224.

Mathew, O.P., Clark, M.L., & Pronske, M.L. (1985). Apnea, bradycardia, and cyanosis during oral feeding in term neonates (letter). *Journal of Pediatrics, 106,* 857.

Miller, A.J. (1986). Neurophysiological basis of swallowing. *Dysphagia, 1,* 91–100.

Miller, A.J. (1987). Swallowing: Neurophysiologic control of the esophageal phase. *Dysphagia, 2,* 72–82.

Monahan, P., & Shapiro, B. (1988). Effect of tube feeding on oral function. *Developmental Medicine and Child Neurology,* Supp. 57:7.

Morris, S.E. (1978). Interpersonal aspects of feeding. In J.M. Wilson (Ed.), *Oral motor function and dysfunction in children* (pp. 106–113). Chapel Hill: University of North Carolina.

Morris, S. E. (1982). *The Normal acquisition of oral feeding skills: Implications for assessment and treatment.* Central Islip, NY: Therapeutic Media.

Morris, S.E. (1989). Development of oral-motor skills in the neurologically impaired child receiving non-oral feeding. *Dysphagia, 3,* 135–154.

Morris, S.E., & Klein, M.D. (1987). *Pre-feeding skills.* Tucson, AZ: Therapy Skill Builders.

Mueller, H. (1972). Facilitating feeding and prespeech. In P.H. Pearson & C.E. Williams (Eds.), *Physical therapy services in the developmental disabilities.* Springfield, IL: Charles C. Thomas.

Mueller, H. (1975). Feeding. In N.R. Finnie (Ed.), *Handling the young cerebral palsied child at home.* New York: E.P. Dutton.

Nelson, C.L.A., & Hallgren, R.A. (1989). Gastrostomies: Indications, management, and weaning. *Infants and Young Children, 2,* 66–74.

Orenstein, S.R., & Orenstein, D.M. (1988). Gastroesophageal reflux and respiratory disease in children. *The Journal of Pediatrics, 112,* 847–858.

Pipes, P.L. (1985). *Nutrition in infancy and childhood.* St. Louis, MO: Times Mirror/Mosby.

Sameroff, A.J. (1968). The components of sucking in the human newborn. *Journal of Experimental Child Psychology, 6,* 607–623.

Schechter, G.L. (1990). Physiology of the mouth, pharynx and esophagus. In C.D. Bluestone & S.E. Stool (Eds.), *Pediatric Otolaryngology* (pp. 816–822). Philadelphia: W.B. Saunders.

Shah, C.P., & Wong, D. (1980). Management of children with cleft lip and palate. *Canadian Medical Association Journal, 122,* 19–24.

Shivpuri, C.R., Martin, R.J., Carlo, W.A., & Fanaroff, A.A. (1983). Decreased ventilation in preterm infants during oral feeding. *The Journal of Pediatrics, 103,* 285–289.

Smith, W.L., Erenberg, A., & Nowak, A. (1988). Imaging evaluation of the human nipple during breast-feeding. *American Journal of Diseases in Children, 142,* 76–78.

Thach, B.T., & Menon, A. (1985). Pulmonary protective mechanisms in human infants. *American Review of Respiratory Diseases, 131,* Suppl. s55–s58.

VandenBerg, K.A. (1990). Nippling management of the sick neonate in the NICU: The disorganized feeder. *Neonatal Network, 9,* 9–16.

Warren, L.R., & Fox, C. (1987). The use of videofluoroscopy in the evaluation and treatment of children with swallowing disorders. In *Problems with Eating: Interventions for Children and Adults with Developmental Disabilities*. Rockville, MD: The American Occupational Therapy Association.

Weber, F., Woolridge, M.S., & Baum, J.D. (1986). An ultrasonographic study of the organization of sucking and swallowing by newborn infants. *Developmental Medicine and Child Neurology, 28*, 19–24.

Wilson, J.M., Ed. (1977). *Oral-motor function and dysfunction in children*. Chapel Hill: Division of Physical Therapy, Department of Medical Allied Health Professions, University of North Carolina.

Wilson, S.L., Thach, B.T., Brouillette, R.T., & Abu-Osba, Y.K. (1981). Coordination of breathing and swallowing in human infants. *Journal of Applied Physiology, 50*, 851–858.

Wolf, L.S., & Glass, R.P. (1992). *Feeding and swallowing disorders in infancy: Assessment and management*. Tucson, AZ: Therapy Skill Builders.

Wolff, P.H. (1968). The serial organization of sucking in the young infant. *Pediatrics, 42*, 943–955.

9

⬜ ⬜ ⬜
⬜ ⬜ ⬜
⬜ ⬜ ⬜

Parent–Child Relations: Interaction and Intervention

Jodie Redditi Hanzlik, PhD, OTR

The importance of the parental effect upon child development has never been questioned. It has only been recently, however, that active parent involvement and participation has become a standard component in early intervention programs. Since a positive parent–child relationship is vital to optimum child development, it is clear that if the goals of an intervention program are for long-term, maximum benefits, facilitation and support of a positive parent–child relationship should be an integral part of the program. Parental styles of behavior that have traditionally been associated with positive parent–child relationships in populations of typical children include behaviors such as sensitivity to child cues, contingent responsiveness, and affection and warmth during interaction (Ainsworth & Bell, 1973; Baumrind, 1967, 1971; Clarke-Stewart, 1973). These behaviors have also been associated with positive parent–child relationships in populations of children with disabilities (Mahoney, Fors, & Wood, 1990).

Parental styles of behavior are not, however, the only factors contributing to the child's development. Characteristics of the caregiver and the child influence each other and, ultimately, control the composition of their relationship and their interactions. Parent–child interactions are conceptualized as bidirectional, the parent and the child mutually affecting each other's behavior (Bell & Harper, 1977), as opposed to the traditional unidirectional view in

Work reported in this chapter was supported, in part, by grant #H029F20026 from the U.S. Department of Education, Office of Special Education Programs and by grant #MCJ-009105 from the Department of Health and Human Services, Bureau of Health Care Delivery and Assistance, Maternal and Child Health Training Program.

which the parent controls the child's behavior. In addition, the child's development is also affected by the continuous and cumulative effects of the interactions between the developing individual and her environment (Sameroff &
Chandler, 1975; Sameroff & Fiese, 1990). The environments of a child range
in complexity from the child's inanimate (physical) and animate (family)
surroundings to the cultural-political systems of our world (for further details
on the ecological perspective see Bronfenbrenner, Moen, and Garbarino [1984]
and Garbarino [1990]). Factors that serve to directly influence the quantity
and quality of the child's interactions within her family environment are as
diverse as marital satisfaction of the child's parents (Maccoby & Martin,
1983); births and number of siblings in the family; family socioeconomic
status, education, and support systems (Dunst & Trivette, 1988); and the
child's own competence (Ainsworth, 1973). Factors that serve to indirectly
influence interactions are as far-reaching as corporate and political decisions
of companies and nations (Garbarino, 1990). It is clear that at birth, the child
enters a complex environment of competing relationships. For the child to
be a successful member of that environment, she too must compete—particularly for attention from her primary caregiver.

According to social learning (Bandura, 1977) and ethological attachment
(Ainsworth, 1973) theorists, the competitive behavior that the child must
demonstrate to elicit and to maintain her caregiver's attention (given the
caregiver's capability to effectively or competitively interact) is the ability
to engage in reciprocal turn taking or jointly regulate the dynamics of the
caregiver–child behavior with the caregiver. What happens, however, to the
caregiver–child dyad if one of the dyad members is not competitive? More
specifically, what are the effects on the dyad's interactional patterns when
the child has difficulty participating as a joint regulator of interactions and
the dyad's behavior becomes asynchronous (e.g., reciprocal turn taking does
not occur)?

This chapter begins with a selected overview of the transactional patterns
that parents and their children with disabilities engage in, elucidating the
asynchrony of these dyads during interaction. Next, there is discussion of
controversial issues surrounding parent–child interaction. The chapter concludes with a review of intervention techniques that have been used to support
positive parent–child interactions.

Parent–Child Interactions

The acknowledgment of the basic importance of parent–child
interaction has resulted in increasing amounts of research in this area. The
majority of the research has been conducted on mothers. The few investigators

that have reported paternal interaction patterns (Levy-Shiff, 1986; Maurer & Sherrod, 1987; Stoneman, Brody, & Abbot, 1983) have indicated that the interactive patterns of mothers and fathers of children with developmental disabilities are similar. Both groups direct more (Maurer & Sherrod, 1987) and play less (Stoneman, Brody, & Abbot, 1983) with their children in comparison to parents of children who are typical. Parenting roles between parents of children with and without disabilities, however, were parallel. Regardless, of the status of the child, mothers took the role of manager in family groupings while the fathers deferred to the mothers' control.

Researchers who have studied mothers and their children with disabilities during play have indicated that they engage in a wide variety of interaction styles, which are represented on a continuum from optimum to less than optimum, just as the interaction patterns of mothers and their children with disabilities are represented (Crawley & Spiker, 1983; Mahoney, 1988). In addition, like children without disabilities, children with disabilities also elicit behaviors from their mothers that match their levels of development. Groups of mothers and their children with and without disabilities have a variety of behaviors in common.

Nevertheless, researchers have also indicated that there are some patterns of interaction that appear to characterize the interactions of a large number of mothers and their children with disabilities. These mothers have been presented as being more directive (Barrera & Vella, 1987; Hanzlik, 1989; Hanzlik & Stevenson, 1986; Kogan & Tyler, 1973) and as initiating more interactive turns (Mahoney, Fors, & Wood, 1990; Vietze, Abernathy, Asche, & Faulstich, 1978) than mothers of children without disabilities. Children with disabilities have been presented as being less responsive and as taking fewer interactive turns than their counterparts under a variety of subject-matching conditions (Kogan & Tyler, 1973; Mahoney, Fors, & Wood, 1990; Tannock, 1988). Though there are other behaviors for both mothers and children that discriminate between these groups, the discriminating behaviors generally appear to reflect a greater amount of maternal directives and initiation of interaction and a lesser amount of child initiation and responsiveness.

Controversial Issues of Parent–Child Interaction

There are two basic issues related to parent–child interaction that are controversial. The first issue questions the cause of directiveness as a maternal interactive or communicative technique. The second issue questions whether directiveness is the most effective communication technique to facilitate optimum child interaction and development.

Maternal Directiveness

Researchers have postulated that the maternal interactive directiveness associated with mothers of children with disabilities is the result of a variety of factors. One interpretation suggests that mothers are more directive because they intend to enhance their children's behavior (Davis, Stroud, & Green, 1988; Eheart, 1982). Another notion proposes that mothers are more directive to compensate for the relative passivity of their children (Maurer and Sherrod, 1987; Tannock, 1988). Still another explanation emphasizes a social systems perspective (Dunst & Trivette, 1988) and the effects that family and personal issues have on maternal interactive behavior. Examples of the variables that affect the mother's interactions are socioeconomic status, presence or absence of a support system, parent education, and child diagnosis.

Bell and Harper (1977) have proposed that the interactional patterns of behavior produced by mother–child dyads result from the unique behavioral contributions of each partner and the effect those behaviors have on each partner. They have also proposed that a mother's interactional behavior is affected by the expectations she has of her child's behavior relative to the intensity, frequency, or situational appropriateness of the child's behavior. In addition, Bell and Harper (1977) have suggested that the maternal expectations for the child's performance are dependent on the continuous and cumulative effects of the mother's life experiences (e.g., personal or family issues to subcultural or political issues). Accordingly, the mother's own individual assimilation of all of life's forces shapes her expectations for her child's behavior and provides her with a frame of reference for her own behavior. Against this background, Bell and Harper (1977) have proposed that a child's passive or inactive behavior will elicit a hierarchy of maternal control behavior intended to influence the child's behavior to meet individual maternal expectations. Maternal control behavior, however, will only be elicited if there is a discrepancy between the mother's expectations and perceptions of her child's behavior.

In support of Bell and Harper's proposal related to maternal interaction style, empirical research has consistently indicated that there is a cluster of low-activity–related child behavior that differentiates between children with and without disabilities. Specific findings have indicated that children with disabilities engage in fewer positive gestures, which results in the attainment or direction of the mother's attention (Marfo & Kysela, 1988) and fewer face-to-face interactions (Barrera & Vella, 1987; Hanzlik, 1990). Compared to their peers, they were also less likely to initiate and sustain interactions and more often were delayed or silent in response to their mother (Mahoney, Fors, & Wood, 1990; Maurer & Sherrod, 1987). Consequently, mothers do not receive as much interactive stimulation or information from their children as they could. The low amount of face-to-face interaction that occurs between mother—child dyads (specifically in dyads that include children with cerebral palsy and cognitive delay) exemplifies the loss of important interactive information for the pair. These mothers and children are unable to take advantage of the rich nonverbal cues of eye contact or facial expressions that, if observed, would have the potential to add to and more sensitively direct the dyads' communication.

Maternal behavior patterns are also empirically consistent with the behaviors predicted by Bell and Harper. The behavior that has differentiated between mothers of children with disabilities and mothers of children without disabilities is primarily verbal directiveness. Mothers of children with disabilities have been reported to be more verbally directive, to take more turns (Tannock, 1988), and to request more actions of their children than mothers of children without disabilities (Mahoney, Fors, & Wood, 1990). In addition, mothers of children with disabilities more frequently monitored their children visually (Marfo & Kysela, 1988), and asked their children to attend to information that was not directly related to their children's current focus of attention (Mahoney, Fors, & Wood, 1990) in contrast to their counterparts. Some of the behaviors that are naturally demonstrated by the mothers of children with disabilities appear to increase the opportunity for and to cause a spiraling of maternal directiveness. For example, if mothers make a high number of difficult requests, the form and the type of maternal interactions could potentially increase child-processing time requirements, making the child appear passive to the mothers and, thus, increasing the chances of eliciting more maternal directives.

Other maternal behaviors besides verbal directiveness are consistent with the underlying principles developed by Bell and Harper (1977); specifically, maternal physical contact and physical directives. Mothers of children with cerebral palsy and cognitive delay have been shown to engage in more physical contact than mothers of children with either no delays or a diagnosis of developmental delay (Brooks-Gunn & Lewis, 1984). These mothers have also been shown to engage in more holding and physical directives than mothers of children with no delays (Hanzlik, 1990). Perhaps the physical disabilities of the children with cerebral palsy are influencing factors in these differences. Since some children with cerebral palsy are unable to easily initiate age-appropriate fine motor or gross motor movement patterns, their mothers may have attempted to elicit more physical behavior from them. What effect does maternal directive behavior, verbal or physical, have on child behavior? Is it inhibitory or facilitory?

Facilitation of Optimum Child Behavior

A group of researchers have supported the frequent maternal directives, characteristic of mothers with children with disabilities, as facilitory of child behavior during interaction (Crawley & Spiker, 1983; Tannock, 1988). They have suggested that if directives are used in a supportive fashion (e.g., following a child's lead or responding to a child's interests) as opposed to an intrusive one (e.g., redirecting a child's focus), directives may produce a positive communicative effect for the child with developmental delays (Davis, Stroud, & Green, 1988). It has also been suggested that mothers of children with disabilities primarily use directives in this fashion (Tannock, 1988).

Intuitively, it would seem that verbal or physical directives would stimulate active responsiveness. Researchers have indicated that parents of all children use directive language when they are instructing their children (Cunningham, Reuler, Blackwell, & Deck, 1981; Davis, Stroud, & Green, 1988). Some have reported that mothers of children with disabilities were even more directive in a teaching situation than they were in free play (Cunningham, Reuler, Blackwell, & Deck, 1981) while others have reported that they maintain the same level of directiveness in both situations (Davis, Stroud, & Green, 1988).

Early intervention programs have also adopted the practice of using directives in the instruction of children. Popular curricula, such as the Hawaii Early Learning Profile (HELP) (Furuno, et al., 1983) and the Carolina Curriculum for Handicapped Infants and Infants At-Risk (Johnson-Martin, Jens, & Attemeier, 1986), use this strategy, but as suggested, there is little evidence to guide the application of this concept. Do the reported behavior patterns provide evidence that maternal directives have influenced child behavior to the current levels reported? It is possible; however, research has indicated that as mothers have been instructed to engage in true reciprocal interaction and decrease the number of their nonverbal-physical and verbal directives, their children have increased their verbal and nonverbal activity levels (Girolametto, 1988; Hanzlik, 1989; Mahoney & Powell, 1988). In fact, when groups of mothers who had children with and without disabilities have been compared, a number of behavioral patterns have been demonstrated as a result of maternal nonverbal-physical directives used during interaction.

Hanzlik (1990) has reported that mothers of infants without disabilities decrease both their physical contact and their directive physical guidance with their infants as their cognitive skills or mental ages increase; mothers of infants with cerebral palsy do not decrease their physical contact or guidance. Although mothers of infants with cerebral palsy do decrease their physical contact as their infants' motor skills increase and their severity levels decrease, the observation remains that mothers of infants with cerebral palsy do not adjust their physical contact and their directive physical guidance based on the infant's mental age. The nonverbal behaviors they engage in with their infants are not related to their infants' cognitive level of maturity. Consequently, the effect that these nonverbal patterns of maternal communication could have on the developing infant with cerebral palsy must be addressed. It is typical to expect more physical contact to occur between infants with cerebral palsy and their mothers, excessive physical contact and controlling behaviors have been shown to decrease the infant's competence and levels of independence (Levy, 1943). Beckwith (1976) has suggested that excessive holding of the older infant may restrict the infant's exploratory behavior and activity level, which are related to cognitive growth. It appears that though moderate amount of physical contact is necessary for normal development, physical contact and direction may not facilitate optimum interaction for mother–infant dyads.

Relative to maternal verbal directives, Mahoney, Finger, and Powell (1985) and Mahoney and Powell (1988) have shown negative correlations between maternal directiveness and child development/responsiveness, respectively. The interactional level of the child, not apparently affected by the frequency of maternal directives, has been positively affected by maternal responsivity or sensitivity to child communication and a focus on child-oriented topics (Mahoney, 1988; Mahoney, Fors, & Wood, 1990).

Crawley and Spiker's findings (1983) have indicated that in a free play situation maternal sensitivity, elaborateness, and qualitative stimulation of the child were positively related to child play maturity and social responsivity in children with disabilities. Qualitative stimulation refers to maternal behavior that combines maternal directive and elaborative strategies in a fashion sensitive to the child's involvement to produce optimum cognitive stimulation for the child. Directiveness, however, was not specifically related to any of the variables reflecting child competence. Directiveness was related to play; mothers who were directive and insensitive had children who were less interested in play than mothers who were directive and sensitive.

Much of the controversy surrounding the effects of maternal directiveness seems to be embedded in the classic works of Baumrind (1967, 1971). In those works, she reported that the parental behavior most conducive to purposeful and responsible behavior in children appears to be rational control, inductive discipline, positive encouragement, sensitivity, and strong nurturing (authoritative control). Her findings also indicated that parents whose child-rearing skills were characterized by the use of power assertive or passive techniques had children who were not as mature or socially competent as their counterparts. Baumrind's findings have additionally indicated that no single dimension of parental behavior is responsible for all aspects of child behavior. Consequently, maternal directiveness is meaningful only when we are aware of its usage within the entire behavioral repertoire of the mother. For example, the effects of maternal directiveness combined with a high degree of maternal sensitivity would produce a much different pattern of child behavior than maternal directiveness combined with a high degree of maternal insensitivity.

Just as it is necessary to view mother–child interactions as a result of all of the possible factors imposing upon the interaction, it is also necessary to view the verbal and nonverbal interactions of a mother and her child with disabilities within the context of a 24-hour day. As others have suggested (Mahoney, Fors, & Wood, 1990; Rosenberg & Robinson, 1988), the key to the effects of opposing views regarding maternal directiveness may be dependent on maternal sensitivity. Yet, it may also be relevant to consider the effects of directiveness as they occur within the day-to-day verbal and nonverbal environments of the child. It is apparent that children with disabilities are the recipients of maternal direction in both free play and instructional situations, which could include any educational, therapeutic, or daily living activities. These activities may make up the majority of their time during the day. Consequently, if it is true that sensitive maternal directiveness does promote learning and the child learns only to respond within a context of directiveness, what will be the long-term effects of maternal directives, verbal and nonverbal, on the child's life? How would the child's behavioral repertoire be affected?

When children are constantly directed, they do not have many opportunities to make choices. Consequently, they seldom experience situations that allow them to learn from their behavior or to learn that their behaviors have an effect upon their environments. Cline and Fay (1990) have attributed the self-reliant behavior and good decision making skills demonstrated by some children to a parenting style that encourages children to make choices and take responsibility for their own behavior. When children are seldom allowed to make choices or act independently, in effect, they become passive recipients of uncontrollable events that occur in their environment. Seligman (1975) has theoretically described this phenomenon as learned helplessness. He has proposed that such learning undermines the incentive to respond and is accompanied by feelings of failure and the inability to cope with future events. On a more empirical note, task-oriented play of typical children has been reported to be more competent and persistent when maternal behavior includes sensitive reactions to child initiations and *watchful attentiveness* as opposed to interactions of any other form. Work by Mahoney and Powell (1988) also supports the notion that maternal behavior that is sensitive, less directive, and child-oriented is an effective means of promoting the development of a child with disabilities.

Perhaps a child with developmental delays or disabilities, by definition, requires more external support to perform than a typical child. But how much more support and encouragement is needed and when does more support become too much? It appears that mothers of these children may have to work within a more limited zone of optimal stimulation for their children in comparison to their counterparts. Guidelines must be developed that establish what the child's behavioral cues are when he is in or out of his optimal zone for stimulation of behavior. The answer to the effects of directiveness—positive, negative, or neutral—on mother–child interactions can only be resolved through further research that more closely analyzes the effects of directives versus nondirectives on behavior within the *total* context of the child's life. Nevertheless, there are still a variety of techniques that have been shown to encourage the interactive behaviors of children.

Intervention

Occupational therapists have consistently evaluated and provided intervention for almost all aspects of child development in intervention programs: sensorimotor development, language development, cognitive development, self-help skills, and play. Yet, for some reason, parent–child interaction has not been a traditional focus. Because parent–child interaction is so basic to all other aspects of child development, it is important that occupational therapists offer parents the option of addressing parent–child interaction patterns during intervention sessions. Therapists must also consistently monitor how their more traditional recommendations related to such areas as positioning and self-help reflect the underpinnings of positive verbal and nonverbal interaction patterns. Therapists must remain cognizant of the unique and individual characteristics of each parent–child dyad that affect parent–child interaction (Crawley & Spiker, 1983; Mahoney, Finger, & Powell, 1985). Group instruction can be potentially harmful to those who do not demonstrate normative behaviors but fulfill all of the typical demographic or diagnostic characteristics of the group. Consequently, as suggested by the standard assessment model that is used in the evaluation of sensorimotor development, or self-help skills, it appears that parent–child interaction should also be evaluated on an individual basis resulting in dyad-specific treatment information.

Both Dunst et al., (1987) and MacDonald and Gillette (1988) developed holistic models in order to provide individualized evaluations and dyad-specific treatment. Both of the models focus on facilitating reciprocity between dyad members with respect for the developmental level of the child as it fits within the interactive conventions of our culture. These researchers defined the parameters of successful interaction and proposed that each dyad be evaluated accordingly. From this evaluation information, the therapist can provide the individualized information that each dyad requires. If behavioral mannerisms, which negatively affect the interaction, are present or lacking in the dyad's repertoire, a variety of techniques can be used to mitigate the behaviors.

The techniques these models have suggested for use during intervention are similar to techniques used in the limited intervention research that has been reported. Some of the most frequently used intervention techniques are listed as follows.

- balanced turn taking between dyad members
- parental imitation of child verbal and nonverbal behavior
- face-to-face positioning
- use of adaptive positioning and equipment
- interactive match
- instruction to include fewer verbal and nonverbal directives and more praises, statements, and exclamations

All of these techniques, directly or indirectly, serve to empower the child. The techniques are focused to allow the child to acquire a sense of command over his life and his environment. Table 9-1 provides more specific definitions of techniques, rationale for their use, and specific references.

Mahoney (1988) has organized most of the techniques in Table 9-1 into the context of an intervention program by categorizing the techniques into two instructional paradigms. The first paradigm is turn taking. Turn taking is defined as interactive participation in the transactional experience of the dyad. The first goal is for dyad members to achieve balanced turn taking. The second goal is for each dyad member to have an equal opportunity to focus the dyad's activity during their interaction. Mothers are limited to directing the child's activities no more than 50% of the mother's turns; they must respond to at least 50% of the activities initiated by their child. Specific strategies are used to facilitate the turn taking paradigm. Mothers are instructed to take short turns, to take one turn and wait for the child to respond, gesture to the child to take a turn, and physically prompt turns. Strategies used to facilitate maternal responsiveness include imitation of the child's behavior or following the child's lead, sensitizing mothers to the number of directives and questions they use, and requesting a reduction of those behaviors.

The second instructional paradigm, Mahoney (1988) has organized into his intervention program is interactional matching. Interactional matching helps parents adjust their behavioral style to the child's in the areas of pace, tempo, and complexity levels. Strategies used to facilitate interactional matching include the following behaviors: (1) the mother's interactional style must be compatible with the child's, (2) the topic of communication must be representative of the *child's current* interests, (3) the complexity of the mother's behavior must be within the child's limits of cognitive processing, and (4) the level of the activity must be within the child's limits of comprehension. It is clear that such an intervention program would require a thorough evaluation and understanding of the child's behavioral and cognitive skills in order to provide interaction at the appropriate level.

Table 9-1   Summary of Parent–Child Interaction Intervention Techniques

Technique	Usage Rationale	Instructions	Reference
Parent–child turn taking during interaction	• Is an instrumental skill in our society • Promotes interactive dialogue, which provides the basis for the development of contingency awareness, and controllability and predictability of events • Allows the child to learn that her actions can have a potent effect upon social and nonsocial events • Trains the child to be active instead of passive	• Initiate interaction, wait 5 to 10 seconds for child's response. If there is no response: 1. Signal the child to take a turn with nonverbal cues (e.g., nodding the head, pointing at child). Wait 5 to 10 seconds. If no response, 2. Physically and/or verbally prompt the child to take a turn depending on the context of the situation. Or, 3. If the child has not responded, initiate a new interaction.	Hanzlik, 1989 Dunst, Lesko, Holbert, Wilson, Sharpe, & Liles, 1987 Mahoney & Powell, 1988 MacDonald & Gillette, 1988 Girolametto, 1988
Parental imitation of child behavior	• Helps to slow parents down • Is easily interpreted by the child making the original movement • Is a way to simplify maternal behavior and make interaction age-appropriate for the child	• Take short turns. • Imitate all verbal and nonverbal actions of child.	Field, 1982 MacDonald & Gillette, 1988 Mahoney & Powell, 1988

(continued)

Table 9-1 *Continued*

Technique	Usage Rationale	Instructions	Reference
Face-to-face interaction (especially for children with cognitive delays and cerebral palsy)	• Eye contact is a social releaser and important to attachment and socialization processes • Facilitates more sensitive communication by providing cues from eye and facial expressions	• Find a position with or without adaptive equipment that allows face-to-face interaction. (See Finnie, 1975: pp. 218–219.)	Hanzlik, 1989 Finnie, 1975
Use of adaptive positioning and adaptive equipment that includes face-to-face positioning (especially for children with cognitive delays and cerebral palsy)	• Allows for face-to-face interaction • Decreases the need for physical support from the mother while simultaneously allowing for close proximity between mother and child • May facilitate the separation process in an overly dependent dyad • May facilitate independent motor function, thus no longer requiring as much maternal physical assistance or directiveness • May cause the child to appear older and more competent if child is moved from infant-like position on floor to upright sitting or standing position	• Use therapeutically appropriate positions whether or not you use equipment that also facilitates mother–child, face-to-face interaction.	Hanzlik, 1989

	• Inhibits excessive physical contact and control. Excessive physical contact and control inhibit independent behavior, one's feelings of competency, and self-sufficiency • Use of adaptive positions provides children alternative therapeutic positions for parents to use during their daily routine without using equipment		
Decrease verbal directives and increase praise, statements, and exclamations	• Allows children choice and independent decision making • Provides children with other forms of language stimulation	• Make statements and exclamations, give praises, and imitate your child as you communicate with him. Try not to verbally direct your child all the time. For example, if the child is looking at the ball, say, "The ball is red," and wait for the child's response. Make your next comment after the child responds or after you wait for 10 seconds for the child to respond.	Hanzlik, 1989 Tyler & Kogan, 1977 MacDonald & Gillette, 1988 Mash & Terdal, 1973
Decrease physical directives	• Allows children choice and independent decision making	• When playing with toys with your child give her a chance to physically respond to the toys independently before you assist her in manipulating them. For	Hanzlik, 1989

(continued)

Table 9-1 *Continued*

Technique	Usage Rationale	Instructions	Reference
		example, before you show your child a toy, make sure she is in a good position that allows her to be in maximum control. Then allow her to play with the toy. If she does not respond in 10 seconds or so, demonstrate how the toy works. If the child does not respond again, physically prompt her and wait for a response. If still no response, physically assist the child in playing with the toy.	
Interactive match	• Helps parents adjust their behavioral style to the child's in the areas of pace and tempo • Helps parents to be aware of how they can choose play activities that are within the child's current, rather than potential developmental skills • Helps parents follow child's lead and respond to the child's current interests (sensitivity to child's cues)	• Interactions should be paced to maintain the child's tempo. • Interactions should only occasionally challenge or stretch the child's skills. For the most part, statements and questions referring to the play activity, and the activity itself, should be at the child's current level of functioning. • Interactions should follow the child's lead. Do not redirect the child to different activities.	Mahoney & Powell, 1988 Rosenberg & Robinson, 1988

The intervention techniques used in research have been applied within a variety of contexts. The home (home-based) (Hanzlik, 1989) and the clinic (center-based) (Seitz & Hoekenga, 1974; Tyler & Kogan, 1977) have been the locations for treatment, while interventions have emphasized both verbal and nonverbal interaction patterns. Intervention approaches have included formats ranging from direct instruction and modeling (Hanzlik, 1989) to bug-in-ear coaching (Tyler & Kogan, 1977) for mothers of children who were cognitively delayed with or without cerebral palsy.

The variation in context and technique of the intervention studies have had little effect on their results. Findings have indicated that parent–child interactions, both verbal and physical, could be enhanced through a variety of intervention approaches, and the general effect included at least a short-term decrease in maternal directiveness, an increase in child initiations or activity level, and an improved balance in turn taking between dyad members. Some intervention studies have documented long-term retention of these patterns. Another finding from the intervention research (Hanzlik, 1989) has indicated that mothers applied the intervention information more easily when it was of a *physically doing* or concrete nature (e.g., mothers were told to use adaptive positioning and equipment) as opposed to a *verbally telling* or more abstract nature (e.g., mothers were told to use other forms of communication, such as statements, exclamations, and praise, besides directives during inter- action).

Intervention studies have also used common basic strategies; their in- struction was directed at the mothers. It appears that, to a great extent, the configuration of the interaction is controlled by the mothers. In other words, ·the change in maternal patterning of interaction appeared to be the stimulus necessary to enhance the child's patterns of interactions. These findings could be interpreted to mean that more normalized styles of interaction are within both the child's and mother's repertoire of behaviors, yet due to an apparent interactive breakdown these behaviors are not elicited.

The majority of the intervention studies conducted have addressed the traditional parental styles of behavior associated with positive parent–child relationships in the interventive techniques they have taught to the mothers (e.g., contingent responsiveness and sensitivity). Although parental warmth has been a characteristic that has figured importantly in optimum parenting behavior (e.g., Baumrind 1967, 1971; Clarke-Stewart, 1973) for typical chil- dren, it has not yet been studied in-depth in relation to intervention research for mothers and their children with disabilities. One interesting finding noted by Mahoney and Powell (1988) in their intervention research with mothers and their children with developmental delays was that the effects of the intervention (e.g., increased reciprocity in interaction and interactive match) did not appear to positively affect parental behaviors related to warmth. Nevertheless, the effectiveness of the intervention program appeared to be moderated by the affective manner in which parents used the intervention techniques. Of the parents who implemented the intervention techniques most effectively, children whose parents engaged in high-affect behavior attained developmental gains that were greater than those of children whose parents engaged in low-affect behavior. The need to further examine parental affect and its relation to child outcomes during interactions with their children is evident. In addition, the malleability of parental affect as a personality trait should also be examined.

The intervention literature reviewed here has shown that all mother–child dyads benefit from intervention programming focused toward improving mother–child verbal interaction during play. It has also shown that verbal interaction intervention alone is inadequate to meet the comprehensive needs of mothers and their children who have cerebral palsy. The physical disability of the child with cerebral palsy appears to place an additional burden on mother–child interaction, which has dictated an intervention approach that attends to both the verbal and the physical interaction patterns of the dyad.

The intervention research findings have also indicated that intervention focused on enhancing mother–child interaction patterns during play can simultaneously include other dimensions of behavior as goals. For example, Hanzlik (1989) also emphasized social and physical development by focusing on such areas as positioning with and without equipment and face-to-face interaction, while Seitz and Hoekenga (1974) concentrated on improving each child's language skills and social development. Such examples indicate that the play environment of the child has the potential to be used as the context to facilitate many areas of development at the same time. There is no evidence in the literature that indicates that each area of child development must be treated in isolation.

Accordingly, it is time to integrate the information and techniques from a variety of intervention programs to produce a comprehensive approach to meet the needs of the total child and his family. Treatment approaches must be developed to demonstrate how play can be used as the basis of intervention programs that include the ongoing facilitation of sensitive, reciprocal mother–child interaction, while also addressing the child's needs in areas such as activities of daily living and sensorimotor, language, and cognitive development.

Summary and Application

Parent–child interaction is one of the most potent effectors of child development and parent–child relations. It is for this reason that the focus must be directed toward the psychosocial performance component as well as sensorimotor and cognitive performance components that occupational therapists have traditionally addressed during their intervention sessions. As therapists work with infants and young children and plan, with their families, for their needs over the continuum of their lives, the importance of interaction skills that develop during the early years must be emphasized. Interaction skills lay the foundation for the development of relationships with family, friends, and acquaintances. Consequently, interaction skills also dictate success or failure in the many environments, such as home, school, and community, that require interaction with others.

Several techniques can be used to enhance interactions between children and all the people with whom they communicate (see Table 9-1). Interactions can also be evaluated, on a very informal basis, according to whether the use of these techniques are present or absent in everyday communications. The knowledge acquired from such informal evaluations can then be used to individualize specific intervention information for parents, siblings, friends, relatives, teachers, physical therapists, speech pathologists, and so forth. Such information must be presented in a manner that empowers and enables all communicative partners of the child, so that the child is ultimately competent in all aspects of his life (Dunst, Trivette, & Deal, 1988). Clearly, the environment must consistently expect and reinforce an empowered style of communication from the child.

References

Ainsworth, M. (1973). The development of infant–mother attachment. *Child Development Research, 3,* 1–93.

Ainsworth, M., & Bell, S. (1973). Mother–infant interaction and the development of competence. In C. Connolly & J. Bruner (Eds.), *The growth of competence* (pp. 97–118). New York: Academic Press.

Bandura, A. (1977). *Social learning theory.* Englewood Cliffs, NJ: Prentice Hall.

Barrera, M., & Vella, D. (1987). Disabled and nondisabled infant's interactions with their mothers. *American Journal of Occupational Therapy, 55,* 168–172.

Baumrind, D. (1967). Child care practices anteceding three patterns of preschool behavior. [Monograph]. *Genetic Psychology Monographs, 75,* 43–88.

Baumrind, D. (1971). Current patterns of parental authority. *Developmental Psychology Monographs, 4*(1, Pt. 2).

Beckwith, L. (1976). Caregiver–infant interaction and development of the high risk infant. In T. Tjossem (Ed.), *Intervention strategies for high risk infants and young children* (pp. 119–139). Baltimore: University Park Press.

Bell, R.Q., & Harper, L.V. (1977). *Child effects on adults.* Hillsdale, NJ: Lawrence Erlbaum.

Bronfenbrenner, U., Moen, P., & Garbarino, J. (1984). Families and communities. In H.R. Parke (Ed.), *Review of child development research* (pp. 251–278). Chicago: University of Chicago Press.

Brooks-Gunn, J., & Lewis, M. (1984). Maternal responsivity in interactions with handicapped infants. *Child Development, 55,* 782–793.

Clarke-Stewart, K. (1973). Interactions between mothers and their young children: Characteristics and consequences. *Monographs of the Society for Research in Child Development, 38,* (6–7, Serial No. 153).

Cline, F., & Fay, J. (1990). *Parenting with love and logic.* Colorado Springs, CO: NavPress.

Crawley, S., & Spiker, D. (1983). Mother–child interactions involving two year olds with Down syndrome: A look at individual differences. *Child Development, 54,* 1312–1323.

Cunningham, C.E., Reuler, E., Blackwell, J., & Deck, J. (1981). Behavioral and linguistic developments in the interactions of normal and handicapped children with their mothers. *Child Development, 52,* 62–70.

Davis, H., Stroud, A., & Green, L. (1988). Maternal language environment of children with mental retardation. *American Journal of Mental Retardation, 93,* 144–153.

Dunst, C., Lesko, J., Holbert, K., Wilson, L., Sharpe, K., Liles, R. (1987). A systematic approach to infant intervention. *Topics in Early Childhood Special Education, 7*(2), 19–37.

Dunst, C., & Trivette, C. (1988). Determinants of parent and child interactive behavior. In K. Marfo (Ed.), *Parent–child interaction and developmental disabilities* (pp. 3–31). New York: Praeger.

Dunst, C., Trivette, C., & Deal, A. (1988). *Enabling and empowering families.* Cambridge, MA: Brookline.

Eheart, B. (1982). Mother–child interaction with nonretarded and mentally retarded preschoolers. *American Journal of Mental Deficiency, 87,* 20–28.

Field, T. (1982). Interaction coaching for high risk infants and their parents. *Prevention in human services, 1*(4), 4–24.

Finnie, N. (1975). *Handling the young cerebral palsied child at home.* New York: E.P. Dutton.

Furuno, S., O'Reilly, K., Hosaka, C., Inatsuka, T., Allman, T., & Ziesloft, B. (1983). *Hawaii Early Learning Profile: Activity guide.* Palo Alto, CA: Vort.

Garbarino, J. (1990). The human ecology of human risk. In S. Meisels & J. Shonkoff (Eds.), *Handbook of early childhood intervention* (pp. 78–96). New York: Cambridge University Press.

Girolametto, L. (1988). Developing dialogue skills: The effects of a conversational model of language intervention. In D. Marfo (Ed.), *Parent–child interaction and developmental disabilities* (pp. 145–162). New York: Praeger.

Hanzlik, J. (1989). The effect of intervention on the free-play experience for mothers and their infants who have developmental delay and cerebral palsy. *Physical and Occupational Therapy in Pediatrics, 9*(4), 33–51.

Hanzlik, J. (1990). Nonverbal interaction patterns of mothers and their infants with cerebral palsy. *Education and Training in Mental Retardation, 25,* 333–343.

Hanzlik, J., & Stevenson, M. (1986). Interaction of mothers with their infants who are mentally retarded, retarded with cerebral palsy, or nonretarded. *American Journal of Mental Deficiency, 90,* 513–520.

Johnson-Martin, N., Jens, K., & Attemeier, S. (1986). *The Carolina curriculum for handicapped infants and infants at risk.* Baltimore: Paul H. Brookes Publishing Co.

Kogan, K., & Tyler, N. (1973). Mother–child interaction in young physically handicapped children. *American Journal of Mental Deficiency, 77,* 492–497.

Levy, D. (1943). *Maternal overprotection.* New York: Columbia University Press.

Levy-Shiff, R. (1986). Mother–father–child interactions in families with a mentally retarded young child. *American Journal of Mental Deficiency, 91,* 141–149.

Maccoby, E., & Martin, J. (1983). Socialization in the context of the family: Parent–child interaction. In E.M. Hetherington (Ed.), *Handbook of child psychology: Vol. 4. Socialization, personality and social development* (pp. 1–101). New York: John Wiley & Sons.

MacDonald, J., & Gillette, Y. (1988). Communicating partners: A conversational model for building parent–child relationships with handicapped children. In K. Marfo (Ed.), *Parent–child interaction and development disabilities* (pp. 220–242). New York: Praeger.

Mahoney, G. (1988). Enhancing the developmental competence of handicapped infants. In K. Marfo (Ed.), *Parent–child interaction and developmental disabilities* (pp. 203–219). New York: Praeger.

Mahoney, G., Finger, J., & Powell, A. (1985). The relationship of maternal behavior style to the developmental status of mentally retarded infants. *American Journal of Mental Deficiency, 90,* 296–302.

Mahoney, G., Fors, S., & Wood, S. (1990). Maternal behavior revisited. *American Journal of Mental Retardation, 94,* 398–406.

Mahoney, G., & Powell, A. (1988). Modifying parent–child interaction: Enhancing the development of handicapped children. *The Journal of Special Education, 22,* 82–96.

Marfo, K., & Kysela, G. (1988). Frequency and sequential patterns in mothers' interactions with mentally handicapped and nonhandicapped children. In K. Marfo (Ed.), *Parent–child interaction and developmental disabilities* (pp. 64–90). New York: Praeger.

Mash, E., & Terdal, L. (1973). Modification of mother–child interactions. *Mental Retardation, 12,* 44–49.

Maurer, H., & Sherrod, K. (1987). Context of directives given to young children with Down syndrome and nonretarded children: Development over two years. *American Journal of Mental Deficiency, 91,* 579–590.

Rosenberg, S., & Robinson, C. (1988). Interactions of parents with their young handicapped children. In S. Odom & M. Karnes (Eds.), *Early intervention for infants and children with handicaps: An empirical base* (pp. 268–286). Baltimore: Paul H. Brookes Publishing Co.

Sameroff, A., & Chandler, M. (1975). Infant casualty and the continuum of infant caretaking. In F. Horowitz, E. Hetherington, M. Siegel, & S. Scarr-Salapatek (Eds.), *Review of child development research* (Vol. 4, pp. 17–34). Chicago: University of Chicago Press.

Sameroff, A., & Fiese, B. (1990). Transactional regulation and early intervention. In S. Meisels & J. Shonkoff (Eds.), *Handbook of early childhood intervention* (pp. 119–149). New York: Cambridge University Press.

Seitz, S., & Hoekenga, R. (1974). Modeling as a training tool for retarded children and their parents. *Mental Retardation, 4,* 28–31.

Seligman, M.E.P. (1975). *Helplessness: In depression, development, and death.* San Francisco: W.H. Freeman.

Stoneman, Z., Brody, G., & Abbot, D. (1983). In-home observations of young Down's syndrome children. *American Journal of Mental Deficiency, 87,* 591–600.

Tannock, R. (1988). Mothers directiveness in their interactions with their children with and without Down syndrome. *American Journal of Mental Retardation, 93,* 154–165.

Tyler, N., & Kogan, K. (1977). Reduction of stress between mothers and their handicapped children. *American Journal of Occupational Therapy, 31,* 151–155.

Vietze, P., Abernathy, S., Asche, M., & Faulstich, G. (1978). Contingent interactions between mothers and their developmentally delayed infants. In G. Sackett (Ed.), *Observing behavior, theory, and applications in mental retardation* (pp. 69–94). Baltimore: University Park Press.

10

Sensory Integration: Assessment and Intervention with Infants

Susan Stallings-Sahler, MS, OTR

Sensory integration refers to the overall process by which the brain receives, registers, and, in most instances, combines sensory input for use in generating adaptive responses to the surrounding environment. A child with a sensory integrative dysfunction has symptoms that are thought to reflect a disorder in the central neural processing of sensory input. Such a disorder leads to disorganized, maladaptive interactions with the environment from which faulty internal sensory feedback is produced, further perpetuating the problem (Ayres, 1972). However, the clinical picture is not unitary. Difficulties can occur in both the severity and the configuration of factors that comprise each child's individual picture. Sensory dysfunction in one child may ultimately result in learning disabilities, which may result in academic failure (Ayres, 1968, 1969, 1972). In another child, it may be reflected in frustrating clumsiness and a constant struggle to acquire daily living skills that others take for granted. Some children may display fundamental disorders in the modulation of incoming sensations, appearing to be hypersensitive to seemingly ordinary stimuli (Ayres, 1972, 1979; Greenspan & Greenspan, 1985, 1989; Wilbarger & Wilbarger, 1991). Or conversely, a child may fail to orient and to respond to the presence of novel sensory inputs, such as a puff of air to the back of the neck (Ayres & Tickle, 1980). Sensory processing deficiencies frequently lead to poor social adaptation, an inability to form close intimate relationships, and difficulty with expressing and interpreting socioemotional cues (Greenspan & Greenspan, 1989). (See Holloway, Chapter 6.)

Led by the pioneering work of the late A. Jean Ayres, occupational therapists have examined and developed treatment strategies for sensory integrative
dysfunction in the school-age child population since the early 1970s (Ayres,
1972, 1974a, 1981, 1983, 1985; Ayres & Mailloux, 1981; Ayres & Tickle,
1980; Fisher, Murray, & Bundy, 1991). However, as therapists have become
more conscious of the signs of sensory integrative problems and as information
about sensory integration has reached consumer awareness, identification of
possible sensory processing disorders at an increasingly younger age has become possible (DeGangi & Greenspan, 1989; Jirgal & Bouma, 1989; Parham,
1987). A major contribution to therapists' ability to identify these problems
in infants has been enactment of PL 99-457, a federal law mandating early
intervention services to the 0 to 3 at-risk population. This legislation names
occupational therapy as a direct provider of these services; thus, therapists
are now logistically in a better position to detect and treat all types of developmental disorders in both infants and toddlers. Sensory integration deficits are
one aspect of that multidimensional picture.

Much of what has been learned about the early signs of sensory processing
problems has been gleaned from interviewing the parents of older children
to whom services are provided. Many of these parents retrospectively report
that they noticed that things weren't right from the beginning. For example,
their newborn may have had difficulty with the oral-motor demands and
sensory experiences of feeding. Some parents recount, "She had her days and
nights mixed up for a long time," suggesting disruption of normal circadian
rhythms of sleep and wakefulness. Lack of characteristic neonate cuddling
postures may also be mentioned, as well as irritability and colic. Extreme
negative reactions to various types of sounds, tactile experiences, or other
sensations may also be reported. Such infants quickly and effectively convey
their aversion to being handled and, in extreme cases, to visual contact with
the faces of their caretakers (Als, 1982; Jirgal & Bouma, 1989; Wilbarger &
Wilbarger, 1991). During an intake interview with the author, one mother
pulled down the collar of her blouse to reveal a series of scars on her neck
and shoulders where her infant son (now 10 years old) had scratched and
bitten her in response to her attempts to hold and comfort him.

As the infant grows older, motor, social, and self-care milestones may
lag in several areas. The toddler may seem lacking in normal curiosity about
the environment, or have a pattern of environmental exploration that is
disorganized, destructive, and frustrating to her. Past the age range when such
abilities are acquired, she may have trouble figuring out basic whole body
movements, such as how to climb into a chair, or, after ascending the stairs
on all fours, how to climb back down. She also may not be able to formulate
appropriate body signals and gestures to communicate her desire for affection,

food, or a favorite toy (Greenspan & Greenspan, 1989). At age 2 or 3, the child may display difficulty in, as well as avoidance behavior toward, acquiring the simple aspects of basic daily living skills, such as donning and doffing loose clothes, shoes, and coats. Inappropriate handling of toys or other objects or the continued use of repetitive, immature play patterns may be observed. A pattern of spectator play may begin to emerge, with the toddler (approaching preschool age) avoiding manipulative or skilled gross motor play in preference for more sedentary activities, such as watching television or looking at books. Bright children may conceal motor planning inadequacies through make-believe play that emphasizes imagination and social interaction over object manipulation or body coordination.

Early Development of Sensory Integration

There has been surprisingly little research on the early development of sensory integrative and practic functions per se. It is known that the vestibular system is the first sensory system to develop in utero, fully myelinated at 27 to 29 weeks, and mature at birth (Moore, 1978; Ornitz, 1983). Efferent impulses from the vestibular centers flow to the muscles of the embryo and fetus, probably driving the first twitching movements of the unborn child. These movements gradually develop into fairly coordinated patterns, which the tiny fetus can use to propel itself around the womb. Through ultrasonographic observations of in utero behavior, Ianniruberto and Tajani (1981) and Milani-Comparetti (1981) have filmed 14- to 16-week-old fetuses climbing up the uterine wall and over the umbilical attachment at the placenta. Eviatar, Eviatar, and Naray (1974) concluded that the vestibular responses of pre- and postrotary nystagmus are a sensitive and reliable indicator of central nervous system (CNS) maturity in infancy.

The somatosensory system also develops early in the prenatal period, supplying the fetus with the ability to withdraw from potentially harmful stimuli, as well as to take in the protecting warmth and closeness of the womb (Bronson, 1982). Discriminative tactile functions emerge gradually throughout infancy and early childhood (Ayres, 1964, 1972; Kravitz, Goldenberg & Neyhus, 1978). Research in the last decade has revealed that auditory perception matures in the last trimester to a much greater degree than previously thought, sufficiently enough that a newborn infant will show a preference for infant-directed speech over adult-directed speech (Cooper & Aslin, 1990) and for the mother's voice over that of adult female strangers (DeCasper & Fifer, 1980). The visual system is also capable of much more at birth than was previously thought. Within the first month, babies can discriminate between the face of their mother and that of a strange adult female (Bushnell, Sai, & Mullin, 1989).

Infant and child development research documents relatively predictable patterns of increasing behavior organization in the areas of motor, language, adaptive, and social performance (Bayley, 1969; Knobloch & Pasamanick, 1974; Uzgiris & Hunt, 1975). A normally developing infant engaged in everyday situations can easily be observed in order to analyze the constant sensation gathering, creating, and processing of sensations, which occur consistently as the infant grows older. Initially random movements of the newborn utilize the sensory input they create to gradually differentiate into more refined adaptive responses. Many of these early adaptive responses are geared toward survival and protection, and are part of the infant's nervous system hardwiring (Ayres, 1972). The inherent capacity and need for sensory integration appears to actually drive the infant's movements and exploration (Ayres, 1972; Yarrow, Rubinstein, & Pedersen, 1975.) This initiation of effort within the environment gradually becomes more goal-oriented and self-reinforcing.

Control over movement appears to proceed generally in a cephalocaudal (head-to-toe) direction. It is interesting to note that control of the head in the newborn has been found to include not only efforts to orient the head in space, but also imitational skills, such as head movements, tongue protrusion, lip widening, and lip pursing (Ikegami, 1988; Reissland, 1988). Differentiation of patterns and increasing ability to isolate movements appears to mature in a proximal-to-distal pattern. This conceptualization of movement maturation is primarily heuristic. The progressions are not strictly linear in nature, but have been more accurately described as spiraling. Case-Smith, Fisher, and Bauer's review of the literature (1989) found no substantiation for the proximal-to-distal explanation in terms of actual neuron growth or myelination. However, they did concur that the apparent dependency of distal development on maturation of proximal responses was a functional, biomechanical relationship that was most evident when upper extremity actions required reaching in space. The simultaneously emerging discriminative functions of the tactile system most certainly contribute to the refinement of movement by the extremities, especially of the arms and hands (Ayres, 1964, 1972, 1985; Kravitz, Goldenberg, & Neyhus, 1978).

Greenspan and Porges (1984) describe emerging levels of experiential organization, the earliest being sensorimotor, which evolves into what they term affective-thematic organization, and finally differentiates into representational organization. Greenspan and Greenspan (1985) state:

> The capacity to experience the world as richly and deeply as possible through one's own senses is also a foundation for *emotional develop-*

ment. . . . You can help orient your baby toward a world that is rich and deep by helping him regulate his senses and by providing him with opportunities to experience a wide range of feelings. (pp. 15–16)

The importance of normal sensory processing to the emergence of ego functions and self-concept is only beginning to be understood (Frick, 1982; Stallings & Lewin, 1985).

Assessment of Sensory Integration Dysfunction in Infants and Toddlers

One of the first aspects of sensory processing to address in an at-risk infant or toddler is that of *sensory modulation.* This phenomenon can be likened to a river dam, where the openings in the dam can be adjusted to allow varying amounts of water to flow through or to change the pattern of the flow. Modulation mechanisms in the CNS serve to control the level of intensity and configuration of incoming sensations and to influence the registration of those inputs. This control comes from a balance and fine-tuning of inhibition and excitation at several levels of the brain (Greenspan & Greenspan, 1989; Royeen & Lane, 1991; Wilbarger, 1984; Wilbarger & Wilbarger, 1991).

Until recent years, formal testing of sensory integrative functioning was possible only in children who were 4 years, 0 months through 8 years, 11 months of age, via the Sensory Integration and Praxis Tests (SIPT) [or its forerunner, the Southern California Sensory Integration Tests (SCSIT)] (Ayres, 1972, 1989). These instruments were designed to identify and to quantify the contribution of brain stem- and midbrain-level sensory processing to the mechanisms by which "the brain learns how to learn" (Ayres, 1972). The test includes measures of vestibular, proprioceptive, and somatosensory processing; visual-perceptual/motor integration; integration between the two sides of the body (hypothesized to reflect interhemispheral communication); and many of the components of the intricate behavioral construct known as praxis. Of the latter, the SIPT measure postural imitation; motor planning in response to a verbal request; motor sequencing ability; imitation of oral movements; graphic reproduction; and three-dimensional block construction (Ayres, 1985, 1989; Ayres, Mailloux, & Wendler, 1987). Collectively, these measures assist us in analyzing the multiple factors involved in sensory integrative function.

Other aspects and measures of praxis have been mentioned in the research literature, including the ability to imitate gestures of tool use, such as brushing one's teeth with a toothbrush and hammering a nail with a hammer (Cermak, Coster & Drake, 1980; Kaplan, 1968; Overton & Jackson, 1973), and ideomotor praxis, or the ability to perform a familiar gesture on command, such as saluting the flag (Kimura, 1977). In adults, ideational praxis refers to the ability to use common objects correctly, such as a key (Rapin, 1982). This is observed in children as the development of strategies for using objects and the generalization of those strategies to other similar objects.

Despite the fact that the SIPT cannot be used to measure sensory processing directly in infants and toddlers, a wealth of diagnostic information has been learned from that test (and from the SCSIT) about (1) the classification of some sensory integrative disorders into clusters, (2) the nature of individual behaviors or abilities that combine to form those clusters, (3) developmental trends that can be identified in many sensory integration performance areas, and (4) sensory system functions that combine to impact behavior and skills in one area as opposed to another (Ayres, 1972, 1974b, 1976, 1989).

With increased attention being focused on the infant and preschool populations, occupational therapists have been instrumental in developing assessments that attempt to examine sensory processing and its contribution to other areas of early development. The DeGangi-Berk Test of Sensory Integration (DeGangi & Berk, 1983) is a criterion-referenced test that was developed to primarily test vestibular-based sensory integrative functions of postural control, bilateral motor integration, and reflex integration in 3- to 5-year-olds. The Miller Assessment for Preschoolers (MAP) (Miller, 1982) is a standardized test for children ages 2 years, 9 months through 5 years, 8 months, which examines sensory and motor abilities from both sensory integrative and neurodevelopmental perspectives. Information from other domains tested by the MAP, such as the verbal and nonverbal indices and the complex tasks index, combined with the foundations and coordination indices, allow the evaluator who has knowledge of the sensory integration theory to infer how the child's sensory integrative functioning contributes to his ability to perform more cognitively complex developmental tasks (Stowers & Huber, 1987). The test also provides sheets for recording behavioral and clinical observations that aid the interpretive process.

Another recent contribution to the assessment of sensory processing in infants is DeGangi and Greenspan's (1989) Test of Sensory Functions in Infancy (TSFI). Domains intended for measurement include: (1) reactivity to tactile deep pressure, (2) adaptive motor functions, (3) visual-tactile integration, (4) ocular-motor control, and (5) reactivity to vestibular stimulation. The TSFI is intended for use in the screening and the diagnosis of infants with difficult temperament and developmental delays. However, it is recommended that clinicians read the manual section on psychometric properties to ensure appropriate usage of the instrument. Although its normative data extend down to age 4 months, validity for clinical populations appears limited below 10 months. The test should be administered twice within a week's time to ensure stability of observations. It is interesting to note that although tactile defensiveness is usually associated with light touch, the instrument assesses the infant's response to deep touch. This may be attributable to two factors: (1) response to light touch in infants is usually much more diffuse and generalized, so that borderline negative responses may be difficult to detect, and (2) a negative response to deep touch may be a more reliable indicator of later sensory defensiveness and of an aversion to weight-bearing positions.

Clinical observation, years of experience evaluating and treating all ages of children, and a thorough knowledge of the theoretical underpinnings of sensory integration remain the best tools available to clinicians for assessment of sensory processing, emerging practic abilities, and their effect on the occupational behavior of infants. Frequent observation and handling of normal infants are also vital contributors. It is important to recognize that formal tests are not always necessary or even desirable with infants and young children, as they frequently do not respond well to the structure and demands of a test situation. However, the need to measure change objectively, communicate with parents and physicians, or satisfy institutional standards often necessitates that therapists measure infant behavior via appropriate standardized instruments.

Traditional instruments are replete with items that reflect the early sensory processing and practic abilities essential to the performance of the developmental skill represented by that item. Many of the typical early infancy items of most developmental tests examine the products of sensory registration; that is, orientation and attention. For example, "responds to sound of bell (rattle) (voice)" (Bayley, 1969), "turns eyes to red ring (light)" (Dubowitz & Dubowitz, 1981), "reacts to paper on face" (Brazelton, 1973). Other items tell us about the child's inherent drive to explore, which Ayres hypothesizes is a reflection of ideational praxis. The emergence of ideational capacities through early movement experiences is observed in items that evaluate object permanence, the use of a tool (e.g., a crayon or a stick), and the functional use of objects.

Table 10-1 summarizes an analysis of items that are characteristic of developmental tests and the information that these tests can provide about an infant's sensory processing, coordination, and practic capacities. The developmental ages for which the test items are intended must be kept in mind. The list is not intended to be comprehensive, but represents a sampling. In addition, the opportunity for making clinical observations of related behaviors, such as signs of sensory defensiveness or quality of postural mechanisms (Chandler, Andrews, & Swanson, 1980; Milani-Comparetti & Gidoni, 1967) should not be overlooked. Generally, behaviors and skills in the right column have been listed in their developmental order.

Table 10-1   Analysis of Sensory Processing or Praxis Components in Typical Developmental Test Items and Clinical Observations

Sensory Processing or Praxis Component	Item Topic
State regulation/organization	Autonomic responses to sensory input (changes in respiration, skin color, muscle tone); self-shielding, self-consoling behaviors; clear, robust sleep states; smooth, gradual state transitions
Sensory registration: orientation, attention	Initial response/habituation to sights, sounds, postural changes; alerting, shifting of eyes, and/or head turning toward stimulus; increasingly prolonged attention to and interaction with test objects and toys; emergence of selective attention; ability to divide attention
Vestibular-proprioceptive responsiveness	Response to being picked up; positional tolerance; response to procedures testing labyrinthine and tonic neck reflexes; Moro response; head righting; pivot prone; protective extension; use of equilibrium maintenance strategies; 1- to 2-foot, static balance; ability to position and move with developmentally appropriate base of support
Somatosensory responsiveness: use of tactile input for protection, survival, comforting, exploration, discrimination, and to guide adaptive motor responses	Reaction to paper, cloth, hand on face; cuddling response; play with own hands, feet; reaching for and manipulating objects; fingering own hands, table edge, holes in pegboard; use of tactile cues for formboard completion
Oculomotor coordination	Visual regard of objects, persons; horizontal, vertical and circular following of moving object
Visual-motor integration	Reaching for and grasping red ring, toy; placing pegs, rings; pointing to objects; building block towers; tracing on a line; placing or moving an object or tool through space
Visual space perception: spatial relationships	Container play; placing shapes in formboards; construction (3-D); drawing shapes; understands prepositions (in absence of language disorder)

Table 10-1 *Continued*

Sensory Processing or Praxis Component	Item Topic
Bilateral integration and laterality	Early crawling movements; arm thrusts; symmetry/asymmetry items; crawling/creeping patterns; stair-climbing patterns; jumping off floor, both feet; hopping; catching ball with two hands; hand-to-hand object transfer; all items requiring one hand to hold or stabilize one object, while other hand moves or places objects into or on it (e.g., stringing beads, placing lid on container)
Anticipatory behaviors and adaptive motor responses	Anticipatory excitement; anticipatory adjustment to lifting; preparatory postural movements for catching, kicking ball; reaction to paper, cloth, hand on face
Sequencing	Pulling string to secure toy; putting cubes in a cup; successive peg placement; building cube tower; performing cause-and-effect sequences
Object permanence; ideation	Visual recognition of mother; reaction to disappearance of face; turning head after/looking for vanishing spoon; uncovering hidden toy; fingering holes in pegboard; pushing car along; spontaneous scribbling with crayon; attaining toy with stick; dangling ring by string; rotating object to correct orientation
Praxis on verbal command	Items that involve responding to verbal requests to move body in a certain way
Imitational praxis (not accompanied by verbal cues)	Imitation of: stirring with spoon; patting whistle doll; making crayon strokes; familiar gestures (e.g., waving bye-bye); familiar actions (e.g., pat-a-cake, so-big) vs. unfamiliar gestures or actions
Constructional and graphic praxis	Building 3-D structures with blocks or cubes; mental planning and drawing of specific lines or figures

(*continued*)

Table 10-1   *Continued*

Sensory Processing or Praxis Component	Item Topic
Body scheme	Playing with own hands, feet, toes; mirror image approach; mending broken doll; body part awareness; response to imitative or verbal cues involving placement/position of body parts; awareness of where clothing items go (shoes on feet, hat on head, etc.)

Source: Data from Bayley N, 1969; Brazelton TB, 1973; Dubowitz L & Dubowitz V, 1981; Folio MR & Fewell RR, 1983; Uzgiris IC & Hunt JM, 1975.

Clinical Picture of Sensory Processing Problems in Infants

Sensory Modulation Disorders

Sensory Defensiveness

One of the first indications that an infant has a sensory processing disorder is a parent's report that the baby is hypersensitive to one or more types of sensation. The infant may become upset, even hysterical, when touched or moved during everyday caregiving activities. The infant responds to the face-to-face position with a caretaker by turning her head away from direct eye contact. Battles at feeding time may ensue, with the infant able to accept only the breast or only the bottle and formula, but no spoon or solid food. Oral feeding intolerances may compromise the baby's nutritional needs to the extent that the placement of a gastrostomy tube for hyperalimentary feedings is needed (Wilbarger & Wilbarger, 1991).

The phenomenon of sensory defensiveness in infants and in children is widely unrecognized in the everyday medical community. Outside of the occupational therapy literature, it is mentioned only infrequently and is sometimes referred to as *tactile sensitive behavior* (Greenspan & Greenspan, 1985, 1989). The diagnosis of sensory defensiveness is drawn almost solely from behavioral symptomatology, since the findings from neurophysiological tests are usually negative (Cool, 1990; Wilbarger, 1984; Wilbarger & Wilbarger, 1991). Ayres (1964) first described *tactile defensiveness* in relation to behaviors that may be observed during testing for tactile discrimination in the Southern California Sensory Integration Tests. Tactile defensive behavior, hyperactivity, and distractibility are found in children with learning disabilities (Ayres, 1964, 1972). She defined tactile defensiveness as "feelings of discomfort and a desire to escape the situation when certain types of tactile stimuli are experienced" (Ayres, 1972, p. 88). Older children manifest this desire through verbal objections and by moving away from the source of the discomfort. Small infants would exhibit other avoidance behaviors; for example, cry vigorously and emit motor withdrawal behaviors including arching or the angry waving of arms and legs. Tactile defensiveness has been hypothesized to be related neurophysiologically to pain mechanisms (Bishop, 1980; Fisher & Dunn, 1983; Melzack & Wall, 1965), including the action of substance *P*, a neurochemical believed to operate in pain transmission (Cool, 1990).

Ayres later acknowledged oversensitivity in other sensory modalities, especially auditory (Ayres, 1981, 1983). She described subjective feelings of fear and discomfort during certain types of vestibular-based experience, which she termed *gravitational insecurity* (Ayres, 1983). Behaviors associated with this syndrome are generally observed in response to the head and trunk being tilted backwards (Fisher, 1991).

Wilbarger and Wilbarger (1991) have chronicled hundreds of anecdotal cases of infants, children, and adults who manifest various types and degrees of withdrawing, defending behaviors in response to sensory input. Rather than discussing these problems on the basis of which sensory channel is affected, they have conceptualized the problem into a unitary syndrome. They, along with Knickerbocker (1980), call this syndrome *sensory defensiveness*. It is detected and diagnosed according to parental response to interview questions and to direct observation of the child's reactions to various sensory input presented by the therapist. Severity of the disorder is categorized as mild, moderate, or severe, according to the number of sensory systems affected and the degree to which the disorder interferes with the child's social-emotional adaptation and daily living skills (Wilbarger & Wilbarger, 1991).

Sensory Dormancy and Poor Sensory Registration

Knickerbocker (1980) has referred to another disorder of sensory modulation termed *sensory dormancy*, which she has observed in some children. She felt that these clients were underreactive to sensory input, as opposed to the hyperresponsiveness of the defensive child. At the opposite end of the spectrum from sensory defensiveness, dormancy is explained as a problem of too much inhibition within the nervous system. Ayres referred to a similar condition as simply poor sensory registration. Dormancy is frequently difficult to discretely identify because both defensiveness and dormancy can appear in the same child, but under varying circumstances or in different sensory channels.

Assessment of Sensory Modulation

Sensory Defensiveness

The Test of Sensory Functions in Infancy (DeGangi & Greenspan, 1989), described earlier, assesses infant reactivity to various sensory stimuli. Negative responses as defined on that instrument may indicate a sensory modulation disorder. However, any evidence of such a disorder during standardized testing should be corroborated by additional clinical observations and parental reports of the infant's behavior at home. Frequent negative behaviors such as screaming, crying, withdrawing, or aggression in response to age-appropriate activities suggest sensory defensiveness. Some of these activities are as follows:

- being held or handled in certain positions
- diaper or clothing changes
- being given a bath and towel-dried
- nipple changes, textured foods, or the introduction of spoon feedings
- being moved through the air, riding in a car, or being in a swing
- finger- or toenails being cut
- hair washing, combing, or cutting
- being touched by another child
- intrusive noises, such as the telephone ringing, the doorbell, a reaction toy, or a vacuum cleaner
- level of room illumination normally tolerated by most children

Sensory Dormancy

Infants with sensory dormancy manifest their poor registration of sensory input in several ways. A preponderance of hyporesponsive scores on the Test of Sensory Functions in Infancy (DeGangi & Greenspan, 1989) may provide an objective measure. One infant observed by the author would sit in the middle of the floor, surrounded by inviting toys, and yet remain quiet, uninterested, and static. In his case, a lack of arousal coupled with failure to register incoming visual and auditory information contributed to reduced interest in the environment and a lack of awareness of the potential for pleasurable play and sensory experiences that lay within arms' reach. Other children display varying degrees of dormancy through behaviors such as the following:

- hyporesponsive nystagmus
- sluggish responses to sensory input

- lack of normal response to pain; (e.g., appears oblivious to bumps and bruises)
- delays in responding to verbal request, due to slow auditory processing
- use of excessive force when using tools, pencil, and crayon
- appearance of affective depression
- sensory-seeking behaviors, such as excessive jumping, spinning, rocking, visual staring, or touching
- head banging and self-mutilation (in severe cases)

However, before concluding that dormancy is present in a particular sensory channel, it must be determined whether the child may be seeking one kind of input in order to help modulate defensiveness in another sensory system. For example, a toddler with tactile defensiveness may crave massive amounts of jumping or of crashing play in order to engage the inhibitory influence of the proprioceptive system on the processing of light touch.

Example of Sensory Modulation Disorder

When registration and integration of incoming sensory impressions are poorly modulated within the brain, many infants fail to develop the ideational capacities needed for meaningful interaction with their environment (Ayres, 1981, 1983). Unlike normal two-year-olds, a toddler with poor sensory modulation is unable to perceive the play potential of common objects usually interesting to children or to generalize experiences with one type of object or toy to a similar one.

The case of three-year-old Evan provides an example of a child with a sensory modulation disorder who appears to be predominantly defensive, although he displays poor registration of rotational vestibular input.

Evan came to his initial occupational therapy session in a stroller and was carried into the treatment room in his mother's arms. He was fragile in appearance and seemed frightened by the unfamiliar surroundings and the new faces present. His mother reported that he refused to stand or walk, although pediatricians, neurologists, and orthopedists had examined him and could find no medical or structural reasons to explain this inability. Evan also withdrew from touch by anyone, and squinted at the lights in a normally illuminated room. He did not handle objects or toys of any kind. Evan's skin color was sallow and webbed in appearance. He was extremely thin, and his mother reported a long history of feeding difficulties. Evan refused all but smooth, pureed foods. He did not masticate or lingually manipulate food within his mouth prior to swallowing, seeming to want to get the food out of his oral cavity as quickly as possible. He also did not tolerate having his teeth brushed.

Upon observation of his modes of mobility, it became quickly evident that Evan avoided weight-bearing positions both with his upper as well as lower extremities, causing even his creeping patterns to appear awkward and disorganized. When placed in a standing position, he began to cry as if in pain, and it was noted that he had developed shortened hamstrings from his self-imposed positional restrictions. Evan cried at sudden or loud noises, such as people laughing or the sounds made by a vacuum cleaner or a doorbell. After a few treatment sessions, he did allow the therapist to rotate him in a suspended cocoon swing in order to observe the duration of his postrotary nystagmus, which was only about two seconds.

This basic difficulty with sensory modulation pervaded every aspect of Evan's development and his family's attempts to care for him. His mother appeared depressed. She expressed that she felt rejected by her own child, and doubted her maternal abilities and instincts.

Adaptive Movement Response Disorders

Adaptive movement responses are intended to reflect both those motor behaviors that are the result of postural development and those that reflect more complex, midbrain-cortex–mediated motor planning, since during the first year these two domains may be difficult to separate. As is true with the older children found to have sensory integrative problems, one infant may manifest mild hypotonia, developmental delays in postural and equilibrium reactions, and problems with midline integration, but perhaps have no, or an insignificant degree of, motor planning deficits. A more clinically involved child displays a similar picture of postural mechanism immaturity, which is compounded by early signs of dyspraxia. Given these two general cases, the child with dyspraxia is generally identified much sooner, having more problems with play and with functional skills acquisition.

Vestibular-Proprioceptive–Based Posture and Bilateral Integration Problems

The likelihood of early identification of a child with postural dysfunction (but not dyspraxia) may be accelerated if inattention, hyperactivity, or sensory modulation problems are present to prompt a parent to seek help. In the absence of distressing behavioral issues, these children probably will not be identified until entering school, if even then. An astute parent or professional may observe postural tendencies, such as the child's inclination toward inactive positions and sedentary activities, W-sitting, problems with balance; difficulties with bimanual tasks, or the fact that the child is not showing any particular hand preference. Protective, righting, and equilibrium responses are unreliable or incomplete. Immature gait patterns may be noted, such as use of a wide base with lateral weight-shifting of the lower extremities. In order to compensate for low extensor muscle tone in the upper body, shoulder girdle positioning may be marked by scapular retraction, shoulder elevation, and high-guard arm posturing. While these postures are typical of the toddler, they indicate atypical postural instability in the 2- to 3-year-old.

The process of integration and coordination of the two sides of the body begins early in infancy and forms the foundation for the organization of motor behaviors involving the extremities (Ayres, 1972; Gilfoyle, Grady, & Moore, 1991). This ontogenetic process is the physical manifestation of the emerging organization of cognitive functions in the cerebral cortex, which begins in a relatively (not completely) symmetrical state and proceeds to become more lateralized and asymmetrical (Njiokiktjien, 1988). It is important to note that consistent anatomical asymmetries between the cerebral hemispheres have been noted as early as the second trimester in utero (Galaburda & Habib, 1987). Ayres (1972, 1976) hypothesized that in normal development, vestibular and proprioceptive sensory processing contribute to the efficiency of inter-hemispheral communication and, thereby, enhance bilateral integration. Central to the discussion of bilateral integration and coordination is the body midline, around which the extremities, eyes, and ears are symmetrically arranged (Cermak, Quintero, & Cohen, 1980). The midsagittal plane is believed to be a key component in the development of body scheme (Schilder, 1951), spatial orientation (Goody & Reinhold, 1952), and directionality (Benton, 1955), as well as bilateral integration and lateralization (Ayres, 1972). All of these principles are of great significance in our treatment of children who show signs of delayed emergence of bilateral integration.

Refinement of sensory integrative theory since the introduction of the Sensory Integration and Praxis Tests has illuminated a component of postural preparation and movement called *projected action sequence*, which appears to be related functionally to bilateral integration and coordination (Ayres, 1989; Fisher, 1991; Goldberg, 1985). Projected action sequence refers to the individual's ability to anticipate the spatial parameters of an impending action progression involving her body and a stable object, or with a more mature response, in relation to a moving object (Brooks, 1986). Organization of such responses requires efficient integration of visual, vestibular, and proprioceptive sensory intake, and reflects the use of feedforward processing (Schmidt, 1988). Some examples would be running to catch a fly ball at the appropriate point in its trajectory or letting go of a trapeze bar just as one's body has swung out over the center of the pillow. This construct of motor control in the older child has its developmental precursors in the subtle preparatory postural adjustments observed in infants and in young children, such as getting the head, trunk, and extremities ready to be picked up; positioning the body and legs to be placed in a stroller or high chair; and holding out the arms in order to catch a gently thrown or rolled ball. Skills such as the latter, which require the child to move synchronously with a moving inanimate object, should be expected to be performed with only moderate competency by about age 30 to 36 months. However, total absence of postural preparation for retrieving a moving object may indicate a deficit in the feedforward mechanism.

Assessment of Postural Dysfunction

Potential problems in the area of postural adaptation can be observed during performance of certain typical items from standardized infant developmental tests (see Table 10-1). Such items include

1. postural responses while being picked up, held, and handled; later, more mature postural responses, such as shifting weight in preparation for kicking a ball or positioning the upper body for catching a ball
2. observations of protective, righting, and equilibrium reactions
3. observations related to bilateral integration and laterality (e.g., early crawling movements, arm thrusts, symmetry/asymmetry items, crawling or creeping patterns, stair climbing patterns, jumping and hopping, ability to use hands together at midline, catching a ball with two hands, hand-to-hand object transfer, and holding an object with one hand while manipulating with the other)

The preschooler with hypotonia and difficulties with equilibrium, postural mechanisms, and bilateral integration may be identified via certain items of the Miller Assessment for Preschoolers (Miller, 1982). These items are Romberg, stepping, kneel-stand, walks line, and rapid alternating movements, depending on the age of the child and normative expectations. Three-year-olds at risk for postural and bilateral integration deficits will experience difficulty on the DeGangi-Berk Test of Sensory Integration (DeGangi & Berk,

1983) with items that test co-contraction, symmetrical movements, and rapid alternating movements.

Early Signs of Developmental Dyspraxia

Children may display behaviors suggestive of developmental dyspraxia in various ways and for different reasons. An infant with mental disabilities may exhibit dyspraxia by reason of, and in proportion to, his cognitive impairment, although it is possible that sensory processing deficits may overlie and compound the cognitive delay. *Somatodyspraxia* refers to deficits in praxis that are the result of inefficient processing of tactile-kinesthetic, proprioceptive, or vestibular sensory input within the body (Ayres, 1989; Cermak, 1991). Two general categories of movement conceptualization and planning may be observed in the infant. The first involves his mastery over whole body, goal-directed movements in the environment. (The absence of neuromuscular impairment is assumed.) The second category generally comprises movements required to act on objects or to relate two or more objects to one another.

Assessment of Dyspraxia

Difficulty in executing purposeful movements within proximal body space is often observed early in development; for example, the infant may fail to remove a piece of masking tape placed loosely on the back of her hand, an item from the Test of Sensory Functions in Infancy (DeGangi & Greenspan, 1989). The infant must first feel and see the tape on her skin. She must then have the curiosity and desire to explore or remove it. The infant's ability and efficiency in organizing the response of bringing that hand toward the midline or in reaching with the contralateral hand toward the taped area reveals the basic core of praxis. Once the two hands are approximated, the perseverance with which the infant attempts to grasp and to remove the tape suggests the degree of sustained attention of which she is capable. Infants and children with dyspraxia often appear unable to master a task because they lack the ability to stay with a new task long enough to problem solve what is to be done.

Other examples of body-centered dyspraxia, which an ambulatory infant may manifest, include difficulty with tasks such as turning around to sit down in a chair or getting out of one, not knowing how to climb to obtain a toy that is out of reach, and failure to assist with dressing by holding out an arm or foot and placing it into clothing. Inability to imitate simple gestures modeled by an adult, such as pat-a-cake, bonsai! (arms up in the air), or waving hello and good-bye, also suggests a basic practic impairment. Items on the

Miller Assessment for Preschoolers (Miller, 1982) to observe, according to the child's age, include imitation of postures and the previously mentioned postural items (e.g., rapid alternating movements, kneel-stand, walks line, and stepping), which require the child to follow the demonstration of the examiner. A vital aspect of differential diagnosis between dyspraxia and a postural disorder without dyspraxia is the ability to imitate. Many, perhaps most, children with dyspraxia have postural dysfunction that contributes to their poor motor planning. Children with postural dysfunction only retain the ability to imitate static postures (Ayres, 1972, 1983).

The practic ability of effectively acting on the environment and relating objects to one another in space can be observed in the child's interest and age-appropriate proficiency in learning to use common utensils and play tools, such as eating utensils, toothbrush, hairbrush or comb, hammer, scooping or pouring implements, crayons, and containers. Constructional praxis may seem a long time in coming for the typical toddler who is more interested in mastering her environment by taking apart, pulling out, and tearing down. Eventually, this drive diminishes and interest in putting together, assembling, and building takes over. A 30-month-old or older child who appears to be stuck in a destructive mode may be showing early signs of constructional dyspraxia. Standardized test items to observe include tower, sequencing, block designs, and puzzle from the Miller Assessment for Preschoolers (Miller, 1982), although the contribution of visual space perception will need to be considered. Other useful developmental test items that may be used to assess praxis are listed in Table 10-1.

Sensory Integration Treatment Principles as Applied to Infants Zero to Three Years of Age

Most of the more familiar principles of the sensory integrative treatment approach are relevant to treatment of infants and young children. The central axiom involves the provision of controlled sensory input through activities presented by the therapist in order to elicit adaptive responses from the child, thereby improving brain organization. That unfolding process should reflect the normal developmental sequence as closely as possible. While treating infants, the therapist attempts to heighten the current developmental experiences of the child, thus influencing development as it is occurring. The goal of the therapist's techniques is usually to elicit responses from the child that require processing at subcortical levels of the brain, while the child's goal is to master the challenges within the play activities structured by the therapist.

Intervention to Facilitate Sensory Modulation

The first developmental task that an infant must achieve is internal control over his physiological systems given a variety of environmental demands. This basic coping capacity requires the ability to modulate incoming sensory information while engaged in feeding, face-to-face interactions with family, bathing and diapering, or just being held.

If the infant or young child appears to be over- or underregistering sensory input in one or more channels, this must be the initial focus of therapy. Otherwise, this problem will only impede attempts to facilitate the child's meaningful interaction with his family and with the environment. Because the child's intolerance of sensations incidental to normal caregiving has a potentially detrimental effect on parent–child relationships, improved sensory modulation becomes a therapy priority. The occupational therapist must design, and together with the family, implement a sensory diet that emphasizes the types and patterns of input that are known to have an inhibitory or excitatory effect on the overall modulation of sensation, depending on what is needed (Wilbarger, 1984).

In the previous case of Evan, the occupational therapist recognized one of the child's primary problems as a sensory modulation disorder and explained the concept of sensory defensiveness to his mother. The therapist designed a controlled sensory diet for Evan to be used in therapy, which could also be implemented in the home and in his early childhood classroom. Tactile and proprioceptive input was regularly provided using a surgical scrub brush and manually applied joint compression (Wilbarger & Wilbarger, 1991). In addition, several other methods for reducing tactile defensiveness were recommended, such as placing a sheepskin mattress cover on his bed to provide constant total body tactile input during sleep and placing swaddling in a soft blanket for overall pressure-touch and calming. For all home procedures taught, the therapist instructed the family to provide a consistent pattern of input and to observe Evan's appearance and behavior for signs of autonomic stress. In the clinic, Evan's therapist used a lamp with a low-watt incandescent bulb to light the treatment area, rather than the standard office fluorescent lighting (natural lighting though preferable, was not available).

In conjunction with the interventions for improving somatosensory modulation, the therapist gently swung Evan in a cocoon-like swing lined with lambskin, using predominantly linear patterns of stimulation. In the early stages of intervention, linear-directional movement input seems to promote integration and to have an organizing effect on the nervous system. Since Evan displayed many signs of poorly functioning inhibitory mechanisms in his nervous system, rotation was used only if he initiated it. Evan was observed carefully for changes in skin color, breathing, and expressions of distress that might signal that his ability to modulate sensations was being overtaxed. Many of the signs and symptoms of stress identified by Als (1986) apply to infants and toddlers, as well as newborns. (See Table 10-2.)

The intermediate results of Evan's occupational therapy treatment were reported as follows:

> Evan's modulation of somatosensory, visual, and auditory input began to show signs of normalizing almost immediately. He began allowing his family and therapists to handle him more frequently, and began to tolerate other stimuli that had previously seemed noxious to him. His affect changed from a scowling somberness to smiling and blowing kisses at the other therapists at their desks as he passed by. He began to crawl more normally, and to tolerate standing and walking.

In therapy with an infant who fails to appropriately orient to sensory input, the therapist is challenged with breaking through what appears to be the child's wall of complacency or oblivion to the sensory environment. Ayres and Tickle (1980) found that autistic children who displayed poor orienting to sensory stimuli tended to respond less well overall to sensory integrative procedures. However, Slavik, Kitsuwa-Lowe, Danner, Green, and Ayres (1984) found that specific vestibular input in the form of rapid, horizontal oscillations significantly increased visual attention in a small group of child clients with poor sensory registration. Ayres observed this effect clinically with similar children and hypothesized that, through integration with proprioceptive information from the muscles and joints and perhaps even indirect connections with the limbic system via the reticular formation and cerebellum, the therapeutic utilization of horizontal or vertical acceleration can heighten sensory registration. The therapist should be aware that many children display fluctuating patterns of sensory modulation and registration, or differences among modalities—for example, tactile defensiveness coexisting with auditory hyporesponsiveness (Ayres, 1979, 1983).

Holloway (1985) suggests that the occupational therapist may become a kind of environmental consultant, by examining what composition of surrounding sensory input obtains the optimum balance of arousal, motoric, and physiological adaptation from the infant. This information can be used to help the family to understand their child's signals of optimum coping or stress, and to modify their interactions and home environment accordingly.

Table 10-2   Signaling Behaviors of Young Infants as Defined by Als

Defensive Behaviors Signaling Stress	*Behaviors Signaling Self-Regulation and Approach*
Autonomic signals:	Autonomic signals:
Respiratory irregularity, pause, holding breath	Smooth, regular respirations
Seizures	Pink, stable color
Skin color changes: webbed, mottled, cyanotic, gray	Stable viscera
Gagging, choking, spitting up, gasping	Motor signals:
Hiccuping, coughing, sneezing, yawning, sighing	Well-regulated tone, smooth, coordinated movements
Motor stress:	Use of organizing postural strategies
Facial, truncal, or extremity flaccidity	Use of efficient self-regulating strategies
Hypertonicity in extension:	Hand, foot clasping
Arms—salute, airplane, high-guard	Finger folding, hand holding
Legs—bracing, sitting on air	Hand-to-mouth maneuver
Trunk—opisthotonus, arching	Grasping of caregiver finger, washcloth roll, pacifier
Extremities—finger-, toe-splay	Hands to midline
Facial—grimacing, squinting, tongue protrusion	Oral searching and sucking
Hypertonicity in flexion: fetal tuck, fisting of hands	Ability to assume flexion tuck
General frantic activity	Regulation of state and attention:
Tremulousness, twitching	Well-defined, robust sleep states
State-related stress signs:	Vigorous, rhythmical crying
Diffuse, poorly regulated sleep/awake states	Effective, spontaneous self-quieting; consolability by caretaker
Roving eye movements, staring, frequent gaze aversion, glassy eyes, closing of eyes (but in alert state)	Focused alertness, bright eyes; animated facial expressions; frowning, cheek rounding; mouth makes "ooh" expression; cooing; responsive smiling, imitation of caretaker facial expression
Straining to maintain alertness; drowsy alertness	

Sources: Als H: A synactive model of neonatal behavioral organization: Framework for the assessment of neurobehavioral development in the premature infant and for support of infants and parents in the neonatal intensive care environment. *Physical and Occupational Therapy in Pediatrics*, 1986, 6, 3–24, and Als H: Toward a synactive theory of development: Promise for the assessment and support of infant individuality. *Infant Mental Health Journal*, 1982, 3, 229–243.

Intervention to Enhance Postural Mechanism and Bilateral Integration

In general, the therapist's goals for assisting a young child who appears to be at risk for postural and bilateral integration deficits usually will include several of the following:

1. enhancing integration of vestibular-proprioceptive processing
2. facilitation of more normal muscle tone, especially around proximal joints and trunk flexor, oblique, and extensor groups
3. elicitation of protective extension patterns if they have not yet emerged
4. elicitation of mature righting and equilibrium reactions, including the components of weight shifting and trunk rotation with extension in response to postural challenges
5. elicitation of mobility patterns that utilize reciprocal movements of arms and legs during crawling or creeping, or if ambulatory, enhance bipedal standing or walking balance
6. enhancement of midline hand function, increasing the frequency with which hands come together in the body's central space to hold objects; concurrent stabilization and manipulation of toys with two hands; and increasing tendency of the preferred hand to spontaneously cross the midsagittal plane into contralateral space
7. facilitating the emergence of hand preference

In most normal children, hand preference emerges gradually after the first year, although a stable dominance pattern may not set in for several years (Caplan & Kinsbourne, 1976). A clear hand preference within the first year may be reflecting abnormal asymmetry indicative of CNS dysfunction. The occupational therapist should be careful to rule out the presence of any distinct upper motor neuron disorder that would make the diagnosis of bilateral coordination deficit inappropriate. Also, any perinatal or congenital condition, such as intraventricular hemorrhage or hydrocephalus, in which damage to, or malformation of, the anterior forebrain commissures are associated with deficits in bilateral motor coordination (Nelson, 1988; Preilowski, 1972). The treatment implication of these types of conditions is that, due to the presence of identifiable cortical-level damage, sensory integrative procedures alone will have limited impact. However, occupational therapy using other methods may still be indicated in order to ameliorate the negative impact on daily living skills development.

Central to Ayres' suggestions for treating postural and bilateral integration problems is the incorporation of guided vestibular and proprioceptive input. This can be done through use of the physioball and suspended equipment as moving surfaces with which to present graded challenges to the child in maintaining a stable posture in relation to gravity and direction of movement. If general muscle tone is somewhat hypotonic, as it frequently is in these children, the use of linear, fast, nonrhythmic patterns of input has a facilitatory effect on muscle tone, especially the extensors via the vestibulospinal tracts (Ghez, 1981). To stimulate tone more specific to certain muscle groups (e.g., abdominals, upper thoracic area, etc.), using physioball surfaces of various sizes, facilitating transitional movements of the child, and placing the therapist's hands over specific muscle groups may be more effective and developmentally appropriate. Physioball activities are generally safer than suspended equipment, especially for infants who do not have the strength or control to hang on to suspended equipment. Some three-year-olds may be able to hug a small bolster swing lying prone for a few seconds or to possibly perform the activity in supine underneath (for fewer seconds) in order to facilitate total body flexion toward the midline. Straddling a small vertically suspended inner tube provides similar results, but in a less demanding sitting position.

To reinforce weight-bearing and lateral or diagonal weight-shifting over the extremities, a rectangular-shaped platform swing is ideal for all ages of infants or young children, as it permits the therapist to sit on the swing, control its movements, and handle the child at the same time. For example, if the goal is to facilitate a diagonal weight shift in quadruped, the therapist may place the child in a four-point position on the swing and guide the swing to move so that a weight shift occurs over the contralateral hand and knee in either direction. Anteroposterior and lateral weight shifts can similarly be accomplished, as well as other types of weight-bearing (prone, kneeling, standing). Depending on the age and the size of the child, an inner tube placed in the swing or side bars can provide additional upper extremity support, if needed.

The use of the two hands together during play on suspended equipment will facilitate bimanual coordination (a supported trunk may be necessary with younger clients). Other examples of activities to facilitate bilateral coordination include holding a handle with both hands while pulling oneself (or being pulled) on a swing or scooter board or catching a beach ball while lying prone in the sling swing.

With children who show weak or no lateral preference, Knickerbocker (1980) recommends a technique she refers to as *dominance exploration*, wherein the child is allowed to engage in a unilateral heavy-work activity, such as pounding with a hammer. By trying the activity with each upper extremity and switching occasionally between the two, one arm (and the postural background patterns that support it) eventually comes to feel more competent. Knickerbocker hypothesizes that, through the intensive proprioceptive input received by the joints of each arm and communicated to the contralateral cerebral hemispheres, the lateralization process is facilitated. Activities that use this treatment principle are easily incorporated into the toddler's home and preschool play environments.

Intervention for Young Children with Dyspraxia

Since most children with dyspraxia manifest many signs of postural dysfunction, many of the therapeutic activities described in the previous section support the development of praxis in a young child. Additional considerations relevant to assisting children with dyspraxia in using their bodies and external objects effectively in the environment are included in this section.

Eliciting Adaptive Responses

Of primary importance to the occupational therapist is whether the treatment situations presented elicit optimum adaptive responses from the child and whether they cause neurophysiological stress. This has been a primary criticism of therapeutic techniques (such as some of those mentioned previously) that appear to supply passive stimulation to the child's CNS, but which do not require the child's active engagement. In the infant or child with a sensory modulation problem, it may be necessary to begin by preparing the CNS to be able to accept and to process the normal levels of sensation that are found in everyday activities. This, in itself, is a physiological adaptive response. As stated previously, during and for some time after these types of procedures, it is essential that the therapist closely monitor the infant or child for signs of autonomic stress, signalling overstimulation.

When working with the older infant or toddler, the astute therapist continually assesses the child's emergent attempts to react purposefully to his surroundings as opportunities to assist him in successful interaction. As soon as this level of responding begins to appear, the therapist should begin to upgrade the therapeutic activities so that higher level postural adaptation and praxis are required. At the same time, passively imposed sensory input that does not require an adaptive response on the part of the child is gradually eliminated from the therapy repertoire. The feedback created by adaptive responses helps to forge the CNS connections that will become neuronal models, which serve as the foundation for complex adaptive behaviors (Ayres, 1981, 1983, 1985). Returning to Evan, it can be seen that as Evan became more acquiescent and was presented with a variety of opportunities for engaging in simple adaptive responses, the severity of his dyspraxia became evident. When placed prone over the rim of an inner tube swing, Evan hung limply and seemed to have no idea of what he might do there. When given a small trapeze bar to hold, while being pulled on the rectangular platform swing, he let go after two seconds. He was not able to remain sitting on a bolster swing without moderate trunk support from the therapist. He was able to hold on to toys and tools, but did not use them in a meaningful way. Evan also displayed immature postural and equilibrium responses, failure to cross the body midline, and no sign of emerging hand preference.

When approaching an infant or toddler like Evan who has low adaptive response capacity, the occupational therapist must reason on at least three levels.

Normalization of Sensory Processing

If there is a problem, how can sensory modulation or registration be normalized for this particular child? What channels and patterns of sensory input generate the excitatory or inhibitory influence needed? Poorly modulated sensation will not provide the feedback necessary to formulate neuronal models of the body or the environment. In Evan's case, praxis could not be assessed and probably had not developed because of his intolerance for sensory input generated through his own movements.

Simple Adaptive Responses

What is the child's repertoire of simple adaptive and postural responses? Some examples might be standing, rolling, creeping, or simply the ability to maintain a quadruped weight-bearing position. How can each of these behaviors be elaborated upon in treatment? The therapist should identify which pieces of equipment present in the clinic can be utilized by the child with the simple adaptive responses that he cannot perform. For example, a 3-year-old who can alternately flex and extend his legs may be able to jump while hanging in the inner tube swing. What new opportunities for simple somatomotor adaptation can be presented that are likely to be completed successfully? In Evan's case, jumping off a low chair into a big pillow provided a new movement experience, but with a simple demand on motor skill.

Organization of Behavior

There are roughly four stages of emerging ability to organize complex adaptive responses. In the first, the infant or toddler may have little or no initiative and, thus, must be put through the required movements of the activity by the therapist. (Though seemingly passive, this does generate some kinesthetic feedback that may aid sensory registration.) An example might be the child sitting on the therapist's lap in a swing, with the therapist's hands over the child's who is holding pull-handles. Later, the child may be able to follow the lead of another person and imitate the therapist or another child performing the action. In this instance, the child may sit next to another client, each pulling on separate handles. If ideation becomes sufficiently established for the task, the child may then be able to initiate it independently without a model present. This is due to the development of patterned memory traces, which are a representation of an experienced stimulus configuration, called a *neuronal model*. Neuronal models need to be established for both the child's awareness of her own body as an effective agent of self-actualizing, purposeful activity, and for the physical world with its many opportunities for interaction and mastery (Ayres, 1981, 1983; Pribram & Maginnis, 1975).

Finally, as the child's neuronal models of her body, the environment, and experiences with both become more complex, she will begin to create new play schemes or apply familiar approaches to unfamiliar objects (Ayres, 1983). The child may devise ways to pump other types of swings, using different types of handles, or experiment with her body in various positions.

The knowledge and use of principles of the neurodevelopmental treatment approach (Bobath, 1980) are valuable in working with infants and toddlers at risk for sensory integrative and practic dysfunction. As has been stated, postural mechanisms and developing movement components are among the earliest somatomotor adaptive responses. An essential aspect of putting our small patient through the motions must include the therapist's own hand placement over muscle groups the child needs to activate or to inhibit in order to respond adaptively. The therapist must assess muscle tone, points of postural instability, relative balance between flexor and extensor muscle groups, and presence or absence of rotational components in the child's body. Normal postural mechanisms, too, must be painted in to become a part of the neuronal models for emergent praxis. Often, a child may not have sufficient postural responses to mount or to maintain postural stability while swinging on a piece of suspended equipment. Preparation of her trunk, using neurodevelopmental treatment techniques, may enable the child to take full advantage of the sensory integrative treatment activity.

Regarding the use of vestibular input to influence postural mechanisms and praxis, Ayres has suggested that semicircular canal input (axial or rotatory in direction) serves a more specific purpose of regulating oculomotor function during head movement and, hence, may have a less important role in trunk and limb-related postural motor development and praxis (Ayres, 1981, 1983, 1985). However, Roberts (1978) suggests that the semicircular canals are also important in the mediation of transient head movements, which precede phasic equilibrium responses. Therefore, activities that combine linear and rotational vestibular input, as well as proprioception, may be facilitative toward developing postural mechanisms. A combination of fast and slow movements in the horizontal or vertical linear planes, can be accomplished using the bolster swing, rectangular platform swing, or scooter board. Asking the child to adapt posturally, while sitting atop a slowly moving physioball or barrel, assists the child in developing and sustaining antigravity equilibrium reactions.

Providing opportunities to receive tactile sensory input, integrated with active body movement, is a vital aspect of developing praxis. The use of a toddler swimming pool filled with plastic bubble balls in which to jump, splash, and swim provides an ideal experience of moving, total body, tactile input that facilitates the development of the body scheme and motor planning. As with older children, movement activities on thick-pile carpet or textured fabrics provides incidental tactile input, which some children might not accept otherwise. Play with foods should be encouraged given the rich variety of textures and shapes the child can experience during food play.

Summary

Infants and young children with sensory integrative dysfunction show a disorder in the central processing of sensory input. This dysfunction may lead to disorganization of the child's own internal states, as well as poorly organized attempts to interact with objects and people in the environment. As therapists have become more astute at recognizing and measuring sensory integrative problems, identification of sensory processing disorders at increasingly younger ages has become possible. When assessing the behavior of infants and young children, the therapist first examines the developmental appropriateness of the child's ability to regulate his own autonomic responses to ambient and imposed environmental stimuli. Dysfunction in this area must be the initial focus of treatment. The child's age-relevant ability to evince whole body adaptive motor responses of a postural-bilateral nature should also be examined, as well as anticipatory responses to impending movement by an approaching person or object. In a toddler or young preschooler, difficulty with imitating simple gestures and actions, with problem-solving how to move the body in familiar daily activities, and with acquiring basic tool and toy use may indicate developmental dyspraxia. In addition, preschoolers with dyspraxia may display immature, disorganized, or destructive play patterns. Treatment of children with problems in adaptive movement responses should focus on providing opportunities for intake of sensory information from their own body actions, on facilitating the emergence of more normal movement patterns, and on enhancing complex interactions with the environment through creative play in all aspects of therapy.

References

Als, H. (1982). The unfolding of behavioral organization in the face of a biological violation. In E. Tronick (Ed.), *Human communication and joint regulation of behavior.* Baltimore: University Park Press.

Als, H. (1986). A synactive model of neonatal behavioral organization: Framework for the assessment of neurobehavioral development in the premature infant and for support of infants and parents in the neonatal intensive care environment. *Physical and Occupational Therapy in Pediatrics, 6*(3/4), 3–53.

Ayres, A.J. (1964). Tactile functions: Their relation to hyperactive and perceptual motor behavior. *American Journal of Occupational Therapy, 18,* 6–11.

Ayres, A.J. (1968). Sensory integrative processes and neuropsychological learning disabilities. *Learning Disorders, 3,* 41–58.

Ayres, A.J. (1969). Deficits in sensory integration in educationally handicapped children. *Journal of Learning Disabilities, 2,* 160–168.

Ayres, A.J. (1972). *Sensory integration and learning disorders.* Los Angeles: Western Psychological Services.

Ayres, A.J. (1974a). Development of the body scheme in children. In A. Henderson et al. (Eds.), *The development of sensory integrative theory and practice: A collection of the works of A. Jean Ayres.* Dubuque, IA: Kendall-Hunt.

Ayres, A.J. (1974b). The factor analytic studies. In A. Henderson et al. (Eds.), *The development of sensory integrative theory and practice: A collection of the works of A. Jean Ayres.* Dubuque, IA: Kendall-Hunt.

Ayres, A.J. (1976). *Interpreting the Southern California Sensory Integration Tests.* Los Angeles: Western Psychological Services.

Ayres, A.J. (1979). *Sensory integration and the child.* Los Angeles: Western Psychological Services.

Ayres, A.J. (1981). *Aspects of the somatomotor adaptive response and praxis.* [Audiotape material]. Torrance, CA: Sensory Integration International.

Ayres, A.J. (1983). Sensory integration theory and treatment. Unpublished lecture material. University of Southern California, Los Angeles.

Ayres, A.J. (1985). *Developmental dyspraxia and adult-onset apraxia.* Torrance, CA: Sensory Integration International.

Ayres, A.J. (1989). *Sensory Integration and Praxis Tests.* Los Angeles: Western Psychological Services.

Ayres, A.J., & Mailloux, Z.K. (1981). Influence of sensory integration procedures on language development. *American Journal of Occupational Therapy, 35*(6), 383–390.

Ayres, A.J., Mailloux, Z.K., & Wendler, C.L. (1987). Developmental dyspraxia: Is it a unitary function? *Occupational Therapy Journal of Research, 7,* 93–110.

Ayres, A.J., & Tickle, L.S. (1980). Hyper-responsivity to touch and vestibular stimuli as a predictor of positive response to sensory integration procedures by autistic children. *American Journal of Occupational Therapy, 34*(6), 375–381.

Bayley, N. (1969). *Bayley Scales of Infant Development.* New York: Psychological Corporation.

Benton, A.L. (1955). Right-left discrimination and finger localization in defective children. *Archives of Neurology and Psychiatry, 74,* 583–589.

Bishop, B. (1980). Pain: Its physiology and rationale for management. Part I. Neuroanatomical substrates of pain. *Physical Therapy, 60*(1), 13–37.

Bobath, K. (1980). A neurophysiological basis for the treatment of cerebral palsy. *Clinics in Developmental Medicine, No. 75.* Philadelphia: J.B. Lippincott.

Brazelton, T.B. (1973). *Neonatal Behavioral Assessment Scale.* Philadelphia: J.B. Lippincott.

Bronson, G.W. (1982). Structure, status and characteristics of the nervous system at birth. In P.M. Stratton (Ed.), *The psychobiology of the human newborn.* London: John Wiley & Sons.

Brooks, V.B. (1986). *The neural basis of motor control.* New York: Oxford University Press.

Bushnell, I.W.R., Sai, F., & Mullin, J.T. (1989). Neonatal recognition of the mother's face. *British Journal of Developmental Psychology, 7,* 3–15.

Caplan, P., & Kinsbourne, M. (1976). Baby drops the rattle: Asymmetry of duration of grasp by infants. *Child Development, 47,* 532–534.

Case-Smith, J., Fisher, A.G., & Bauer, D. (1989). An analysis of the relationship between proximal and distal motor control. *American Journal of Occupational Therapy, 43*(10), 657–662.

Cermak, S.A. (1991). Somatodyspraxia. In A. Fisher, E. Murray, & A. Bundy, (Eds.), *Sensory integration: Theory and practice.* Philadelphia: F.A. Davis.

Cermak, S., Coster, W., & Drake, C. (1980). Representational and non-representational gestures in boys with learning disabilities. *American Journal of Occupational Therapy, 34*(1), 19–26.

Cermak, S.A., Quintero, E.J., & Cohen, P.M. (1980). Developmental age trends in crossing the body midline in normal children. *American Journal of Occupational Therapy, 34*(5), 313–319.

Chandler, L.S., Andrews, M.S., & Swanson, M.W. (1980). *Movement assessment of infants: A manual.* Rolling Bay, Washington.

Cool, S.J. (1990). Use of surgical brush in treatment of sensory defensiveness: Commentary and exploration. *Sensory Integration Special Interest Section Newsletter, 13*(4), 4–6. Rockville, MD: American Occupational Therapy Association.

Cooper, R.P., & Aslin, R.N. (1990). Preferences for infant-directed speech in the first month after birth. *Child Development, 61*(5), 1584–1595.

DeCasper, A., & Fifer, W. (1980). Of human bonding: Newborns prefer their mothers' voices. *Science, 208*, 1174–1176.

DeGangi, G.A., & Berk, R.A. (1983). *DeGangi-Berk Test of Sensory Integration.* Los Angeles: Western Psychological Services.

DeGangi, G., & Greenspan, S.I. (1989). *Test of Sensory Functions in Infancy.* Los Angeles: Western Psychological Services.

Dubowitz, L., & Dubowitz, V. (1981). *The neurological assessment of the pre-term and full-term newborn infant.* Philadelphia: J.B. Lippincott.

Eviatar, L., Eviatar, A., & Naray, I. (1974). Maturation of neurovestibular responses in infants. *Developmental Medicine and Child Neurology, 16*, 435–446.

Fisher, A.G. (1991). Vestibular-proprioceptive processing and bilateral integration and sequencing deficits. In A. Fisher, E. Murray, & A. Bundy (Eds.), *Sensory integration: Theory and practice.* Philadelphia: F.A. Davis.

Fisher, A.G., & Dunn, W. (1983). Tactile defensiveness: Historical perspectives, new research—A theory grows. *Sensory Integration Special Interest Newsletter, 6*(2), 1–2. Rockville, MD: American Occupational Therapy Association.

Fisher, A.G., Murray, E., & Bundy, A. (1991). *Sensory integration: Theory and practice.* Philadelphia: F.A. Davis.

Folio, M.R., & Fewell, R.R. (1983). *Peabody Developmental Motor Scales.* Allen, TX: DLM Teaching Resources.

Frick, R.B. (1982). The ego and the vestibulocerebellar system: Some theoretical perspectives. *Psychoanalytic Quarterly, 14*, 93–122.

Galaburda, A.M., & Habib, M. (1987). Mechanisms of asymmetries. The first Annett mode. The Levy-Nagylaki model. In P.J. Magistretti (Ed.), *Cerebral dominance: Biological associations and pathology. Discussions in neurosciences, Vol IV.* Geneva: FESN.

Ghez, C. (1981). Introduction to the motor system. In E.T. Kandel & J.H. Schwartz (Eds.), *Principles of neural science* (pp. 271–283). New York: Elsevier.

Gilfoyle, E., Grady, A., & Moore, J. (1991). *Children adapt.* Thorofare, NJ: Slack.

Goldberg, G. (1985). Supplementary motor area structure and function: Review and hypotheses. *Behavioral and Brain Sciences, 8*, 567–616.

Goody, W., & Reinhold, M. (1952). Some aspects of human orientation in space: Sensation and movement. *Brain, 75,* 472–509.

Greenspan, S.I., & Greenspan, N.T. (1985). *First feelings: Milestones in the emotional development of your baby and child from birth to age four.* New York: Viking Penguin Press.

Greenspan, S.I., & Greenspan, N.T. (1989). *The essential partnership: How parents and children can meet the emotional challenges of infancy and childhood.* New York: Penguin Books.

Greenspan, S.I., & Porges, S. (1984). Psychopathology in infancy and early childhood: Clinical perspectives on the organization of sensory and affective thematic experience. *Child Development, 55,* 49–70.

Holloway, E. (1985). Sensory intervention in the NICU. *Sensory Integration Special Interest Newsletter, 8*(4). Rockville, Md: American Occupational Therapy Association.

Ianniruberto, A., & Tajani, E. (1981). Ultrasonic study of fetal movements. *Seminars in Perinatology, 5*(2), 175–181.

Ikegami, K. (1988). Effects of mother's lapping on imitation of mouth openings and tongue protrudings in early infancy. *Japanese Journal of Educational Psychology, 36,* 192–200.

Jirgal, D., & Bouma, K. (1989). A sensory integration observation guide for children from birth to 3 years of age. *Sensory Integration Special Interest Newsletter, 12*(2), 5. Rockville, MD: American Occupational Therapy Association.

Kaplan, E. (1968). The development of gesture. Unpublished doctoral dissertation. Clark University, Worcester, MA.

Kimura, D. (1977). Acquisition of a motor skill after left hemisphere damage. *Brain, 100,* 527–542.

Knickerbocker, B.M. (1980). *A holistic approach to the treatment of learning disorders.* Thorofare, NJ: Slack.

Knobloch, H., & Pasamanick, B., eds. (1974). *Gesell and Amatruda's developmental diagnosis: The evaluation and management of normal and abnormal neuropsychologic development in infancy and childhood.* 3rd ed. New York: Harper & Row.

Kravitz, H., Goldenberg, D., & Neyhus, A. (1978). Tactual exploration by normal infants. *Developmental Medicine and Child Neurology, 20,* 720–726.

Melzack, R., & Wall, P.D. (1965). Pain mechanisms: A new theory. *Science, 150,* 971–975.

Milani-Comparetti, A. (1981). The neurophysiologic and clinical implications of studies on fetal motor behavior. *Seminars in Perinatology, 5*(2), 183–189.

Milani-Comparetti, A., & Gidoni, E.A. (1967). Routine developmental examination in normal and retarded children. *Developmental Medicine and Child Neurology, 9,* 631–638.

Miller, L.J. (1982). *Miller Assessment for Preschoolers.* New York: Psychological Corporation.

Moore, J. (1978). *The vestibular system.* [A workshop]. Dartmouth: New Hampshire Occupational Therapy Association.

Nelson, M. (1988). *Neurodevelopmental outcome of prematurity at 5–8 years of age: A new consensus for continuity of development.* [Lecture material]. Chicago: University of Illinois.

Njiokiktjien, C. (1988). *Pediatric behavioral neurology: Volume I.* Amsterdam: Elsevier-North Holland.

Ornitz, E.M. (1983). Normal and pathological maturation of vestibular function in the human child. In R. Romand (Ed.), *Development of auditory and vestibular system* (pp. 479–536). New York: Academic Press.

Overton, W., & Jackson, J. (1973). The representation of imagined objects in action sequences: A developmental study. *Child Development, 44,* 309–314.

Parham, L.D. (1987). The evaluation of praxis in pre-schoolers. *Occupational Therapy in Health Care, 4*(2), 23–36.

Preilowski, B. (1972). Possible contribution of the anterior forebrain commissures to bilateral motor coordination. *Neuropsychologia, 10,* 267–277.

Pribram, K.H., & Maginnis, D. (1975). Arousal, activation and effort in the control of attention. *Psychological Review, 82*(2), 116–149.

Rapin, I. (1982). *Children with brain dysfunction: Neurology, cognition, language, and behavior.* New York: Raven Press.

Reissland, N. (1988). Neonatal imitation in the first hour of life: Observations in rural Nepal. *Developmental Psychology, 24,* 464–469.

Roberts, T.D.M. (1978). *Neurophysiology of postural mechanisms.* 2nd ed. Boston: Butterworth.

Royeen, C.B., & Lane, S.J. (1991). Tactile processing and sensory defensiveness. In A.G. Fisher, A.C. Bundy, & E.A. Murray (Eds.), *Sensory integration: Theory and practice.* Philadelphia: F.A. Davis.

Schilder, P. (1951). *Brain and personality.* New York: International Universities Press.

Schmidt, R.A. (1988). *Motor control and learning: A behavioral emphasis* 2nd ed. Champaign, IL: Human Kinetics.

Slavik, B.A., Kitsuwa-Lowe, J., Danner, P.T., Green, J., & Ayres, A.J. (1984). Vestibular stimulation and eye contact in autistic children. *Neuropediatrics, 15,* 33–36.

Stallings, S.A., & Lewin, J.E. (1985). *Self-concept in children with sensory integrative dysfunction.* Paper presented at the American Occupational Therapy Association National Conference, Atlanta, Georgia.

Stowers, S., & Huber, C. (1987). Developmental and screening tests. In L. King-Thomas & B.J. Hacker (Eds.), *A therapist's guide to pediatric assessment.* Boston: Little, Brown & Co.

Sullivan, T. (1987). *Toward an operational definition of gravitational insecurity.* Unpublished master's thesis. Chicago, Illinois: Rush University.

Turkewitz, G., & Kenny, P.A. (1985). The role of developmental limitations of sensory input on sensory/perceptual organization. *Developmental and Behavioral Pediatrics, 6,* 302–306.

Uzgiris, I.C., & Hunt, J.M. (1975). *Assessment in infancy.* Urbana: University of Illinois Press.

Weisberg, M.A. (1984). The role of psychophysiology in defining gravitational insecurity: A pilot study. *Sensory Integration Special Interest Section Newsletter, 7*(4), 1–4. Rockville, MD: American Occupational Therapy Association.

Wilbarger, P. (1984). Planning an adequate "sensory diet"—Application of sensory processing theory during the first year of life. *Zero to Three,* 7–12.

Wilbarger, P., & Wilbarger, J. (1991). *Sensory affective disorders: Beyond tactile defensiveness.* Available from Patricia Wilbarger, 642 Island View Drive, Santa Barbara, CA 93109.

Yarrow, L.J, Rubinstein, J.L., & Pedersen, F.A. (1975). Infant and environment: Early cognitive and motivational development. Washington, DC: Hemisphere, Halsted, Wiley.

11

□ □ □
□ □ □
□ □ □

Assistive Technology in Early Intervention: Theory and Practice

Yvonne Swinth, MS, OTR
Jane Case-Smith, EdD, OTR

Assistive technology has always been an important tool for occupational therapists in rehabilitation and in special education. For years, therapists have used different types of low technology, such as adaptive equipment and other handmade devices, to promote the functional independence of their clients. More recently, high technology has become commonly used in the practice of occupational therapy (Smith, 1991). A wide range of technological devices, from simple switches to complex robotics, are used to promote the function of children with developmental disabilities. Such assistive technology opens new doors, creates opportunities for children, and enables occupational therapists to realize functional goals previously unattainable. However, therapists need to be willing to make transitions concurrent with the present advances and innovations in assistive technology.

This chapter discusses the use of assistive technology with infants and young children; yet, many of the principles described apply to clients of any age who may be using or who need technological support. For the purposes of this chapter, the term assistive technology includes computers, electric wheelchairs, adaptive switches, augmentative communication, and environmental controls. A glossary has been provided at the end of the book to aid the reader with unfamiliar terms. (See Appendix B.)

Assistive technology appears to hold unique opportunities for teaching and for advancing the life choices of children with disabilities (Lahm, 1989). Many types of technology are available for young children with disabilities, particularly those with limited motor control. Introducing the appropriate types of technology systems to these children as young as possible may enable them to experience important learning situations that otherwise, because of their disabilities, may not be possible. Lack of learning opportunities for any child may produce passive and unmotivated school-age children who do not have the interest or the skills to interact with the environment (Douglas, Reeson, & Ryan, 1988). When opportunities for integrating basic cognitive and perceptual skills are missed in early childhood, the child does not develop a foundation for learning higher level concepts. Assistive technology can enable the young child to learn basic contingencies, cause-and-effect, discrimination, turn taking, and environmental control, all of which provide foundational skills for higher level conceptual learning. Technology creates exciting opportunities for children with special needs to explore, to interact with, and to function in their environments.

Related Legislation

A number of recent legislative acts have directly affected the availability and use of assistive technology for individuals who have disabilities. The Rehabilitation Act, which was first introduced in 1973 and then rewritten in 1986 (PL 99-506), supports the use of technology for individuals with disabilities to (1) have greater control over their lives; (2) participate in home, school, and work environments; (3) interact with peers who do not have disabilities; and (4) otherwise do acts taken for granted by individuals without any known disability. The enactment of the Education for All Handicapped Children Act of 1975 (PL 94-142) provides support for designing, adapting, and using technology in the education of individuals with disabilities. This act encourages both private and public sectors to market new technology and provide incentives for the dissemination of information regarding technology. The implementation of The Education of the Handicapped Act Amendments of 1986 (PL 99-457) provided guidelines for states to develop family-focused early intervention services for children birth to 3 years of age. By emphasizing the importance of comprehensive services early in the young child's life, the law encourages professionals to evaluate the child's potential use of technology at the earliest appropriate time. It also makes available discretionary funding for technology-related research and development in special education (Behrmann, Jones, & Wilds, 1989).

In 1990, the Individuals with Disabilities Education Act (IDEA) (PL 101-476) amended and renamed the Education for All Handicapped Children Act. This law calls for the provision of assistive technology devices as required to provide a free appropriate public education for children with disabilities. The law defines *assistive technology device* as any item, equipment, and system used "to increase, maintain, or improve functional capabilities of individuals with disabilities." *Assistive technology services* include any service that directly assists a child with a disability in the selection, acquisition, or use of an assistive technology device. Other assistive technology services provided under the law are coordinating and using therapies, training, or technical assistance for individuals with disabilities. Through this language, the IDEA places a powerful emphasis on the importance of assistive technology in the child's education and ability to function in the academic setting and the community. Each of the above legislative acts has improved services to children with disabilities and has brought new options to therapy and to education for both children and their families.

Technology: Linking Theory with Practice

As in all practice, the occupational therapist uses theoretical frameworks to guide recommendations for and application of technology in intervention. Understanding the rationale behind the use of technology with the very young child who has a disability assists the occupational therapist in establishing priorities for the child. It also allows the professional team involved to substantiate the decisions made and forms the basis for future planning. The therapist's recommendations for technology are based on his understanding of early child development, theoretical frameworks of occupational therapy, and the possible consequences of limited motor control during the crucial stages of development.

Guiding Principles in the Application of Assistive Technology

From core theories of occupational therapy practice come several guiding principles that apply to the use of assistive technology with children. These principles and their application are described.

1. The child acquires higher level sensorimotor skills through developmental processes that are genetically determined and through purposeful, goal-directed interactions with the environment (Gilfoyle, Grady, & Moore, 1981). Activities that increase a child's functional independence must be meaningful and purposeful to the child.

In order for technology to elicit an adaptive response, it must match the developmental skills of the child. Before implementing technological support, it is crucial to determine whether the activity does have purpose and meaning for both the child and family.

For example, a young child with severe motor limitations, who requires complex adaptations to access a computer system, may not have the cognitive skill needed to use the system. Task analysis of the activity, information and formal evaluation instruments, past experience, professional judgment, and the resources of other professionals are used by the therapist to evaluate the child's developmental readiness to use assistive technology. Introducing the complex system prior to the development of appropriate skills can be frustrating for both the child and family, and it may discourage their willingness to use assistive technology.

2. Functional skills are achieved through a spiraling, interweaving process of sensory input, motor output, and sensory feedback. In the child with CNS impairment, the spiraling process is disrupted (Gilfoyle, Grady, & Moore, 1981). Intervention with assistive technology can help the child achieve functional skills by providing alternative input or output methods into the sensory-motor-sensory feedback spiral. Technological supports can augment sensory input, adapt the required motor output, and provide alternative sensory feedback for the activity, enabling its successful accomplishment.

Examples of adaptations for *sensory input* are switches with textured surfaces and programs with auditory feedback. Large letters on the keyboard or on the screen are examples of adaptations for children with low vision.

Through assistive technology, the *motor output* needed to accomplish a functional skill is adapted. Mobility can be achieved through pressing a joystick or a head switch of a powered chair. The computer can be accessed through an optic light-scanning system rather than through the use of the standard keyboard.

The *sensory feedback* of an activity can be augmented or adapted using technology. Speech synthesizers and augmentative communication are examples of technology with adapted sensory feedback. The sensory feedback of switch-activated toys reinforces the child's ability to activate the switch and promotes a motor sequence that can be generalized to skills on a keyboard.

3. All human occupation arises out of an innate urge to explore and to master the environment (Kielhofner & Burke, 1980). Fulfillment of this need enhances motivation and initiative. Self-identity and self-esteem emerge from the child's ability to productively play and successfully interact with others.

Adaptive equipment and assistive technology enable the child to successfully master his environment in play and in activities of daily living. Through application of technology, the young child becomes more independent and competent, which positively affects his motivation, initiative, self-esteem, and self-identity.

4. Learned helplessness is a secondary disability that can affect the functional skills and interactions of children with developmental delays. Learned

helplessness is the individual's belief that one cannot exert personal control over outcomes experienced when interacting with the environment (Abramson, Seligman, & Teasdale, 1978; Gargiulo & O'Sullivan, 1986; Maier & Seligman, 1976; Weisz, 1979).

When young children learn that they have little control over outcomes, deficits in motivational, cognitive, and emotional areas result. The child develops low self-esteem, directly affecting how he interacts and performs in the environment. Children with learned helplessness usually show a lack of initiation and an inability to cope with the events around them.

The potentially permanent effects of failure on young children with disabilities suggest that methods to teach and to motivate them early in life are essential. Strategies and adaptations that allow these children the maximum amount of independence possible decrease the chance for them to learn that they have no control over the environment.

According to Goldenburg (1979), parents and professionals working together to increase independence and capitalize on the child's early experiences can improve his potential capabilities and provide a feeling of competence and success. Among the different teaching and learning options that parents and teachers of children with disabilities can use, assistive technology presents one of the most viable and versatile methods.

Assistive Technology: Ethical Dilemmas and Responsibilities of the Occupational Therapist

When considering implementation of assistive technology into the program of a young child, a therapist must consider several ethical questions as well as certain responsibilities. The use of technology may present new issues and dilemmas both in the child's therapy program and at home; therefore, several questions must be addressed to fully evaluate the potential effectiveness the technology may have for the child and family. All children have the right to develop to their fullest potential. Occupational therapists provide options for children to attain this goal. However, although some children may have the potential to use technology, it may not be practical for the family to functionally use within the home or for the instructors to manage in the early childhood program. As part of the decision making process, the occupational therapist examines the practicality and feasibility of the technology being considered. The high cost of assistive technology is one of the most important considerations within the decision making process. The cost of technology includes the ongoing cost for maintenance and for adding software or hardware to the system. Therefore, the family incurs hidden costs that continue long after the original purchase of the device. If an inappropriate device is recommended and then purchased by the family, limited monies are wasted and the child is prevented from receiving needed technology in the future. As a result, the child's functional independence may be limited by the incorrect recommendation, and the family may be discouraged from making additional investments in other devices.

The team addresses these issues and the long-term implications of their recommendations when considering assistive technology for the child. As decisions are made for the child, the team and family consider the following issues:

1. What financial resources are available to the family?
2. When the device or technology is in need of repair, does the family have access to services?
3. Does it significantly increase the child's level of independence and function?
4. Can it be adapted to enable higher levels of function as the child grows and matures?
5. Can a less complex device meet the same needs just as well?
6. Is the technology culturally acceptable?

The team discusses these issues and others unique to each family in deciding whether or not the device is a reasonable and appropriate investment for the family that will result in increasing the child's developmental skills and functional independence. If the child lives in a rural community that is 200 miles from the nearest city, an elaborate computer system with a complex access system may be inappropriate for the family to maintain. High-tech devices usually require frequent repair and servicing. If someone who is knowledgeable in servicing the device is not easily accessible, the family may incur unusual time and financial expense to obtain repairs. When the device malfunctions, it tends to be inoperable for long periods of time. As a result, the child's excitement in learning new skills is replaced with frustration and disappointment that opportunities for interaction are inconsistently available. The family should be presented with objective and realistic information regarding investment in and use of technology. Given a complete description of the options and alternatives, the family makes the final decision as to what technology is implemented and how it is implemented into the child's program. Some rural families may choose to make the long drive for services when the technology malfunctions. They value the increased independence that the technology offers their child to such an extent that they willingly expend their time and resources to maintain that independence.

Therapists who routinely use technology with young children maintain knowledge of the current devices available and the functions and benefits of each device. (Appendix C lists resources for obtaining equipment, software, and information.) Since the technology available is rapidly changing, the therapist must make an ongoing effort to stay abreast of what is available and what technology has become obsolete. Therapists often have the responsibility of assisting the family or teacher in obtaining the recommended device and in integrating the device into the child's daily life. "Microcomputers and the accompanying technology can indeed make a powerful impact on the potential outcomes for young handicapped children, but that impact will be diluted if early childhood personnel do not know about the potential of technology or how to use it" (Kinney & Blackhurst, 1987). By reading the current literature and research that addresses the uses of technology with children, the occupational therapist can effectively match the needs of clients with the available technology and can prepare children and families to use it to its greatest potential.

Strategies for Evaluating, Designing, and Selecting Assistive Technology Systems for Young Children

When considering implementation of any type of technological support as part of a child with a disability's program, the unique needs and strengths of the child are considered. Given two children who have the same disability, devices that work for one child may not work for the other. Recommendations are based on comprehensive evaluations of the child and the environment. The priorities of the child, the family, and the professional team working with them are assessed.

Matching Technology to the Child's Skills

First, the specific needs and strengths of the child are assessed and goals are developed. These goals should reflect both functional and developmental outcomes. From the assessment results and knowledge of the child's present and future environments, the team and family predict the skills the child will need in order to successfully function and manage the demands of those environments. As a result, the team selects assistive technology that meets the child's immediate needs and prepares her to cope with future environments. To best match present and future needs, the team determines the child's present developmental and functional levels, estimates the rate of developmental progress, and then plans the technology that will be appropriate in the near future. Long-term needs (e.g., entrance into school) are also considered, but should not drive the decision regarding the best present solutions for the child.

For example, to teach the concept of cause-and-effect, it may be appropriate to begin working with the child using a single switch-activated toy. If the eventual goal of the child is to begin interacting with a computer, then concurrently the child should be introduced to some computer activities. The therapist may select simple single switch cause-and-effect games on the computer as a method of generalizing the skill. Eventually, the therapist presents high-level computer activities that require choosing one of two or three possibilities and matching a stimulus to one of two choices on the computer.

Several authors have attempted to define specific prerequisite skills when introducing young children to technology. However, empirical studies that quantify or qualify the developmental skills that result in effective use of technology remain limited (Behrmann, Jones, & Wilds, 1989; Bowser, 1989; Symington, 1990). Each child with a disability has unique needs, abilities, and characteristics.

Limited motor control is often one of the greatest challenges faced by an occupational therapist when considering any type of technological support for these children. Other factors and behaviors that can affect the child's performance include cognitive and memory deficits that increase the amount of time needed to learn a task, and postural instability that requires adapted positioning. Visual-perceptual deficits and auditory processing difficulties may also require selected software and adaptations of the computer programs. These factors affect how a child with a disability learns and determine an expected achievement level, given access to technological support. They also influence the child's and family's response to a task or situation (Lahm, 1989).

Different access systems and assistive technology devices should be considered due to the various difficulties experienced by children with disabilities. The complexity of the system determines the cognitive and motor skills needed to use it (Mann & Lane, 1991). The effectiveness of using a complex access system is highly dependent on the match between the child's cognitive, motor, and perceptual skills and the demands of the system. The system, or an adaptation of the system, must fit the child's developmental skills in each of these domains. A child who has the cognitive abilities to understand how to use a specific device may not be motorically capable of independently using the access system that operates the device. For example, a young child with severe cerebral palsy may have the cognitive ability to recognize cause-and-effect relationships and the perceptual skills necessary to use a variety of software programs; however, due to limitations in motor control, the child is unable to use a standard keyboard. Therefore, another access system, such as an adapted keyboard or Light Talker, must be used.

A progression of systems is introduced that follows the developmental progress of the child. Success using simple access systems must precede trial of more complex systems (e.g., single switch use precedes introducing an adapted keyboard). The occupational therapist who is familiar with the software and access systems available can place them in a developmental sequence. By identifying all of the developmental skills required to successfully operate the system, the therapist makes appropriate selections for the child, avoiding the child's frustration and the expense of an inappropriate match of the child and the software.

Many software programs require that the child make specific, discrete responses to visual, auditory, or tactile stimuli. The child must be able to attend briefly and have the interest and motivation to activate a toy or a computer purposefully. Object permanence and cause-and-effect may also be prerequisite skills for a computer program to be used purposefully. However, computer activities and programs can also be used to teach some of these prerequisite skills, such as interest, motivation, and cause-and-effect relationships. Higher level cognitive skills (e.g., discrimination, matching, directionality) are needed if augmentative communication or an electric wheelchair are recommended for the child. Behrmann, Jones, and Wilds (1989) summarize the skills needed to implement technology into four areas, including motor skills, cognitive-language skills, visual-perceptual skills, and social-emotional skills (see Table 11-1). Their list should be viewed as skills that the child can potentially develop while using technology, rather than as required prerequisite skills. For the child with low-level cognitive skills, simple forms of technology are selected. Examples are switches that activate toys with high levels of sensory input, such as a vibration pillow, a strobe light, or a fan. Most of these toys activate using a simple, single switch.

Matching Assistive Technology to Family Goals

When evaluating the use of assistive technology with the very young child who has a disability, the occupational therapist also considers the concerns and resources of the child's family. Therefore, the selected technology considers the family's financial resources and time, as well as their interests and priorities. One family may be most interested in systems that promote preacademic skills, while another family may be primarily interested in assistive technology that will enable their child to play. In the family-centered approach, the family members have both access to and control of needed resources. With objective information about the specific technology, the family makes the decision. Since they are responsible for the daily use and upkeep of the technology, it is particularly important that parents are the ones to select the type of assistive device or technological support for their child.

When the team working with a child begins to consider implementing assistive technology, especially when the technology is expensive, it is important to include the family in discussion and problem solving sessions as early as possible. For some families, technology can be mystifying and overwhelming. The mystique may be eliminated if the team educates the

Table 11-1 Summary of Skills Needed to
Use Technology

Motor skills
• Range of motion
• Strength and endurance
• Press and release
• Reliable and consistent motor movement

Cognitive-language skills
• Cause-and-effect
• Attention span (sustained or selective)
• Object permanence
• Means-ends causality
• Imitation
• One-to-one correspondence
• Intentional behavior (desire to communicate)
• Symbolic representation (recognize pictures)
• Reliable yes and no response
• Receptive understanding of commands
• Making choices

Visual-perceptual skills
• Visual tracking and scanning
• Figure ground
• Form discrimination

Social-emotional skills
• Initiating and terminating interactions
• Turn taking and waiting for turn
• Attending to an object or person
• Following one-step directions

Source: Reprinted from Behrmann M.M., Jones J.K.,
and Wilds M.L., Technology intervention for very
young children with disabilities, *Infants and Young
Children*, Vol. 1 : 4, p. 70, with permission of Aspen
Publishers, Inc., © 1989.

family on the uses of technology and explains the rationale for using it with their child. At times, the parents of a young child with a disability continue to grieve and have not yet come to terms with the disability. The idea of their child having to use assistive devices can increase their grief, because it serves as a visual reminder that their child is not like other children. The technology may also signify defeat; that is, a method of compensation is needed because certain developmental skills may never be achieved. By listening to the parents' concerns and by demonstrating an understanding of their feelings, therapists can aid the family in working through their grief and anxiety. Once the family understands that the devices will help their child interact with the environment and accomplish new skills, their willingness to use them increases. Explaining that technology facilitates the development of skills and compensates for the disability allows the family to positively view devices and computer use.

The family is a system with unique resources and functions. The type of technology that is implemented into the child's life should not only increase the child's independence, but should also meet the needs of the family at home. For example, often children with severe cerebral palsy have limited oral-motor control, which prohibits speech. At a young age, these children and their families communicate through simple yes and no responses, using eye gaze or head movement. For these families, the implementation of an augmentative communication device into the child's program opens a new world of communication and brings new depth to her interactions. Such a device may enable the child to express her feelings to family members for the first time. This not only increases the child's independence, but it fulfills the family's need to communicate with their child at a higher level of understanding. As the child's communication increases, the family is better able to respond to the child and mutual interactions are made possible. Decisions about technology that include the family and consider the child in the context of the family unit are most likely to result in effective application of technology. When decisions are made without the family's input and technology that meets the professionals' needs rather than the family's needs is elected, family members do not have interest or investment in the device. Use of the device in the home is more likely to result in stress and frustration than success.

An Interdisciplinary Team Approach to Using Assistive Technology

As part of an interdisciplinary team, the therapist consults other team members when exploring the different types of assistive technology that may be provided for the child. Decisions based on the input of the entire team and the family are most likely to meet the multifaceted needs of the child. A decision making process that includes the viewpoint of several disciplines, as well as the family's perspective about home life, results in a more comprehensive and appropriate program for the child.

Often the introduction of a technological device, specifically a complex device, changes the team's focus. Each team member's involvement and emphasis with the child is affected when the child begins to use a major technological device. Program time is now spent on training and practice and team members make efforts to integrate use of the device into the child's everyday activities; therefore, development of the skills needed to use the device often become the focus of intervention. For example, if the professional team recommends an electric wheelchair for a child and the family purchases one, every team member may contribute to the initial wheelchair training. Interdisciplinary input is used in designing correct positioning, in training the child to drive the chair, and in problem solving the inevitable difficulties unique to each child (e.g., selection and positioning of the driving system to compensate for motor limitations). Involvement by every member of the team encourages skill generalization in a variety of settings and situations as the child becomes increasingly proficient in driving the chair, both at home and outdoors. The teacher may spend several days working on wheelchair skills rather than academics. Occupational therapy sessions may involve practice with the chair's joystick rather than practice of self-feeding or other fine motor activities. All team members accept the fact that they may need to sacrifice their own discipline-specific goals for the child to the cost of learning a new technological device.

Application of Assistive Technology

A variety of assistive devices can be introduced to infants, toddlers, and young children. Using these devices to provide increased independence as early as possible can decrease the learned helplessness that the child may later develop. Such a device may allow the young child to be included with peers in social and academic environments. The following examples illustrate basic principles in selecting, recommending, and using technology.

Single Switch

The single switch is usually the best device with which to first introduce a child to potential technological devices and access systems. Initially, the switch can activate a simple battery-operated toy. Toys may be adapted using simple equipment (e.g., battery interrupters, copper wiring, soldering irons, and phone plugs) (Burkhart, 1980, 1982; Vanderheiden, Brandenburg, Brown, & Bottorf, 1988) or may be purchased from a variety of catalogues. (See Appendix C for a list of vendors.) Through playing with the switch toy, the child develops basic skills in object permanence and cause-and-effect relationships. The child also learns that she can control the surrounding environment. Since many children with disabilities are unable to independently manipulate toys due to limited motor control, the switch allows children access to toys and play activities similar to their peers without disabilities. These play activities may be used as preliminary training for interaction using augmentative communication devices, navigation of electric wheelchairs, and operation of environmental control devices and computers (Williams & Matesi, 1988). The following example illustrates strategies for implementing a single switch and the benefits that can be realized.

Case Study 1: At 9 months of age, Josh, who had been diagnosed with spastic quadriplegia, entered an occupational therapy program. He was lethargic and did not demonstrate interest in his surroundings. He did not sit independently and his head control was poor. He had great difficulty controlling upper extremity movements. His interest in toys was limited and his attention span was short.

After observing Josh's level of interaction and motor control, the therapist introduced a switch toy as part of her intervention. She found that he responded well to auditory stimuli, therefore, she connected a switch adapter to a toy robot that made noises and moved in circles. To the adapter, she attached a plate switch operated by pressing on its surface. After demonstrating the switch and assisting Josh in activating it, the therapist encouraged him to play with the robot independently. Quickly, Josh learned to consistently press the switch and expressed great delight in the robot's response.

In the therapy sessions that followed, different toys were connected to the switch. Different switches (e.g., lever switches, joysticks) were used and were positioned to enhance upper extremity, head, and trunk control. Over several months, he developed consistent head control, independent sitting, and consistent upper extremity function to grossly manipulate a variety of objects. His vocalizations also steadily increased. His parents began to use adapted switches with battery-operated toys at home. With these prerequisite skills, Josh began to work on simple cause-and-effect computer activities.

Environmental Controls

The single switch can also be used to operate environmental control devices and to access computer systems. With an adapter, or with adaptations to the appliances in a home, the young child can use a single switch to control his home environment (e.g., turning on lights or activating the television). As the child matures, more complex switching devices can be used for environmental control, increasing the child's sense of mastery (e.g., operating more than one device, switching channels, and changing the volume). (See Figure 11-1.)

When considering environmental controls for a child, it is first necessary to determine what is most important for the child to control in the environment. By evaluating the child's environment and daily routine and her functional and motivational capability, the team and family can determine the need for and benefit of an environmental control device.

Case Study 2: Lisa, a 24-month-old child with spinal atrophy, lacks motor control of both her upper and lower extremities. One of Lisa's favorite pasttimes is to listen to her music. Lisa's parents asked her occu-

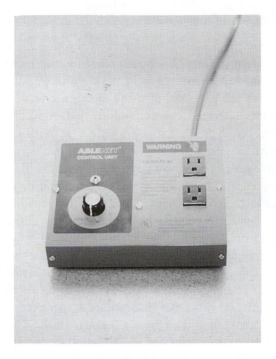

Figure 11-1 This commonly used environmental control device (such as this one marketed by Ablenet AccessAbility, Inc., 1081 Tenth Ave. SE, Minneapolis, MN 55414) has a timer so that the device can be set to keep the appliance on for varying lengths of time. It can also be set so that the appliance operates only while the individual keeps the switch closed.

pational therapist to help them design a method that would allow her to independently turn on the family stereo. Thus, the occupational therapist set up an environmental control system that operated by means of a single switch. Since Lisa's method of mobility was rolling, the family decided to place the switch on the floor by the stereo. When she wanted to turn on the music, she rolled to, and then on top of, the switch. The environmental control system had a timer so that music automatically played for up to 60 minutes. The length of time for the music to play could be adjusted to provide an optimal reward system for Lisa. Both Lisa and her family enjoyed her new independence.

The same system could be wired to other electronic devices in the home and a variety of switches could be used to match the goals and the improving skill levels of the child. The system allowed Lisa more opportunities to explore and master her environment, which in turn increased her motivation to engage in other activities.

Personal Computers

Use of the personal computers with young children is becoming increasingly prevalent in early childhood programs, clinics, and homes. Behrmann (1984) reported that children with the cognitive and physical skills of a 3-month-old have the potential of using electronic learning. In his study, 3-month-old infants activated a switch to hear their mothers' voices. A more realistic guideline is to begin cause-and-effect activities when the child reaches a 7-month cognitive level. The computer can be a motivating tool to help the child learn and develop a large repertoire of skills. Its effectiveness results from its potential for reciprocal interaction and its capability to specifically respond to the child's input. The computer provides simulations of experiences that cannot otherwise be experienced by children with motor disabilities. For example, a child with a disability who lacks independent mobility may experience the concept of directionality for the first time using the computer and appropriate software. The computer is also infinitely patient with drill and practice and can provide the repetition needed for some children to learn. Often software programs incorporate a sequence of activities that teach children to generalize their newly learned skills. The computer may also be a focal activity to encourage socialization between children (Figure 11-2) (Spiegel-McGill, Zippiroli, & Mistrett, 1989).

With a variety of software and input devices, computers provide endless adaptations that ensure success for each child. The level of difficulty and the requirements to operate the system can be adjusted to meet the unique needs of the child. The Adaptive Firmware Card (AFC) (for Apple computers) and the Ke:nex (for the Macintosh) enable the user to enhance the versatility of the system for children with disabilities. The AFC card is installed inside the computer, and the Ke:nex card plugs into the ADB port. Both enable the therapist to individualize computer programs and to provide the user with a variety of access systems. After the AFC is used to program the software, the child can use an expanded keyboard such as a Unicorn Board® (see Figure 11-3) or a switch to operate software that was not specifically developed for children who have disabilities. Individualized methods to access the computer help ensure the child's success in using the computer. For example, with the AFC in place, the therapist can program the Unicorn Board to provide two distinct responses. If the child presses on the left half of the board, the computer software responds in one way; if he presses on the right half of the board, the computer gives a different response. Due to the large size of the Unicorn Board, the child with decreased fine motor control and adequate upper extremity range of motion can successfully make choices on the computer. The AFC can also be programmed so that the computer keyboard is redefined; that is, so that the keys are rearranged, or that programs can be

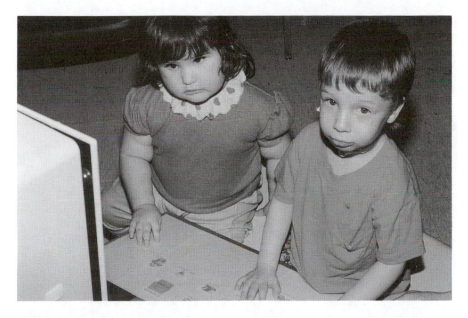

Figure 11-2 Peers interact, using a computer system set-up with a Unicorn Board®.

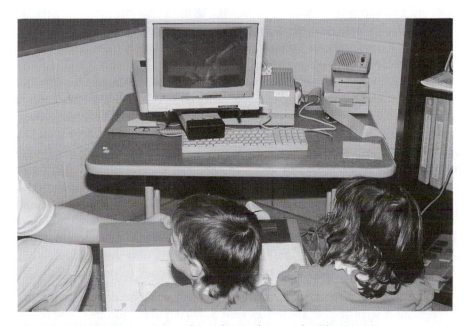

Figure 11-3 The Unicorn Board® replaces the standard keyboard.

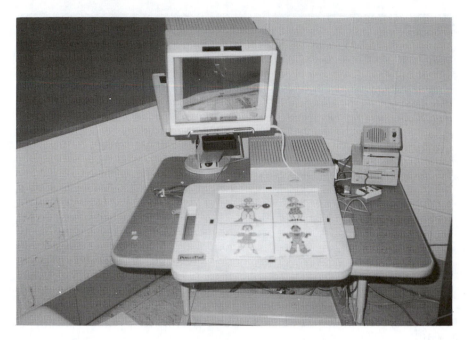

Figure 11-4 The Power Pad® is a versatile input method.

accessed through Morse code or scanning. Other programs and systems are available that operate much like the AFC; for example, programs that decrease the speed of the computer's response or programs that eliminate the repeat function of keys.

The Touch Window® and the Power Pad® (Figure 11-4) are two computer access systems appropriate for and appealing to young children. The Touch Window plugs into the game port of the computer and attaches to the computer screen. By touching its transparent surface, the child activates the computer. For example, a cause-and-effect program can be activated by touching the screen. The Touch Window can also be used on the table similar to a writing pad. The Power Pad is a square tablet that can be used to operate compatible programs. Its function includes use as a game board or as a talking word board. The Power Pad-based programs can be customized to meet the child's individual needs. Another example of an access system for young children is the Muppet Keyboard®. This colorful, uniquely designed keyboard teaches basic skills such as colors, numbers, and letter recognition.

Case Study 3: Computer access systems and software can encourage interaction with the computer, as well as visual attention to the screen. Sara was a 24-month-old child with Down syndrome. In collaboration with the early intervention team, her parents actively sought out methods to enhance her learning. They purchased an Apple IIGS for Sarah at home and were interested in how she might successfully interact with it. The team debated which access system was most appropriate for her, due to her young age, decreased attention span, and high-level distractibility. The team also had limited information regarding her understanding of cause-and-effect, because she seldom interacted with toys. Therefore, the occupational therapist tried a variety of access systems, including the standard keyboard, the Unicorn Board, a toggle switch, the Power Pad, and the Touch Window.

Sara had the motor control to use a standard keyboard, but became easily distracted given a number of choices. She also had difficulty attending to the computer screen. After discussing the options with Sara's parents and the other professionals working with Sara, it was decided that eventually she would be able to independently use a standard keyboard. To improve her focus on the screen, the therapist recommended that she use a Touch Window with occasional opportunities to use the standard keyboard. The occupational therapist also provided recommendations on the type of software to consider purchasing to help Sara's cognitive, social, and fine motor development. After 3 months with the Touch Window, Sara asked to play on the computer by standing near it and vocalizing. She spent up to 5 minutes in independent play. Other children from the neighborhood enjoyed playing with Sara on the computer and it became a positive way for Sarah to interact with her peers. Sara's experiences on the computer taught her that her actions could be purposeful and meaningful. Her success in this activity helped to increase her willingness to try other new tasks both in the classroom and at home.

Augmentative Communication

Augmentative communication can be defined as communication that does not require speech and that can be individualized to the unique needs of the individual. The overall purpose of augmentative communication is to enable an individual to be able to transmit a message through production-based or selection-based techniques (Fishman, 1987). The possibilities for augmentative communication are numerous, including a communication board, the Intro Talker, the Touch Talker® (see Figure 11-5) and the Light Talker (Figure 11-6). The Touch Talker and Light Talker® are electronic communication devices that are programmed with individualized overlays. The board's overlays can indicate as few as 8 and as many as 128 choices to the child. While the Touch Talker is activated by touch, the Light Talker has numerous different selection techniques, including direct selection using an optic light, row-column scanning, direct scanning, and Morse code.

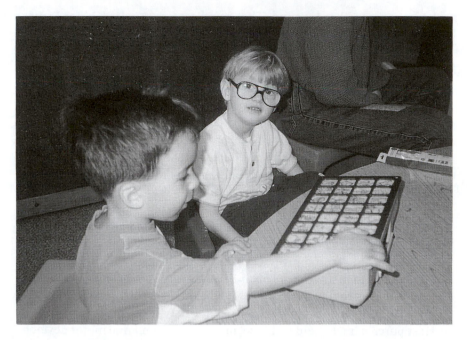

Figure 11-5 Peers interact, using a Touch Talker® with a vocabulary of 32 programmed phrases.

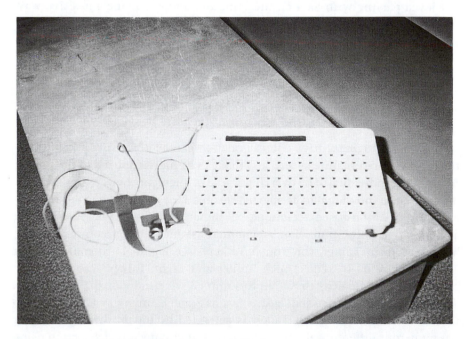

Figure 11-6 A Light Talker® and an optic light.

When an augmentative communication system for a child is considered, the complexity of the system can be a disadvantage as well as an advantage. The range of devices available requires an equally great range of abilities from the user. As with other types of technology, it is important to consider the unique skills of the child in all developmental areas and to solicit the family's priorities before making a final recommendation.

Often, both speech and language therapists and occupational therapists work together to select and to train children to use augmentative communication. Both have unique perspectives and skills to offer in this specialized area. As a member of the augmentative communication team, the occupational therapist helps evaluate and provide training of the fine motor and perceptual motor skills needed to use the device. For example, if the child uses a switch to activate the augmentative communication system, the therapist helps to determine the best placement of the switch. The type of switch and its placement should facilitate success when learning a new system. The child's posture and position when using a communication system are also essential to successful system access. High levels of external support should be given to the child with trunk instability to allow for optimal upper extremity movement and to facilitate concentration on the activity.

In addition, the occupational therapist may assist in evaluating the child's prerequisite skills to determine which communication device is most appropriate. The therapist assists the child in learning prerequisite skills, such as cause-and-effect relationships and object permanence. Therapy can include activities to develop adapted switch use and keyboard skills using a head pointer or other device to access the communication system.

Collaboration among team members is made easier when discipline roles are delineated and are well understood. Understanding the goals of the speech and language therapists enables the occupational therapists to provide appropriate support to the communication goals. Occupational therapists should be familiar with terminology used in the area of augmentative communication, such as single-switch scanning selection, encoding, directed scanning, and direction selection (Angelo & Smith, 1989). Continuing education courses and additional training can familiarize therapists with the terminology and the available hardware and software.

Many parents experience frustration and stress when they attempt to communicate with their child whose speech and communication abilities are severely limited by multiple disabilities. As the child matures, lack of speech can become a more frustrating problem as the child attempts to express his feelings and more complex thoughts.

Case Study 4: Jason is 24 months old and has cerebral palsy with resulting quadriparesis. He seems cognitively aware of his environment. His mother expressed frustration at being unable to interpret Jason's speech when he attempted to communicate at home. The augmentative communication team at Jason's preschool held a meeting to discuss his communication difficulties. The occupational therapist had been working on switch and computer training with Jason during therapy, and he was 90% accurate with a head switch. His speech and language therapist was working on basic concepts with him; however, communication was quite limited, as he did not have a consistent method of communication other than the words yes and no. The team evaluating Jason decided that he could benefit from a Light Talker, which he could use either with direct selection using an optic light, or with scanning using a single switch.

The Light Talker could eventually operate a computer or an electric wheelchair, which were both long-term goals for Jason. Therefore, he could learn one system and then generalize those skills to several areas of daily living and academics. Initially, the team tried both direct selection and scanning methods with Jason. After 3 months, he successfully used the optic light to choose one picture out of four choices that communicated the next activity he wanted to do. Since direct selection allows for more efficient communication than scanning, the team decided to continue working with Jason using the optic light and reevaluate his progress in 3 months.

Eventually, the team planned to expand the number of overlays and the number of choices on each overlay from 8 to 16 on his Light Talker. The long-term goal (of several years) was for Jason to use all 128 choices on each overlay. Jason enjoyed his new-found freedom with communication and demonstrated less frustration. He also began to use his optic light as a pointer to make choices in the classroom and at home. This method of selection has greater accuracy than eye gaze in most situations. Through successful use of his Light Talker and increased opportunities to communicate, Jason demonstrated a greater interest in interaction with his peers and with others.

Powered Mobility

Recent research strongly supports the use of powered mobility for young children with disabilities (Butler, 1986; Chiulli, Corradi-Scalise, & Donatelli-Schultheiss, 1988; Jaffe, Butler, Hays, & Everard, 1986). Douglas and Ryan (1987) found that the introduction of an electric wheelchair into the life of a 3-year-old boy with severe physical disabilities affected his emotional, social, and intellectual state in a positive manner. Butler (1986) demonstrated that children as young as 23 to 38 months could independently drive an electric wheelchair. Research results indicate that motivational, cognitive, and emotional gains are achieved when powered mobility is introduced at young ages (Butler, 1986; Butler, Okamoto, & McKay, 1983; Douglas & Ryan, 1987). Children who use powered mobility at young ages have been observed to be more interested in their environment and seem more likely to be self-motivated. Independent mobility using a powered chair may help prevent the development of learned helplessness. "Onset of this passive, dependent pattern coincided with failure of the normal development of locomotion at about 12 months of age, and was increasingly manifested as inhibited locomotion progressively interfered with normal childhood activities" (Butler, 1986). Other possible goals of implementing powered mobility into a child's life include the development and understanding of such concepts as spatial awareness, speed, distance, directionality, independence, and control of and responsibility for actions (Chiulli, Corradi-Scalise, & Donatelli-Schultheiss, 1988).

In selecting a powered mobility device for a child, an electric wheelchair and other devices should be considered. Due to the high cost of an electric wheelchair, it is prudent for the interdisciplinary team to consider other, less expensive options for children. Less permanent types of powered mobility, such as the Probe Six are available in toy stores (see Figure 11-7). Cost of the Probe Six is approximately one-tenth the cost of an electric wheelchair and

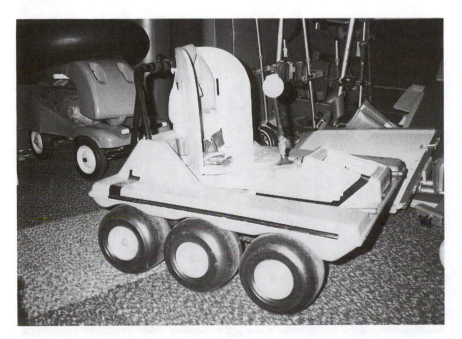

Figure 11-7 A Probe Six® with an adaptive seat and an extended joystick

can be used to achieve the same goals that are attained using more expensive powered mobility devices. At times, these battery-operated toys require adaptations in order to be effectively used by a child with a disability. For example, an adapted seat provides additional support for the child with decreased trunk control.

A child can independently drive a wheelchair in a variety of ways. Children can use joysticks, different types of switches, and computer interfaces to direct the chair. As with the different access systems on a computer, some of these systems are inappropriate for the very young child when the cognitive requirements of the system exceed the child's developmental level. Cognitive and perceptual, as well as motor skills, need to be evaluated prior to making a recommendation for a specific child. A dual-switch system can enable the child with severe motoric disabilities to operate a wheelchair. The head switch system (see Figure 11-8) operates by transmission of pressure from the child's head to the switch plates attached to the headrest of the chair. A light-touch switch placed near the child's hand or foot works with the head switch system. By tapping the light-touch switch, the child can then drive in reverse using the same headrest switch that drove the chair forward. By tapping the touch switch a second time, the headrest switch reverts to its previous function of forward propulsion. Systems such as this give the child with severe motoric limitations the independence and freedom to explore his environment. The

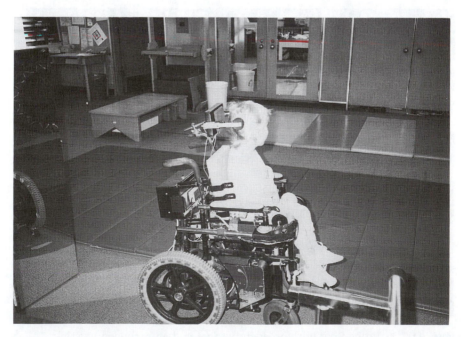

Figure 11-8 A child in a wheelchair that is run by a head switch system

child receives various sensory input, such as visual and vestibular, which may have positive effects on the child's cognitive and motivational development.

The occupational therapist makes unique contributions to the team considering powered mobility for a child with a disability. Seating and positioning are crucial to a child's comfort and success in learning activities. The child's position should encourage maximum function and active use of upper extremities. Often, additional support is required for those children who have poor trunk control and hypo- or hypertonicity. The occupational therapist also helps to determine the child's type of motor control and the best driving system for the mobility device. Many skills attained through the use of powered mobility, such as spatial awareness, understanding of cause-and-effect relationships, and fine motor control, are often program goals that the occupational therapist addresses. Therefore, powered mobility can be one additional modality used to help build upon and strengthen the skills that the child is learning.

> *Case Study 5:* Susie is a 26-month-old with spina bifida. Her parents and doctors were considering using reciprocating gait orthotics (RGOs) for mobility, but Susie had not yet received them. At this time, her parents were resistant to obtaining any type of wheelchair because they did not want to inhibit her motivation to walk. Typically, she was a motivated child who used commando crawling as her primary form of mobility in the classroom and at home. At this time, her teacher noticed that she seemed less interested and motivated in independent mobility. Susie often sat and cried until someone held her and carried her where she wanted to go. Her mother reported an increase in this behavior at home as well. The interdisciplinary team working with Susie recommended that the school's Probe Six® be used with Susie to increase independent mobility until she received her RGOs. Her parents agreed that this recommendation was an acceptable method by which to increase her independence. Adaptations were made so that Susie had a stable base of support when sitting in the Probe Six.® Within 2 weeks, she transferred into and out of the Probe Six® independently and asked for someone to buckle her seat belt. She used a joystick without adaptations to drive the chair. Her family also purchased a Probe Six® for home that the occupational therapist adapted so Susie could go on walks with her family.

This example illustrates how a less expensive, less permanent device can be used to provide powered mobility for a young child with a disability. When the team is uncertain about the appropriateness and practicality of an electric wheelchair or when the parents prefer options other than a wheelchair, battery-powered mobility toys can be adapted to meet the child's needs, at least on a temporary basis.

Summary

Children who use technology at an early age have the advantage of developing with technology and using it to their benefit throughout their lives. Recent advances in technology allow many devices to grow and expand with the child during the developmental years. With the current pace of progress and research, future technology will offer greater ease of use, wider application, assistance in additional areas of function, and more availability due to lower costs.

In particular, a great need exists for further research and development in the use of technology with very young children (Behrmann, Jones, & Wilds, 1989). The potential benefits to the child and family are discussed in this chapter. However, the state-of-the-art has not sufficiently advanced to enable professionals serving children with disabilities to meet the needs easily or adequately (Behrmann, Jones, & Wilds, 1989). One major task of computer software developers is to design programs that match the cognitive skills and interests of young children.

Technology has reached a level of sophistication and affordability that increases its effectiveness with and availability to a wide range of young children (Hannaford & Taber, 1982). The research that has been completed on the use of technology with children suggests exciting possibilities for improving the quality of life through assistive technology (Lahm, 1989). Technology allows children with severe disabilities to become independent in mobility, communication, and control of the environment. It enhances their daily living skills, their interaction with others, and their learning capabilities. Selecting and implementing a technological support system for a child exemplifies the importance of the team and the family in decision making and problem solving. Due to the complexity of the technology available, a solid match to the child's skills and the family's needs and strengths requires the input of each discipline on the team. Technology is effective for a child only when it fits her unique abilities as well as the goals and priorities of the family.

References

Abramson, L.Y., Seligman, M.E.P., & Teasdale, J.D. (1978). Learned helplessness in humans: Critique and reformation. *Journal of Abnormal Psychology, 87*(1), 49–74.

Angelo, J., & Smith, R.O. (1989). The critical role of occupational therapy in augmentative communication services. *Technology review '89: Perspective on occupational therapy practice.* Rockville, MD: AOTA.

Behrmann, M.M. (1984). A brighter future for early learning through high tech. *The Pointer, 28*(2), 23–26.

Behrmann, M.M., Jones, J.K., & Wilds, M.L. (1989). Technology intervention for very young children with disabilities. *Infants and Young Children,* 1(4), 66–77.

Bowser, G. (1989). *Computers in the early intervention curriculum.* Oregon Technology Access Project, Oregon Department of Education.

Burkhart, L.J. (1980). *Homemade battery powered toys and educational devices for severely handicapped children.* College Park, MD: Author.

Burkhart, L.J. (1982). *More homemade battery devices for severely handicapped children with suggested activities.* College Park, MD: Author.

Butler, C. (1986). Effects of powered mobility on self-initiated behaviors of very young children with locomotor disability. *Developmental Medicine and Child Neurology,* 28, 325–332.

Butler, C., Okamoto, G.A., & McKay, T.M. (1983). Powered mobility for very young disabled children. *Developmental Medicine and Child Neurology,* 25, 472–474.

Chiulli, C., Corradi-Scalise, D., & Donatelli-Schultheiss, L. (1988). Powered mobility vehicles as aids in independent locomotion for young children. *Physical Therapy,* 68(6), 997–999.

Douglas, J., Reeson, B., & Ryan, M. (1988). Computer microtechnology for a severely disabled preschool child. *Child Care: Health and Development,* 14, 93–104.

Douglas, J., & Ryan, M. (1987). A preschool severely disabled boy and his powered wheelchair: A case study. *Child Care, Health and Development,* 13, 303–309.

Education for All Handicapped Children Act of 1975 (PL 94-142), 20 U.S.C. Secs. 1400–1485.

Education of the Handicapped Act Amendments of 1986 (PL 99-457), 20 U.S.C. Secs. 1400–1485.

Fishman, I. (1987). *Electronic communication aids.* Boston: Little, Brown and Co.

Gargiulo, R.M., & O'Sullivan, P.S. (1986). Mildly mentally retarded and nonretarded children's learned helplessness. *American Journal of Mental Deficiency,* 91, 203–206.

Gilfoyle, E.M., Grady, A.P., & Moore, J.C. (1981). *Children adapt.* Thorofare, NJ: Slack.

Goldenburg, E.P. (1979). *Special technology for special children.* Baltimore: University Park Press.

Hannaford, A.E., & Taber, F.M. (1982). Microcomputer software for the handicapped: Development and evaluation. *Exceptional Children,* 49(2), 137–142.

Individuals with Disabilities Education Act (PL 101-476), 20 U.S.C. Secs. 1400–1485 (1990).

Jaffe, K.M., Butler, C., Hays, R.M., & Everard, D.H.S. (1986). An innovative motorized wheelchair for young disabled children. *Journal of the Association of Children's Prosthetic-Orthotics Clinics, 21*(3-4), 46–51.

Kielhofner, G., & Burke, J.P. (1980). A model of human occupation: Part one, conceptual framework and content. *American Journal of Occupational Therapy, 34,* 572–581.

Kinney, P.G., & Blackhurst, A.E. (1987). Technology competencies for teachers of young children with severe handicaps. *Topics in Early Childhood Special Education, 7*(3), 105–115.

Lahm, E.A., ed. (1989). *Technology with low incidence populations: Promoting access to education and learning.* Reston, VA: The Council for Exceptional Children.

Maier, S.F., & Seligman, M.E. (1976). Learned helplessness: Theory and evidence. *Journal of Experimental Psychology: General, 105*(1), 3–46.

Mann, W.C., & Lane, J.P. (1991). *Assistive technology for persons with disabilities: The role of occupational therapy.* Rockville, MD: AOTA.

Smith, R.O. (1991). Technological applications for enhancing human performance. In C. Christiansen & C. Baum (Eds.), *Human performance deficits.* Thorofare, NJ: Slack.

Speigel-McGill, P., Zippiroli, S.M., & Mistrett, S.G. (1989). Microcomputers as social facilitators in integrated preschools. *Journal of Early Intervention, 13*(3), 249–260.

Symington, L. (1990). Pre-computer skills for young children. *Exceptional Children,* Jan/Feb, 36–38.

Vanderheiden, G.C., Brandenburg, S., Brown, G., & Bottorf, C. (1988). Toy modification note. *Trace Reprint Series,* 1–25.

Weisz, J.R. (1979). Perceived control and learned helplessness among mentally retarded and nonretarded children: A developmental analysis. *Developmental Psychology, 15*(3), 311–319.

Williams, S.E., & Matesi, D.V. (1988). Therapeutic intervention with an adaptive toy. *American Journal of Occupational Therapy, 42*(10), 673–676.

A

Observation Guidelines for Sensorimotor Development

I. General Appearance of Movement
   A. Physical appearance
      1. Is there anything unusual about the child's body?
      2. When plotted on a chart, are the child's height and weight age-appropriate?
   B. Motor activity
      1. Is the child able to get from one play area to another alone?
      2. What is the child's primary means of moving during play (crawling, walking, running, etc.)?
      3. Does the child appear to move more often or less often than other children?
      4. What positions does the child choose for play?
      5. How often does the child use each position for play?
      6. Are there any motor skills that the child seems to avoid?
II. Muscle Tone/Strength/Endurance
   A. Features of normal muscle tone
      1. Do body parts on the right and left side look and move the same?
      2. Does the child assume a wide variety of positions?
      3. Does the child look coordinated when moving from one position to another?

Adapted from Hall S. Observation guidelines for sensorimotor development. In T. Linder (Ed.), Transdisciplinary play-based assessment: A functional approach to working with young children. Baltimore: Paul H. Brookes Publishing Co., 1990, pp. 231–236, reprinted with permission.

B. Common feature of unusual muscle tone
   1. What behaviors indicate the presence of low tone?
      a. Does the child have difficulty holding the head up?
      b. Is the child's posture slumped?
      c. Is there a wide base of support?
      d. Is there a tendency to lock joints?
      e. Is there a tendency to lean against supports?
      f. Is there a tendency to "W" sit?
   2. What behaviors indicate the presence of high tone?
      a. When the child moves, does the body get stiffer?
      b. At rest, do the arms or legs appear to be stiff?
      c. Is there fisting in one or both hands?
      d. Does the child stand or walk on the toes?
      e. Does the child have balance problems?
   3. What behaviors suggest the presence of fluctuating tone?
   4. Can any pattern of unusual tone be detected?
      a. Does one side of the body appear to be stiffer than the other?
      b. Do the legs appear to be stiffer than the arms?
C. Strength and endurance
   1. Does the child get tired if a motor activity is performed over and over?
   2. Are there indicators of decreased cardiovascular function?
      a. Skin changes?
      b. Blue lips and fingernails?
      c. Breathing difficulty?
III. Reactivity to Sensory Input
   A. Touch
      1. Does the child respond to tactile stimuli?
      2. Does the child seem to have a pleasurable reaction to tactile input?
   B. Movement
      1. Does the child respond to movement?
      2. Does the child seem to have a pleasurable reaction to movement?
   C. Auditory
      1. Does the child respond to auditory stimuli?
      2. Does the child seem to have a pleasurable reaction to auditory stimuli?
   D. Visual
      1. Does the child respond to visual stimuli?
      2. Does the child seem to have a pleasurable reaction to visual stimuli?
   E. Does the child demonstrate a sensory preference?
      1. Visual preference—the child attends longer to the visual features of objects or to objects that have strong visual features

2. Auditory preference—the child attends longer to toys with auditory features
3. Tactile preference—the child attends longer to toys that provide strong tactile input
4. Vestibular preference—the child attends longer to activities that provide movement or vestibular input

IV. Attention Span
   A. Attention preferences
      1. What is the average length of time the child spends per activity?
      2. What activities engage the child for the longest time?
      3. What activities engage the child for the shortest time?

V. Stationary Positions Used for Play
   A. Prone (lying on the abdomen)
      1. Is the child able to raise the head in prone?
      2. Can the child prop on the forearms?
      3. Can the child bring the hands together and look at them while propped on the forearms?
      4. Can the child reach for a toy and play with it while lying on the stomach?
      5. Are the legs spread wide apart or close together?
   B. Supine (lying on the back)
      1. Can the child maintain the head in midline and turn it to both sides?
      2. Does the child bring the hands together on the chest?
      3. Does the child reach above the chest for objects? with one or both hands?
      4. Are the legs together or apart?
      5. Can the child play with the feet (e.g., put the hands on the knees, play with the feet, or bring the feet to the mouth)?
   C. Sitting
      1. Does the child need to be held in sitting?
      2. How much support does the child need when held in sitting?
      3. Is the child able to hold the head up?
      4. Is the child able to freely turn the head? to both sides, up and down?
      5. Is the back rounded or straight?
      6. Is the child able to sit by propping on the arms?
      7. Does the child sit independently without support?
      8. Can the child bring the hands together in front of the body?
      9. Can the child use the arms and hands to play with toys in sitting?
      10. Does the child turn the upper body to reach for or watch objects, keeping the lower body stationary?

11. Is the child able to cross the center of the body with the arms when reaching for a toy?
12. Does the child use the arms to catch herself when falling (forward, sideways, or backwards)?
13. Are the legs spread wide apart or maintained more close together?
14. How many different sitting positions are used?
15. When sitting in a chair, does the child's body droop forward?
16. Does the child's bottom slide forward in a chair?

D. Hands and knees
1. Can the child hold the head up when playing on hands and knees?
2. Can the child reach for a toy while on hands and knees?

E. Standing
1. Does the child need to be held to stand?
2. How much support is needed when held in standing?
3. Can the child hold the head up in standing?
4. Does the child stand alone at a low table or support, steadying by leaning against the table?
5. Can the child stand without support, and for how long?
6. How far apart are the legs when standing?
7. Are the arms in high guard?
8. Do both sides of the body appear to function equally well?

VI. Mobility in Play
A. Movements in prone and supine
1. In stomach-lying, can the child roll onto the side or over to the back?
2. In back-lying, can the child roll onto the side or over to the stomach?
3. Does the body appear rigid during rolling ("log roll")?
4. Does the trunk twist during rolling, so that the hips and shoulders do not move as a unit?
5. Does the child's body arch backwards during rolling?
6. Does the child roll toward both the left and the right?
7. Can the child control rolling, stopping at any point in the sequence?
8. Is the child able to move forward while lying on the stomach?

B. Movements in sitting
1. Does the child pivot in a circle in sitting?
2. Does the child scoot on his bottom in sitting?
3. Does the child move in and out of sitting alone?
    a. From stomach to sitting and sitting to stomach?
    b. From sitting into hands and knees and vice versa?
    c. To both sides (to the right and to the left)?

C. Movements in the hands-and-knees position
1. Does the child rock back and forth while on hands and knees?
2. Does the child move forward while on hands and knees?
3. How mature is the child's creeping pattern?
   a. Do the arm and leg on the same side of the body move forward simultaneously?
   b. Do the arm and leg on the opposite side of the body move forward simultaneously?
4. How does the child move from hands and knees into sitting?
   a. Does the bottom drop straight back, between the thighs?
   b. Does the bottom drop to one side, into side sitting?
   c. Does the child move in both directions, to the right and to the left?
5. Can the child rise from hands and knees into a kneeling position?

D. Movements in standing
1. Does the child bounce up and down when held in standing?
2. Is the child able to pull up into standing by holding onto furniture?
3. When pulling up, do both legs push together or does the child plant one foot and come up through half-kneel?
4. Can the child walk sideways while holding onto furniture?
5. Does the child demonstrate the ability to walk without support?
   a. Are the arms in high guard or down by the child's side?
   b. How far apart are the legs?
6. Is the child able to rise to standing from the floor, without the use of furniture? (Does the child need to place the hands on the floor for support when rising to standing?)
7. Can the child squat in play?
8. Is the child able to lower to the floor from standing?
9. Is the child able to run?
   a. Is there a moment when both feet are off the ground?
   b. Are the arms in high guard?
   c. Does running appear stiff and awkward, or coordinated?
   d. Can the child stop quickly, avoid obstacles, and change directions?
   e. Can the child run on varied surfaces (grass, gravel, or tile)?

VII. Prehension and Manipulation
A. Muscle tone and strength
1. Muscle tone
   a. Does the opposite arm get stiff while one hand plays with a toy?
   b. Does the tongue move or come out of the mouth when the child is concentrating?

    c. Is the mouth open or closed when the child is concentrating?

    d. Are the hands generally open or closed?

  2. Strength

    a. What is the child's ability to lift heavy objects?

    b. Is the child able to pull apart and push together resistive toys?

    c. Is the child able to pull up a zipper or pull off tube socks?

    d. Does the child demonstrate fatigue with increasing repetitions of the same activity?

B. Head and trunk control during prehension and manipulation

  1. Is the child able to keep the head and trunk upright when playing with objects?

  2. Does the child use the arms for support when reaching?

C. Reaching skills

  1. Accuracy of reach

    a. Does the child overreach?

    b. Does the child go directly to the target, or use wide, sweeping motions or corralling of the object?

  2. Visual guidance of reach

    a. Does the child look before reaching?

    b. Does she watch the hand or the object while reaching?

    c. Does she look away while contacting the object?

  3. Is the child able to position the hand and the arm, accommodating them to an object's orientation?

D. Grasping skills

  1. Is the total hand or fist being used?

  2. Is the thumb involved?

  3. What are the actions of the fingers?

    a. Do all the fingers move as a unit?

    b. Is the child able to point or poke with one finger?

  4. What is the grasping action of the thumb and the index fingers?

    a. Mostly at the side of the index?

    b. Pads of the index and the thumb contact?

    c. Very tips of the index and the thumb contact?

  5. Is the child able to grasp more than one object at a time?

E. Releasing skills

  1. Is the child able to release objects by transferring them from one hand to the other (left to right and right to left)?

  2. In order to release with one hand alone, does the child need to support the arm on a surface or press down with the object?

  3. Is the child able to smoothly release objects in free space?

F. Bilateral development

  1. Is the child able to bring both hands together in front of the body?

2. Can the child reach across the front of the body to get a toy on the other side?
3. Is there a preference for one hand?
   a. No difference?
   b. Strong dominance?
4. If there is a preference, is the nonpreferred hand also readily used (i.e., to stabilize a toy)?

G. Manipulative prehension
   1. When holding an object in one hand, is the child able to reposition it within the hand?
   2. What is the quality of the child's motor control when coloring?
   3. Does the child attempt to color within a confined space?
   4. What other examples of higher level tool use are demonstrated (e.g., cutting with scissors, turning key on a shape sorter, or unscrewing lids)?

Glossary

Adaptive Firmware Card (AFC): This RAM-based card for the Apple II computer series fits into the computer and provides alternative access for individuals who have difficulty using the standard keyboard. It allows an individual to adapt Apple software and use a keyboard emulator.

Augmentative Communication: Any techniques or devices used to supplement an individual's speech. Techniques that require use of a device are termed "aided"; techniques that do not use a device, such as signing, are termed "unaided." Electronic communication devices may be dedicated systems that only serve augmentative communication purposes. Computers may also be adapted to provide augmentative communication functions. Typical features are synthesized voice output, print output, and keyboard emulation.

Direct selection: An access method in which the child simply touches or points to his choices on the keyboard or communication board. Letters, words, sentences, phrases, or pictures may be directly selected.

Encoding: A technique for increasing the number of selections possible from a limited number of input options. Encoding uses symbols such as numbers, colors, or letters to represent words (e.g., Morse Code). Encoding techniques require the least motor output, but the greatest cognitive skills.

Ke:nex: A full access system for the Macintosh (similar to the AFC for the Apple computers) that allows an individual to program adaptive routines, which the card provides as alternative access for individuals who have difficulty using the standard keyboard.

Light Talker: An electronic communication device that is programmed with individualized overlays and activated by an optic light attached to the user. The Light Talker has numerous different selection techniques, including direct selection, row-column scanning, direct scanning, and morse code.

Light Touch Switch: With a light touch, this switch closes a circuit for activation of a toy or device. Any body part can activate this switch with minimum pressure.

Muppet Keyboard: A touch-sensitive input device that allows users to access the computer without using the keyboard.

Power Pad: A touch-sensitive alternative input device that allows users with special needs to use the computer without the limitations of the keyboards.

Scanning: A selection technique used to make choices on computers or communication systems. Scanning involves moving sequentially through a given set of choices and making a selection by stopping the scanning mechanism when the desired choice is reached.

Touch Talker: An electronic communication device that is programmed with individualized overlays and activated by touch. The user has an option of using as few as 8 and as many as 128 choices.

Touch Window: This device allows individuals to select choices directly on the computer screen through a clear touch screen that attaches to the monitor.

Unicorn Board: An alternative to the computer keyboard for users who need larger definable keys. The Unicorn Board has 128 touch-sensitive keys that can be used individually or grouped together to form larger keys.

Resources for Equipment, Software, and Information

Ablenet
1081 Tenth Ave., SE
Minneapolis, MN 55414
1-800-322-0956

Adaptive Communication Systems, Inc.
354 Hookstown Grade Road
Clinton, PA 15026

Apple Computer
Office of Special Education
20525 Mariani Ave.
Cupertino, CA 95014

Closing the Gap
Route 2, Box 39
Henderson, MN 56044

Communication Aids for Children and Adults
Crestwood Company
6625 N. Sidney Place
Milwaukee, WI 53209
1-414-352-5678

Communication Skill Builders
3830 E. Bellevue
PO Box 42050-E
Tucson, AZ 85733
1-602-323-7500

This is not an exhaustive list, nor does it represent any endorsement.

ComputAbility Corporation
101 Route 46
Pine Brook, NJ 07058
1-201-882-0171

Don Johnson Developmental Equipment
PO Box 639
1000 N. Rand Rd., Bldg. 115
Wauconda, IL 60084
1-312-526-2682

Dunamis
3620 Hwy. 317
Suwanee, GA 30174
1-800-828-2443

Edmark Corporation
PO Box 3903
Bellevue, WA 98009-3903
1-800-426-0856

Hartley Learning Services
1203 Willamette St.
PO Box 10636
Eugene, OR 97440-2636
1-800-877-WEST or 1-800-877-EAST

Kidware
MOBIUS Corporation
405 N. Henry St.
Alexandria, VA 22314
1-703-684-2911

Laureate Learning Systems, Inc.
110 East Spring St.
Winooski, VT 05404-9980
1-800-562-6801

Marblesoft
21805 Zumbrota N.E.
Cedar, MN 55011
1-612-434-3704

Oregon Technology Access Project
Oregon Department of Education
Division of Special Education
1871 NE Stephens
Roseburg, OR 97470
1-503-440-4791

Peal Software
3200 Wilshire Blvd.
Suite 1207, South Tower
Los Angeles, CA 90010

Prentke Romich
1022 Heyl Road
Wooster, OH 44691
1-800-262-1984

RJ Cooper Shareware
24843 Del Prado
Suite 283
Dana Point, CA 92629
1-714-240-1912

Sunburst Communications
101 Castleton St.
Pleasantville, NY 10570-3498
1-800-628-8897

Trace R & D Center
Reprint Service
S-151 Waisman Center
1500 Highland Ave.
Madison, WI 53705

UCLA/LAUSD
1000 Veteran Ave.
Suite 23-10
Los Angeles, CA 90024

Index

DATE DUE

SEP 1 0 1996		
ill:9480952		
dd: 2/16/98		
APR 2 1 1998		
DEC 0 3 1998		
OCT 1 8 1999		
MAY 1 2 2000		
GAYLORD		PRINTED IN U.S.A.